Prosthetic Treatment of the Edentulous Patient

Prosthetic Treatment of the Edentulous Patient

Fifth Edition

R.M. Basker

OBE, DDS Birm, BDS Lond, FDSRCS Edin, MGDSRCS Eng, LDSRCS Eng
Emeritus Professor, University of Leeds, UK
Formerly Consultant in Restorative Dentistry, Leeds Teaching Hospitals NHS Trust
Formerly External Examiner in the Universities of Birmingham, Bristol, Dundee, London, Malaya
Manchester, Newcastle upon Tyne, Sheffield and Wales, University College Cork,
Universiti Kebangsaan (Malaysia)
Examiner, MGDS of the Royal College of Surgeons of England

J.C. Davenport

PhD Birm, BDS Brist, FDSRCS Eng, RBSA
Emeritus Professor, University of Birmingham, UK
Formerly Consultant Dental Surgeon, Southern Birmingham Community Health NHS Trust
Formally External Examiner in the Universities of Amman (Jordan), Dublin, Glasgow, Leeds, London
Manchester, Newcastle upon Tyne, University College Cork and Wales

J.M. Thomason

PhD Ncl, BDS Ncl, FDSRCS Ed
Professor of Prosthodontics and Oral Rehabilitation, Newcastle University, UK
Visiting Professor and Adjunct Professor, McGill University, Montreal, Canada
Consultant in Restorative Dentistry, Newcastle upon Tyne Hospitals NHS Foundation Trust
Formally External Examiner in the Universities of Dublin, Glasgow, Manchester, King's College
London, Hong Kong
Examiner in MRD and MFDS examinations of the Royal College of Surgeons of Edinburgh

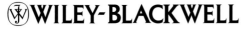

A John Wiley & Sons, Ltd., Publication

This edition first published 2011
© 1976, 1983, 1992 by R.M. Basker, J.C. Davenport and H.R. Tomlin
© 2002 by Blackwell Munksgaard
© 2011 by R.M. Basker, J.C. Davenport and J.M. Thomason

Blackwell Publishing was acquired by John Wiley & Sons in February 2007. Blackwell's publishing program has been merged with Wiley's global Scientific, Technical and Medical business to form Wiley-Blackwell.

Registered office: John Wiley & Sons Ltd, The Atrium, Southern Gate, Chichester, West Sussex, PO19 8SQ, UK

Editorial offices: 9600 Garsington Road, Oxford, OX4 2DQ, UK
       The Atrium, Southern Gate, Chichester, West Sussex, PO19 8SQ, UK
       2121 State Avenue, Ames, Iowa 50014-8300, USA

For details of our global editorial offices, for customer services and for information about how to apply for permission to reuse the copyright material in this book please see our website at www.wiley.com/wiley-blackwell

The right of the author to be identified as the author of this work has been asserted in accordance with the UK Copyright, Designs and Patents Act 1988.

Library of Congress Cataloging-in-Publication Data
Basker, R.M.
   Prosthetic treatment of the edentulous patient / R.M. Basker, J.C. Davenport, J.M. Thomason. – 5th ed.
    p. ; cm.
   Includes bibliographical references and index.
   ISBN 978-1-4051-9261-3 (pbk. : alk. paper) 1. Complete dentures. 2. Edentulous mouth.
I. Davenport, J. C. (John Chester) II. Thomason, J. M. III. Title.
   [DNLM: 1. Denture, Complete. 2. Mouth, Edentulous. WU 530]
   RK656.B338 2011
   617.6′92–dc22

                                                       2010040959

A catalogue record for this book is available from the British Library.

This book is published in the following electronic formats: ePDF [978-1-4443-9324-8]; ePub [978-1-4443-9325-5]

Set in 9.5/12 pt Palatino by Aptara® Inc., New Delhi, India

Printed and bound in Singapore by Markono Print Media Pte Ltd

1 2011

To our families
And to the memory of Bob Tomlin

Contents

Foreword to the First Edition

This addition to prosthetic literature must be widely and warmly welcomed. For a number of years there has been a shortage of British texts for students concerning the edentulous patient. The authors have, correctly, stressed the serious problems that more and more frequently present themselves now that life expectancy is on the increase and the average age of the edentulous is advancing. The dental profession is becoming aware of the particular geriatric situations it now has to face and this book will undoubtedly help in solving many prosthetic geriatric problems.

Emphasis has been placed more upon general principles than upon the minutiae of clinical or technical operative detail. Given a sound basic understanding of the principles to be observed in the treatment of the edentulous, chairside experience rapidly perfects each individual's manipulative skills.

Being not unfamiliar with the labours involved in producing textbooks, one is conscious of the time and effort that have gone into the preparation of this book. It should achieve all the success that these efforts of one's former colleagues deserve.

John Osborne
Shalfleet, Isle of Wight, 1975

Foreword to the Fifth Edition

The breakthrough of implant-supported and/or -retained prostheses has revolutionised dental treatment. A great part of the programmes at current prosthodontic conferences includes presentations based on high-tech implant treatment for partially and totally edentulous patients. So successful have the clinical outcomes with implant treatment been that many clinicians have come to believe that implants can solve all problems related to tooth loss. This is of course not true, confounded as it is not only by unfavourable oral situations but also by a number of non-dental factors. Of these, the greatest obstacle is undoubtedly economic. Viewed in a global perspective, poverty is still extremely widespread, and it exists even in many industrialised countries. Sadly, a majority of edentulous people will never be candidates for any type of implant therapy and complete dentures will remain their sole option.

The declining prevalence of edentulism would seem to indicate a reduction in the number of people in need of complete dentures. However, when epidemiological and demographic data are combined, the ongoing large increase in the number of the elderly will counteract the diminishing rate of edentulism. It is therefore likely that the need to rehabilitate edentulous patients will remain considerable for many more decades. Complete dentures will continue to play a central role in the rehabilitation of edentulism; thus, teaching and training in complete denture prosthodontics must continue.

This successful textbook has reached its fifth edition. It combines a straightforward description of well-proven principles and methods for the treatment of an edentulous patient with modern evidence-based examples of solutions for problems and complicated situations. The text is easy to read and the illustrations give excellent explanations of principles and techniques described. The book will therefore be of great value in both undergraduate and postgraduate education, and it deserves a place in the office of any dentist who treats adult and older patients.

Gunnar E. Carlsson
Gothenburg, Sweden, November 2010

Preface

Two of us have had the particular pleasure of welcoming Mark Thomason to the authors' team. His presence has ensured not only that the text has been brought up to date in a number of important areas, but also that writing a new edition has continued to be a pleasurable and stimulating experience.

Thirty-four years ago, we commented in the preface to the first edition that it was important to adopt a flexible approach to the formulation of treatment plans and to the application of clinical techniques. This opinion was based on the fact that as there is a great deal of variation in the condition of our patients and their mouths a 'one size fits all' approach is not appropriate. We see no reason to change this view. Indeed, the recently published work of Professor Gunnar Carlsson (Carlsson 2009) strengthens our opinion. He has drawn the profession's attention to the lack of randomised controlled trials in many aspects of complete denture provision and has highlighted the fact that there is often a poor correlation between a clinician's assessment of denture quality and the level of patient satisfaction with a prosthesis. There is surely considerable scope for further research to help to improve the reliability of clinical decision making in this area. In the meantime, we hope that the clinical approaches adopted in this book will play a part in clarifying that choice.

During the last 8 years, there has been an explosion in the number of published papers dealing with implant-supported complete dentures. This development is highly relevant to the all-important stage when decisions have to be made on how to manage the transition from what remains of the natural dentition to the totally artificial one. We have expanded the chapters dealing with this critical period.

Another major change in the UK since the publication of the fourth edition has been the formal registration of two further members of the dental team – the clinical dental technician and the dental technician. The clinical dental technician is a qualified dental technician who is able to provide complete dentures directly to patients. Patients with natural teeth or implants must see a dentist before the clinical dental technician can begin treatment. The dental technician makes dentures to a prescription from a dentist or clinical dental technician. The educational programmes for both newly registered members of the dental team are formally recognised.

We are strongly of the view that there must be good communication between dentist, clinical dental technician and dental technician – the right hand must know what the left is doing or is planning to do. Published work suggests that the level of communication between surgery and laboratory still leaves something to be desired (Juszczyk et al. 2009). At the end of chapters dealing with the clinical stages of denture construction, we have again included short sections on 'communication with the dental technician' and 'quality control and enhancement'. We hope that they will encourage the development of clearer communication.

Throughout the book, the description 'clinician' refers to dentist and clinical dental technician.

We have taken the opportunity of thoroughly revising the text and, with the encouragement of our publishers, of introducing colour into the book.

Although there has been a major reduction in total tooth loss in many countries, the edentulous population is living longer. Thus, the demand for prosthetic care will remain at a significant level for the foreseeable future, and the challenges this presents to the clinician will increase in difficulty as the patients become older.

Leeds, Birmingham and
Newcastle upon Tyne, 2010
RMB, JCD and JMT

References

Carlsson, G.E. (2009) Critical review of some dogmas in prosthodontics. *Journal of Prosthodontic Research*, 53, 3–10.

Juszczyk, A.S., Clark, R.K. & Radford, D.R. (2009) UK dental laboratory technicians' views on the efficacy and teaching of clinical-laboratory communication. *British Dental Journal*, 206, E21.

Acknowledgements

We are most grateful to the many friends and colleagues whose support over the years has encouraged and influenced our thinking on the care of the edentulous patient. We are also indebted to our students and young colleagues in training who have challenged our ideas, shaped our thinking and shared our learning.

Our grateful thanks are extended to Professor John McCabe, Professor Jim Ralph, Dr Chris Watson, Mr Francis Nohl and Mr Stewart Barclay for the generous loan of photographs, to Dr Rachel David and Mr Simon Littlewood for their most helpful comments on those sections of the book dealing with speech and orthodontics respectively, and to Professor Damien Walmsley for helpful discussion.

We would like to acknowledge the friendly expertise of the staff of the British Dental Association's Information Centre in helping with the literature searches.

We are most grateful to the members of the Medical and Dental Illustration Unit of the University of Leeds and the Photographic Department of the Dental School at the University of Birmingham for their skill over the years.

We are most grateful to Lucy Nash and Nick Morgan at Wiley-Blackwell and Amit Malik at Aptara for their support, understanding and encouragement throughout the production of this book.

We acknowledge with thanks the permission of the Editor of the *British Dental Journal* to reproduce figures which have appeared in that journal.

An Appraisal of the Complete Denture Situation

Total tooth loss

Perhaps the most fundamental question to ask in the first chapter of a book on complete dentures is: 'What is the demand for such treatment?' Fortunately, more and more evidence has become available to provide an increasingly accurate answer and one which enables future trends to be determined with reasonable confidence. Particularly notable are the series of in-depth studies of adult dental health in the UK that have succeeded in painting a detailed picture over a period of more than 30 years. There are also data from Sweden and Finland and parts of Germany that allow some statistical modelling of the current trends (Mojon et al. 2004).

The most detailed picture comes from the UK and the information that follows is based upon decennial surveys, the most recent one undertaken in 1998.

The situation at the end of the twentieth century

Whilst we await the publication of the survey outlining the state of adult dental health dur-ing the first decade of the twenty-first century, let us first look at total tooth loss within adults in the UK in 1998 (Fig. 1.1) (Steele et al. 2000). Overall, 13% of all adults were edentate, and it can be seen that the condition was strongly correlated with age. Total tooth loss was a rarity up to the mid-forties age group, after which there was a steady climb to the age group 75 and over where the majority had lost all their teeth.

Total tooth loss is related not only to age but also to other variables such as social class and marital status. When multivariate analyses were undertaken, any association between tooth loss and gender disappeared. The differences that are apparent in the UK may be illustrated by comparing extremes. To quote from Steele et al. (2000), women from an unskilled manual background living in Scotland were 12 times more likely to have no teeth at all than men from a non-manual background in the south of England. Of those who had lost their remaining teeth in the previous 10 years, 59% stated that they visited the dentist only when troubled whilst 29% said that they had attended their dentist on a regular basis. This pattern of attendance was almost the complete

Prosthetic Treatment of the Edentulous Patient, Fifth Edition, © R.M. Basker, J.C. Davenport and J.M. Thomason
Published 2011 by Blackwell Publishing Ltd.

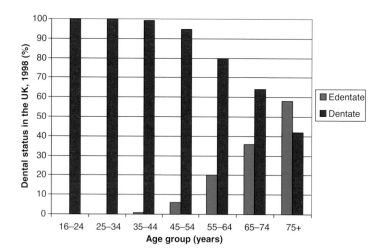

Figure 1.1 The proportion of dentate and edentate people, by age, in the UK in 1998 (with acknowledgements to Steele et al. (2000)).

opposite to that of people who still had their own teeth. What is of particular relevance is the change in the rate at which people lost their remaining teeth in the last 10 years of the twentieth century. It has been a much more gradual process than previously. Whereas in 1968 two-thirds of those who were rendered edentulous had 12 or more teeth extracted at the final stage, in 1998 the proportion had gone down to one-quarter. One possible reason for this change is that both patient and dentist wanted to keep some natural teeth for as long as possible. We are fully supportive of this philosophy and enlarge on the topic of transition from the natural to the artificial dentition in Chapter 3.

As people increasingly wish to function with their natural teeth rather than with dentures, one would expect mental barriers to be erected against the latter. This indeed appears to be the case when we consider that, in 1998, over 60% of those people who relied only on natural teeth stated that they would be very upset if they had to function with complete dentures. This attitude seems to have strengthened as we have moved into the twenty-first century. As the number of edentate patients falls, a 'tipping-point' appears to have been established, which results in a range of concerns being raised, including the social acceptability of

being edentulous. Whilst edentulism was previously thought to be almost inevitable, and thus an 'acceptable' option for patients with dental disease, this is no longer the case in many areas of society. As the number of edentulous patients falls, this smaller population becomes more manageable and allows the possibility for this group of people to be offered other treatments. For example, when there is little chance of maintaining a functional natural dentition, first-line treatment options have increasingly moved towards the preservation of some tooth roots and the use of overdentures. When this is not possible, then the use of implant-supported overdentures as the 'standard of care' has been proposed (Feine et al. 2002; Thomason et al. 2009).

These changes of emphasis on how one may manage the progression from the dentate state to complete dentures are important, especially as most of the complete denture treatment in the future will inevitably be undertaken on older patients. It is imperative that the dentist is aware of the various treatment opportunities, of the need to explore acceptable alternatives and to move into much longer-term treatment planning whilst the patients still have a functional dentition. This longer-term planning may be best regarded as treatment 'mapping' as

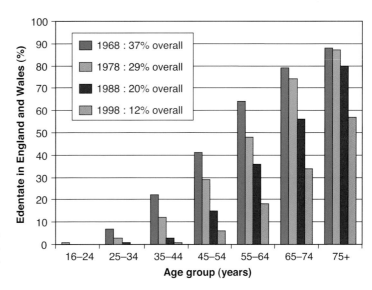

Figure 1.2 The relationship of total tooth loss to age over the period 1968–1998 (with acknowledgements to Steele et al. (2000)).

the absolute plan may need to be more flexible than is commonly the case in many treatment plans.

The past

So much for the 'snap-shot' of total tooth loss in 1998. A fascinating picture emerges when examining the trends that have developed over the 30-year period during which there have been four studies of adult dental health in England and Wales – 1968, 1978, 1988 and 1998. The relationship of total tooth loss to age is presented in Fig. 1.2. The first point to make is that dental health, as measured by total tooth loss, has improved dramatically. In 1968, 37% of adults in England and Wales had lost all their natural teeth. This figure had gone down to 12% in 1998. This improvement reflects the poor state of oral health before and after World War II when the main thrust of treatment, at the inception of the UK's National Health Service, had to be an attack on the high levels of neglect, pain and sepsis existing in the community. Once this battle was won, the pattern of extractions and dentures gave way to a desire to restore the teeth and, eventually, to

prevent further disease. We are perhaps now seeing the next phase where alternatives and longer-term strategies of management and rehabilitation of what remains can be realistically considered.

The very high percentage of those aged 75 and over who had lost all their teeth at the time of the earlier surveys (Fig. 1.2) is of course a reflection of the high levels of dental disease many years earlier. For example, in 1968, 64% of all those in the age group 55–64 were edentate. That same group of people continued to lose their natural teeth until, 20 years later, 80% of them (now in the 75 and over age group) were edentate.

Referring again to Fig. 1.2, we can see how the huge improvement in oral health of the younger members of the population a few years ago is now influencing the figures as these people enter their middle years. Looking again at the 55–64 age group the percentage that had lost all their teeth has dropped from 64% in 1968 to 18% in 1998. More dramatic still is the reduction in the 45–54 age group – down from 41% to 6% in the same period. As these people grow older, it is reasonable to expect that they will, in 20–30 years time, bring down a lot further the current 57% of those 75 and over who are edentate.

The future

With the mass of information which has been accumulated over the last 30 years, it has become possible to predict future trends with reasonable confidence. If the current trends continue, it is calculated that, by 2018, only 5–6% of the UK adult population will be edentate; let us not forget, though, that 5–6% equates to four million people in the UK. We will need to wait for the results of the 2008–2009 UK Adult Dental Health Survey to see if the UK is still on course for these predicted improvements. On a more salutary note, it has been suggested that the effect of having an ageing population will mitigate against the rate of reduction in the overall prevalence of edentulism in the population. Indeed, in the US it has been predicted that far from decreasing, the need for complete denture treatment will actually increase over the first 2 decades of the twenty-first century (Douglass et al. 2002). The authors argue that the ageing 'baby boomers' will more than compensate for the falling prevalence of edentulism. Modelling these changes on European data has suggested that in the UK there will be a reduction in edentulism of the order of 60% over the first 30 years of the century, but it will then remain stable. The mean prediction for Finland follows a similar picture to the UK but the spread of the data is very wide and so is inconclusive (Mojon et al. 2004).

Total tooth loss in other countries

An investigation into the oral health of adults in the Republic of Ireland was undertaken in 1989–1990 (O'Mullane & Whelton 1992). The level of total tooth loss was very similar to that in England, Wales and Northern Ireland in 1988. There had been a considerable decline in the level of edentulousness compared with 10 years earlier.

Table 1.1   The percentage of people aged 35–44 years and 65 years and over with no natural teeth (data from WHO (1991)).

Country	35–44 years	65+ years
Albania	3.7	69.3
Czechoslovakia	0.7	38.3
Denmark	8.0	60.0
Finland	9.0	46.0
Ex-GDR	0.5	58.0
Germany, Federal Republic	0.4	27.0
Hungary	0.3	30.0
Ireland	4.0	49.0
Italy	0.3	18.0
The Netherlands	9.4	65.4
Norway	1.0	31.0
Romania	15.0	55.8
San Marino	1.3	40.7
Sweden	1.0	20.0
Turkey	2.7	75.0
United Kingdom	4.0	67.0
(Former) Yugoslavia	0.6	33.0

The relationship of total tooth loss to age is a worldwide phenomenon, as shown in Table 1.1, where the percentage of edentulous individuals for two age groups in a number of countries is shown. The amount of total tooth loss recorded in or around 1990 varies considerably between countries (WHO 1992). Whilst most EU countries do not have national survey data, in France a recent survey in the region Rhone-Alpes reported that in 1995, 16% of the 65–74 age-band was edentulous compared with 36% for the UK and 34% for the region of Pomerania in Germany (Mojon et al. 2004).

The prospects for the future may be summarised as follows:

• It is unlikely that the edentulous state will disappear, but there probably will be a fall in those requiring complete dentures so that there will be around 60% of the current number required.

- More people will retain a functional natural dentition into old age, but this dentition will not last a lifetime in all cases.
- As the public's expectations for oral health continue to rise, a larger proportion of those who lose their teeth will be very upset about the prospect of having to wear complete dentures and this will influence their response to treatment. Therefore, it will be critical to consider alternative treatment strategies for these patients.
- Most complete denture treatment will be centred on older people and is, therefore, likely to become more complex and demanding. The opportunities to consider retaining teeth as overdenture abutments or to provide osseointegrated implants as overdenture abutments for this group of patients are likely to increase and decisions will have to be made at an appropriate time in the planning cycle.
- Dentists will continue to need complete denture skills, which will have to be of a high order (Steele et al. 2000). Nevertheless, there will be less opportunity for the majority of dentists to practise these skills on a regular basis and some parts of this treatment provision are likely to move into the realm of the specialist.

In the remainder of this book, we endeavour to deal with all these points.

The limitations of complete dentures

The limitations of complete dentures are highlighted when one compares the difference between functioning natural teeth, intimately connected to and embedded in living tissues, with the removable prosthesis which replaces them, constructed of an artificial material simply resting on vital living (and often delicate) tissues. Between these two extremes is the complete overdenture. Whilst having many of the characteristics of the conventional complete denture, it retains elements of functioning teeth in the form of roots. These roots retain a vital periodontal organ and are, therefore, intimately attached to and function with the alveolar bone. Support is provided through this intimate link with the rest of the body and retention can be provided through the use of attachments between the root surfaces and the prosthesis. A similar and better researched area of clinical practice is the use of the dental implant which provides support and retention for the complete overdenture. Clearly, once teeth have been extracted, the use of implants is the only way that overdentures can be made. However, before the last teeth are extracted, both treatment options remain available and the use of natural teeth as overdenture abutments is certainly a less expensive alternative than the implant-supported prostheses.

The resorption and prosthetic replacement of alveolar bone

It is of fundamental importance to remember that the extraction of teeth does not simply mean the loss of the visible crowns. With the loss of the roots, the surrounding alveolar bone resorbs. Whilst it is relatively simple to provide an effective replacement for the natural crowns with a denture, it is frequently difficult, or even impossible, to make good all the lost alveolar bone; the more bone that is resorbed, the greater is the problem.

Atwood (1971) described the continuing resorption of the residual ridges as 'a major oral disease entity'. It occurs in all edentulous patients and proceeds throughout life. Indeed, this would be a major argument in itself for retaining tooth roots as overdenture abutments in that their very presence will reduce the amount of alveolar resorption.

There is, though, considerable individual variation with respect to both amount and rate of loss of bone. Much has been written on the subject, and there has been a comprehensive

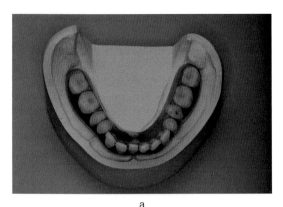
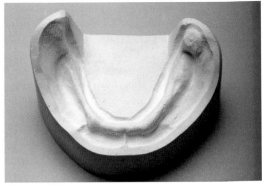

a   b

Figure 1.3 (a) This complete lower denture covers only a small proportion of the available denture-bearing tissue and (b) as a consequence there has been increased resorption of bone and the imprint of the denture can be seen clearly.

review of the literature by Carlsson (1998). A single dominant factor responsible for ridge resorption has not yet been found. There are contradictory reports from investigations into the link between bone resorption and such factors as gender, duration of edentulousness, denture-wearing habits, quality of dentures and systemic influences.

What does emerge is an explanation that, in the early stages of edentulousness, the shape of the residual ridge and the amount of resorption is likely to be influenced particularly by local factors such as the inherent quality and size of the ridge, the technique used to extract the teeth, the healing capacity of the patient and the loads applied to the ridge (Xie et al. 1997a). An example of the latter is shown in Fig. 1.3a, where it can be seen that the lower denture covers only a small part of the area available to support it and, therefore, is not spreading the load sufficiently. This design error results in increased functional stress. The consequence is seen in Fig. 1.3b, where the imprint of the border of the denture can be seen on the residual ridge; the bone has resorbed and the denture has sunk into the underlying tissues. The 'sinking' denture illustrates one of the fundamental advantages of the use of an overdenture compared with a conventional complete denture. Although there has been little conclusive research in this area, it is clinically apparent that supporting complete dentures on tooth remnants as overdentures reduces bone resorption. This may be assumed to be by transferring the usual compressive load of the denture through the mucosa into a tensional load within the periodontium.

It is suggested that the later stages of resorption in the edentulous are likely to be influenced more by systemic factors such as age, nutrition, drug therapy (e.g. corticosteroids) and hormonal factors. There is also a view that severe resorption, particularly of the mandible, is influenced more by systemic factors than by local factors (Xie et al. 1997b).

In spite of the gaps in our knowledge, there would seem to be a sensible way forward. Bearing in mind that a good foundation for complete dentures is such a valuable commodity, and that this foundation is capable of being damaged, it is important to take simple practical steps to reduce the risk. Therefore, the first step to be considered is maintaining some of the last few tooth roots prior to committing a patient to conventional complete dentures. Where this is not possible (and the use of implants as overdenture abutments is precluded), it is wise to encourage patients to reduce the loads on

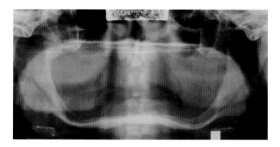

Figure 1.4 This orthopantomograph shows excessive resorption, particularly of the mandible.

the denture-bearing tissues by leaving at least the lower denture out when sleeping, and to ensure that there is no error in denture design which would promote undue resorption. Regular recall and maintenance are also very important so that any developing problems are identified at an early stage before serious damage has been done. All these factors are highlighted elsewhere in this book.

The radiograph reproduced in Fig. 1.4 is an example of extreme resorption; in simple terms, the mandible can be described as 'pencil-thin'. With the loss of skeletal bone comes the loss of support for the facial muscles resulting in the appearance seen in Fig. 1.5. It will be appreciated that to make good this huge volume of lost teeth and bone requires very large dentures. It can become very difficult for the patient to control such substantial foreign bodies. Having lost the opportunity to reduce the resorption by retaining some tooth roots at an early stage of treatment planning, the practical opportunity to avoid further bone loss by the use of osseointegrated implants may also have been lost, as the amount of resorption may no longer leave enough bone into which to place the implants. These plans need to be considered early in the planning cycle to be of maximum benefit.

Restoration of appearance

The limitations of complete dentures in restoring tissue loss, and thus supporting the lips

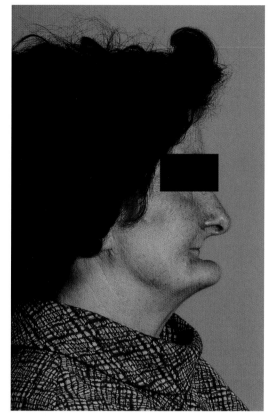

Figure 1.5 Excessive resorption of both jaws has resulted in a dramatic collapse of the lower portion of the face.

and cheeks fully, can contribute to an appearance of premature ageing in the edentulous patient (Fig. 1.6). The facial muscles may lose some of their tone through the ageing process, but loss of tone may also occur because the muscles are unable to function as effectively as before. This is because the underlying artificial supports (the dentures) are only sitting on the mucosa and are not attached securely to the rest of the facial skeleton. In fact, one can liken the difference in oral function between dentate and edentate individuals to that of a person striding briskly along a path rather than moving gingerly over a sheet of ice. The fact that the muscles need

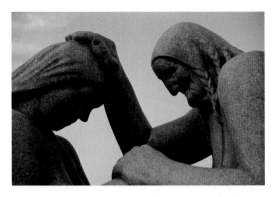

Figure 1.6   This sculpture of age and youth by Gustav Vigeland in Frogner Park, Oslo, illustrates the aged edentulous face well. Bone loss below the anterior nasal spine has occurred and is virtually impossible to replace with a complete upper denture.

a stable surface over which to function further strengthens any arguments in favour of the use of overdenture abutments whether as natural tooth overdenture abutments or in the form of dental implants. A series of studies from McGill University compared patient satisfaction with implant-supported overdentures compared with conventional dentures. Typically, scores for satisfaction with stability of the implant-supported denture were around 30% higher than those for conventional dentures (Thomason et al. 2003). Although there are no data for these differences with natural overdenture abutments, there is little reason to believe that they would be markedly different.

Mastication

Complete dentures certainly help in the control and breaking up of a bolus of food, but their chewing efficiency is considerably lower than that of natural teeth. This is due to the following reasons:

- Natural teeth are firmly attached to the surrounding bone, whereas dentures are merely sitting on the mucosa and, thus, must be actively controlled by the patient.

- The pain threshold of the denture-bearing mucosa is relatively easily exceeded so that the biting force, which is closely correlated with chewing efficiency of complete dentures, is reduced and may be only one-sixth of that of dentate patients.

Although a higher intake of essential nutritional factors is associated with an efficient natural dentition, the wearing of complete dentures does not mean that nutrition will be deficient. Modern food production methods technically enable an adequate diet to be obtained in a form that is readily assimilated despite the most inefficient dentitions. However, as noted later in this chapter, the situation may become critical within certain groups of older people.

Of particular importance is the fact that the enjoyment of eating depends upon the ability to chew, thus making the most of the flavour of the food whilst it is in the mouth. Furthermore, the sense of touch within the oral cavity enables us to distinguish the textures of different foods, a process which heightens the enjoyment of a meal. Such pleasure in eating encourages people to maintain an interest in food. If complete dentures are painful or if their control becomes a problem, eating a meal becomes a chore. In addition, coverage of the palate by the upper denture prevents the full appreciation of the texture and temperature of the food. People with complete dentures are thus more likely to lose interest in eating and switch from such things as meat, fruit and salads to less demanding foods.

People with a natural dentition have been shown to eat more fruit and vegetables than the edentulous. A patient's perception of limitations in chewing ability with complete dentures might be one of the factors influencing this dietary choice, but of greater importance might be the subject's attitude to, and knowledge of, the benefits of an appropriate diet. Indeed, simply improving the quality of a prosthesis does not suddenly cause an improvement in that patient's diet (Moynihan et al. 2000). It may well be that the quality of the denture is important for the personal enjoyment of eating, but to have a good chance of improving the diet of denture-wearers psychosocial factors, as well as perceived chewing ability, must be addressed (Bradbury et al. 2008). There is clear evidence that to make this change a dietary intervention programme is required which ideally runs in parallel with the denture provision (Bradbury et al. 2006).

In spite of the limitations of dentures, the majority of patients manage well and are on the whole relatively happy to have a substitute for what may have been decayed, mobile and painful natural teeth. After all, it must be remembered that the most likely alternative to complete dentures is 'no dentures'.

There are, however, other alternatives that have been alluded to above; overdentures (over tooth roots or implants) or 'fixed' rehabilitations (bridges) constructed on dental implants. Many now regard overdentures supported by two implants to be the most appropriate minimal standard that should be offered to the edentulous in an affluent society (Feine et al. 2002; Thomason et al. 2009) – but there is a long way to go before this concept is universally accepted. There is only poor epidemiological data regarding the prevalence of dental implant treatment. It has been suggested that towards the end of the twentieth century, something like 1/1000 edentulous and partially edentulous patients had been treated using implant-supported prostheses (Carlsson 1998), and the majority of these are likely to have been in the partially edentulous. Sweden probably still has the highest penetration rate of implant treatment in the world (Carlsson 2006), but even here only some 8% of the edentulous population has received any form of implant therapy (Österberg et al. 2000), the other 92% being managed by conventional means. Whilst there is a better alternative to conventional complete dentures, there is still a long way to go before this alternative becomes the 'normal' treatment. The need for this change is clear and

exemplified by the observation that a significant number of people find complete dentures troublesome to the extent that, in one large national survey, over a quarter experienced difficulty in eating and drinking (Walker & Cooper 2000).

One of the fortunate consequences of these developments is that it is becoming increasingly rare that one meets patients whose misguided attitude towards dental disease is that the best approach is to have all the natural teeth extracted electively, when they are restorable, and be replaced by complete dentures. Indeed, bizarre as it now seems, only a few generations ago it used to be a common practice in some areas of the UK for this treatment to be carried out for a bride-to-be in the belief that it would reduce her future dental problems and would avoid saddling her new husband with major dental expenses! Fortunately, this attitude is no longer prevalent and there is rarely any justification for undertaking such a drastic step in early adulthood. Even though the first few years of edentulous life may well be relatively free of problems, it is impossible to predict whether an individual patient will retain an adequate bony foundation and maintain a satisfactory level of comfort and function, or will proceed to a state where denture problems significantly reduce the patient's quality of life.

The older edentulous patient

Earlier in the chapter, it was pointed out that the provision of complete dentures now, and even more so in the future, will largely be directed at the older patient. In recent years, a great deal has been written about this group of people. The purpose of this section of the book is to highlight some of the significant points that relate particularly to complete denture treatment. For a more detailed presentation of the topic, the reader is referred to the bibliography at the end of the chapter, which cites textbooks and papers that were used to compile this summary.

Demographic changes

The life expectancy of those in the developed world has been increasing at the incredible rate of 5 hours per day for the past 200 years. Therefore, it is hardly surprising that we are seeing a change in the age profile of our society, and with it a change in the expectation of those we used to call old. Studies of ageing have brought a generally accepted understanding that ageing is not programmed into each person but comes about by a lifelong accumulation of 'faults' in our cellular make-up. The events causing these faults can be affected surprisingly easily so that delaying damage by reducing exposure to events or boosting our defences will help to postpone the age-related decline which represents old age. This reduced exposure probably explains why the health of our older populations is so much improved – and indeed why the 'old' can now be described as the 'new middle aged'! The improvements in the conditions of our society in terms of housing, nutrition and working conditions may each have contributed to this reduction in accumulated damage and may also go some way to explain the life expectancy differences between better-off and economically deprived areas of our communities.

At one time, an 'elderly person' was commonly defined as someone over the age of 65. Many people have found this label faintly insulting even though the pill may be made rather sweeter if it is pointed out that the label is attached to those who are of pensionable age (Harkins 2002). The term 'older person' has become more acceptable and will be used throughout the rest of the text.

Throughout the world, the older population is growing rapidly. Figure 1.7 shows the proportion of the total population aged 60 years and over living in selected regions. The figures were produced at the World Health Organization (WHO) World Assembly on Aging in 1982. It can be seen that there is a big difference between areas which contain industrialised coun-

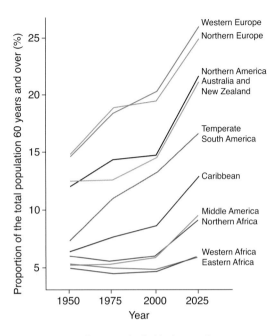

Figure 1.7   The growth of elderly populations in various regions of the world.

tries and those which are composed largely of less developed countries.

It is expected that in the first quarter of the twenty-first century more than a fifth of the population in industrialised countries will be over the age of 65. Those undergraduates reading this book will realise that most of their practising life will be influenced by this pattern. The proportion of edentulous adults in each age cohort will fall during this time, but the effect of the upwards shift in the age profile of our society associated with ageing 'baby boomers' will mean that the number of edentulous adults remaining in our society will remain significant (Mojon et al. 2004). In the UK, the proportion of older people in the population will continue to increase over the next 50 years. The effect of increased life expectancy on the population profile will mean that the greatest increase will be amongst those 85 years and over; their number will almost triple. The increase in the 65–74 and

75–84 age groups will be a little less dramatic (MacMahon & Battle 2002).

The vast majority of older and significantly older people live in the community. A small percentage, estimated at between 12% and 14%, are housebound because of physical or mental handicap. In Northern Europe, between 4% and 7% live in some form of institution. These figures are of particular relevance with respect to the delivery of care. Those people living in some form of institution do have the advantage that their carers are in a position to recognise problems and to seek advice on their behalf. Of course, this presupposes that the carers have some knowledge of prosthetic problems. Those older people who have some form of handicap and are living at home are perhaps the most vulnerable when it comes to dealing with prosthetic difficulties; frequently, the responsibility for initiating help and seeking treatment has not been accepted by any particular person. Valuable guidelines which cover the care of long-stay patients and of those who need treatment on a domiciliary basis have been published (Fiske & Lewis 2000; Fiske et al. 2000).

Some changes seen in older people

This section describes some of the more relevant changes that occur in older people.

Older people typically remain alert and continue to have sound judgement; however, a modest decrease in mental agility occurs. With increasing age there is often seen slight impairment of the abilities to learn and to memorise. With increasing age, there is a progressive loss of neurones and synapses in the cerebral cortex. As a result, there is a slowing of the central processing facility with a consequential lengthening of reaction times and response to sensory stimuli.

Within the sensory system, age brings about a deterioration of the senses of smell and taste, the former being more affected. Hearing is impaired in approximately 25% of people over the age of 65 years and in 80% of those in the age range 75–79 years.

With respect to the motor system, there tends to be impairment of balance and some postural tremor, indicating deterioration of cerebellar function and of the extrapyramidal system. With increasing age, there is less precision in controlling the contraction of muscles, such as the masseter muscles. It takes more time and efforts before new dentures can be controlled automatically. Of course, an older person has a great deal of experience to fall back on, and if a new task is given, which utilises previously acquired skills, difficulties will be minimised. However, problems are more likely to arise if the new task is more demanding than declining abilities are able to cope with. For example, previous denture experience can be of the greatest assistance when having to cope with new dentures, providing that major changes to the design of the dentures have not been introduced (see Chapter 8).

Research has shown that the masseter and medial pterygoid muscles suffer a decrease in cross-sectional area and in muscle density as a consequence of advancing age; the decrease is more apparent in edentulous people (Newton et al. 1993). Such changes might, in individual cases, be responsible for complaints of difficulty in eating and of eating more slowly than the rest of the family. Of course, these problems can be due to the simple fact that eating with dentures is just more difficult than eating with natural teeth anyway!

Age also brings about deterioration of the denture-bearing tissues. The epithelium becomes thinner, the connective tissue is less resilient and the ability of the mucosa to heal is impaired. Osteoporosis is a common problem in older people, particularly affecting postmenopausal women, occurring in about one-third of women over 60 years. Not only is the skeleton affected, but the lower jaw will also show a decrease in bone density. The severity of osteoporosis is related not only to hormonal changes but also to long-term calcium deficiency and to loss of normal function. There is no evidence to suggest that the rate of salivary secretion decreases with age per se, but as will be seen later, normal salivation can be adversely affected by drug therapy.

Systemic disease

The following problems, which commonly occur in older people, can cause complications specifically related to the care and treatment of the edentulous patient.

Psychiatric disorders

Depression is the most common mental disorder in later life. The prevalence of depression requiring clinical intervention in the over 65-year-olds is between 13% and 16% (Banerjee et al. 2002). This condition can result in poor appetite and weight loss and can adversely affect motivation and self-care. It is not a normal consequence of ageing and is treatable. With regard to prosthetic treatment, the condition may reduce the patient's ability to make an effort to accommodate to new dentures.

Dementia is found in 5%–6% of people over the age of 65 and in 20% of those over 80 years old and can result in conditions such as intellectual impairment, a poor memory (particularly for recent events), poor concentration and a reduced level of self-care. The situation can deteriorate to such a level that dentures, particularly the lower, cannot be worn.

Additional problems may arise from the drug therapy given to these patients; they are discussed in the next section and in Chapter 16.

Parkinson's disease

This condition, as well as other tremors that are likely to occur in the older person, can adversely affect the precise control of the mandible, making it more difficult to obtain an accurate recording of the jaw relation-ship. Parkinsonism can also cause difficulty in swallowing, leading to pronounced dribbling, which can be very distressing for the patient.

Cerebrovascular accident

The occurrence of a 'stroke' may result in unilateral paralysis of the facial muscles, making it more difficult for the patient to control dentures, especially the lower denture. The patient may also have difficulty clearing food which has lodged in the buccal sulcus. Speech may be affected, making it difficult for the patient to communicate with the dentist. Ways in which prosthetic treatment can help these patients have been described by Wright (1997).

Angina

Angina can cause pain that is experienced around the left body of the mandible or even the left side of the palate. This usually occurs in association with chest pain and the onset is usually related to physical exertion.

Congestive heart failure, chronic bronchitis and emphysema

Older patients with these conditions are likely to become breathless if the dental chair is tipped back into the supine position.

Diabetes

Type 2 diabetes occurs commonly in later life. It predisposes to infection in the mouth by *Candida albicans*, is a cause of a 'burning mouth' and can result in troublesome dryness of the oral mucosa.

Osteoporosis

Although this condition has already been mentioned with respect to the denture-bearing tissues, it is appropriate to mention that it can lead to a hunched posture, or kyphosis, which requires the dentist to ensure that work is undertaken with the patient in the sitting position with the head and neck adequately supported.

Arthritis

Older patients may suffer from osteoarthritis or rheumatoid arthritis. Either condition may have reached such an advanced state that the patient finds it extremely difficult, or even impossible, to attend the dental surgery. If either of these conditions affects the hands, it becomes increasingly difficult for the patient to clean dentures adequately. The patient can be helped by increasing the thickness of the brush handle so that it can be gripped without discomfort, by providing brushes which can be attached to a washbasin and by recommending an effective cleansing solution which reduces the reliance on mechanical means of plaque removal.

Nutritional deficiencies

Deficiencies of the vitamin B complex, folic acid and iron are not uncommon in the older person. As will be described in later chapters, these deficiencies can lead to pathology of the mucosa and to widespread discomfort or burning.

Drug therapy

It has been reported that older patients are prescribed an average of 2.8 drugs per person. Poor compliance with medication is found in between 50% and 60% of patients; this is a particular problem among older people who are of course taking more drugs and may have some degree of intellectual impairment or poor recall.

The commonest drugs prescribed for older people, in descending order of frequency, are diuretics, analgesics, hypnotics, sedatives, anxiolytics, antirheumatics and beta-blockers. Many of these drugs have side effects that are relevant to the dentist about to undertake prosthetic treatment. Xerostomia is produced by certain antidepressants, diuretics, antihyper-

tensives and antipsychotics, with some drugs having a more profound effect on secretion than others. Lack of saliva adversely affects the retention of dentures, increases the possibility of oral infection, and through the absence of lubrication, can result in generalised soreness or even a burning sensation.

Certain drugs, such as steroid inhalers used in the treatment of asthma, immunosuppressive drugs and broad-spectrum antibiotics used over a long period, can alter the oral flora, thus predisposing to candida infection.

Tardive dyskinesia is a condition characterised by spasmodic movements of the oral, lingual and facial muscles. These uncontrollable movements can make it extremely difficult, or even impossible, to provide stable dentures. The condition is brought on by extensive use of drugs such as antipsychotics and tricyclic antidepressants. It will occur in 20%–40% of patients who have been taking the drugs for longer than 6 months. In approximately 40% of sufferers, the condition is not reversible, even if the drug therapy is stopped.

Psychological changes

Advancing age leads to certain inevitable changes that must be taken into account when treating older patients. For example, the patient finds it more difficult to perform tasks that depend upon rapid movements. Such tasks may well include the need to suddenly control a denture that has become destabilised during normal function. It should also be realised that older people take rather longer to learn to perform new tasks or to remember new information which is not put over clearly or which may not appear to be immediately relevant.

As mentioned earlier, depression is a common condition. One frequent cause is the changing role brought about by increasing age. For example, children are no longer dependent upon the parent, retirement brings about a new life with reduced income, life changes dramatically as a result of the death of the spouse, health deteriorates and the person is less able to care for him or herself. The greater the number of these life events, the more the person has to cope with. Of course, if the person is able to adapt to the changes, there is a reduced risk of depression developing.

Older people are less able to accept new situations, be they a change in denture shape, a new dentist or even the appointment time for treatment. It will be appreciated that the clinician must take many aspects of the life of the patient into account when investigating a complaint. Of course, many problems will be straightforward, but some will be complicated by factors that are far removed from the oral cavity and the existing dentures. Unless their presence is suspected, there is a risk that prosthetic treatment alone will fail to deal with a problem (see Chapter 16).

Nutrition

A great deal has been written on the relationship between nutrition and the efficiency of the dentition, be it natural or artificial. It is not appropriate in this text to rehearse all the arguments. Instead, some of the more important conclusions will be listed.

Although overt malnutrition is relatively rare, it should be pointed out that an inadequate diet can lead to reduced tolerance of the oral tissues to normal wear and tear and that this reduced resistance, in turn, can result in poor adaptation to dentures. Those people more likely to have nutritional problems are the housebound living at home, those with handicaps that make shopping and cooking difficult, alcoholics, people who suffer from mental illness or those who have been recently bereaved. As indicated below, those living in long-stay institutions are a particularly vulnerable group.

Our knowledge of the link between oral health, diet and nutritional status in older people has been improved by the publication of a national diet and nutrition survey of people aged 65 years and over (Steele et al. 1998). In this survey, comparisons were made between those people living at home (the free-living sample) and those in long-term care (the institutional sample). Findings that relate particularly to edentate people are as follows:

- Fifty per cent of the free-living group were edentate as compared with 79% of the institutional group.
- Those living at home wore old dentures with a mean age of 17 years. The complete dentures of the institutional group were older still and had more faults.
- Edentate people reported greater difficulty in eating certain foods than did the dentate. These foods included tomatoes, raw carrots, lettuce, well-done steaks, apples and nuts. The difficulties could be so great that the foods were not eaten at all. Those people who reported dry mouths had greater difficulties with those foods which required chewing. Those living in institutions reported significantly greater restrictions.
- Edentate people had lower plasma levels of vitamins A, C and E than the dentate. Those living in institutions had a disturbingly low level of vitamin C that was at the bottom end of the normal range.

Finally, the point should be made that, in the absence of an effective dentition and an adequate supply of saliva, there is a greater risk of a person choking on a large bolus of food that has not been adequately broken up. Preparation for safe swallowing is an important consideration.

The condition of dentures

Most edentulous people over the age of 65 years are wearing dentures that are more than 10 years old, and as a result, mucosal changes are present in between 44% and 63% of cases. The need for treatment, based on clinical judgement, suggests that 40% of 5-year-old dentures and 80% of 10-year-old dentures should be replaced. However, the picture is not that simple. Need can be measured in a variety of ways:

- 'Normative need' is the need defined by expert or professional opinion.
- 'Felt need' is the patient's subjective desire.
- 'Expressed need' is recorded when the 'felt need' is activated through the patient seeking treatment.

One estimate of 'normative need' has already been described. Others indicate that 70%–85% of older people's dentures require attention and that such need far exceeds the 'expressed need'. Older people are likely to consider that treatment is required as a result of experiencing pain, difficulty in chewing, a deteriorating appearance, or because the existing dentures are broken or have been lost. However, the 'felt need' may not be activated for a variety of reasons, including the following:

- The dental problem is low on the list of priorities compared with other problems.
- Inertia on the part of the patient.
- Ignorance of available services.
- Fear of treatment that may be required. It is important to remember that a large proportion of today's edentulous patients experienced dental treatment in less sophisticated times when pain was a frequent accompaniment.
- Inability to travel to a surgery because of ill health or problems of transportation.
- A feeling that nothing can be done anyway and that the dental problem is just one of the inconveniences of old age.
- Finance.

The effectiveness of some or all of these 'barriers to care' can be gauged from one survey which reported that of a group of 75-year-old people living independently, nearly half had an oral problem, one-third had pain and the majority had not visited a dentist for at least 10 years, and what's more, did not plan to do so.

Caring for the older patient: some practical points

Many of the subsequent chapters of the book refer to modifications to clinical techniques or approaches that may be required to meet the particular needs of the significantly older patient. When dealing with these significantly older patients who may be frail, all members of the surgery team must have a sound understanding of the problems of this older group and be sympathetic to their needs. The sections which follow mention some aspects of management that naturally follow on from the previous discussion.

Mobility

There are many causes of immobility, which may arise from disorders of the musculoskeletal system, neurological disorders, cardiovascular and pulmonary disease, the consequence of drug therapy and psychological problems. The whole story for an individual patient may be quite complex and the consequences may be far reaching. For example, a person's immobility may result in depression, which itself causes loss of appetite, and ultimately, malnutrition (Walsh et al. 1999). It requires little imagination to realise that the added complication of poorly fitting or painful dentures can only worsen the situation.

It should be stressed that to encourage older edentulous patients to attend for dental treatment, it is important to ensure that there is ready access to the surgery. A ground floor location is ideal, and both doors and corridors should be wide enough to provide access for wheelchairs. Once the patient has arrived in the surgery, sufficient time needs to be spent explaining the routine in order to put the patient at his or her ease. When settling the patient in the dental chair, it is important to warn the patient in advance of any movements of the chair that are about to be made and to remember that most older people will be more comfortable in the sitting rather than the supine position.

Communication

It should be recognised that the patient is likely to be anxious and also unclear as to what might be involved at the first visit to the surgery. It is imperative to develop appropriate communication skills so that the patient's problems can be assessed as accurately as possible, a realistic treatment plan evolved, and the patient made fully aware of what will be done and more particularly what may be the limitations of treatment. To this end, it is vital to carry out the discussion in a quiet, unhurried environment, to face the patient when talking and, if the patient has a hearing impairment, to speak slowly and clearly but without undue exaggeration. As the impairment is likely to mean that higher frequencies can no longer be perceived, it is important not to speak too loudly. It is also extremely important to allow plenty of time for listening to the patient's account of any problems so that he or she feels that sufficient opportunity has been given for matters of concern to be adequately explained to the dentist.

When information is being given to the patient, it should be relayed reasonably slowly, in a carefully structured manner, and without distraction or interruption. It is useful to back up verbal comment with written advice, recognising that the print should be large enough for those whose eyesight has deteriorated.

When obtaining a history, it is important to remember that older people have an increasing number of 'aches and pains', but regarding these problems as being a normal consequence of ageing can result in a risk of underdiagnosing. It must also be appreciated that chronic pain and depression commonly go together, so it is important to establish any predisposing factors. For example, widespread pain under a lower denture might be due to a clenching habit which has bruised the mucosa, and which has been initiated by worry at home;

the pain is no less real, whatever the cause. In such circumstances, prosthetic treatment on its own is unlikely to offer long-term success. Effective care is likely to require communication between the dentist and the patient's medical practitioner.

Planning treatment

When deciding upon a course of treatment for an older patient, one must always have the original complaint at the forefront of one's mind and plan a programme of care that can be achieved in the particular circumstances. For example, the request to see the patient may come from a relative who has become increasingly embarrassed that dentures are not being worn on social occasions. The health of the patient may have deteriorated to such an extent that successful control of a new lower denture is clearly out of the question. It may be concluded that realistic treatment is the provision of an upper denture only, which will be worn for appearance's sake rather than for function. In such circumstances, it can be argued that the dentist is treating the relative as well as the patient, a course of action that surely is entirely justified. Although this particular illustration may be thought of as an extreme one, it is by no means uncommon in long-stay care homes and does serve to make the point that successful treatment is the 'art of the possible'.

Postscript

In this section of the chapter dealing with the older and significantly frailer patient, we have drawn attention to conditions that are likely to influence overall care. The reader should not progress to the remainder of the book with the impression that prosthetic treatment of the older patient is invariably going to be complicated by a long list of problems. It is important to put things in perspective by appreciating characteristics of normal ageing. Many of these characteristics are widely recognised but some have been less well accepted. Certain features that are well recognised include the following:

- The majority of older people are *not* senile, nor do they feel miserable for most of the time.
- Most older people can learn new things.
- Older peoples' reaction times tend to be slower.
- Physical strength tends to decline with age, but about 80% of individuals are healthy enough to carry out normal activities.
- The majority like some kind of work to do.

Those features which are less well recognised include the following:

- All five senses tend to decline with age.
- Most older people are not set in their ways; they do, however, take longer to learn something new.
- The majority are seldom bored and are neither socially isolated nor lonely.
- The majority of old people are seldom irritated or angry.

References and additional reading

Anon. (1990) Elderly people: their medicines and their doctors. *Drugs and Therapeutic Bulletin*, 20, 77–9.

Atwood, D.A. (1971) Reduction of residual ridges: a major oral disease entity. *Journal of Prosthetic Dentistry*, 26, 266–79.

Baillie, S. & Woodhouse, K. (1988) Medical aspects of ageing. *Dental Update*, 15, 236–41.

Baker, K.A. & Ettinger, R.L. (1985) Intra-oral effects of drugs in elderly persons. *Gerodontics*, 1, 111–16.

Banerjee, S., Wedgewood, F. & Ha, Y. (2002) Old age psychiatry. In: *Elderly Medicine – A Training Guide* (eds G.S. Rai & G.P. Mulley), pp. 111–25. Martin Dunitz, London.

Bradbury, J., Thomason, J.M., Jepson, N.J.A, Walls, A.W.G, Allen, P.F., & Moynihan, P.J. (2006) Nutrition counseling increases fruit and vegetable intake in the edentulous. *Journal of Dental Research*, 85(5), 463–8.

Bradbury, J., Thomason, J.M., Jepson, N.J.A., Walls, A.W.G., Mulvaney, C.E., Allen, P.F. & Moynihan, P.J. (2008) Perceived chewing ability and intake of fruit and vegetables. *Journal of Dental Research*, 87, 720–5.

Budtz-Jørgensen, E. (1999) *Prosthodontics for the Elderly: Diagnosis and Treatment*. Quintessence Publishing Co., Chicago.

Carlsson, G.E. (1998) Clinical morbidity and sequelae of treatment with complete dentures. *Journal of Prosthetic Dentistry*, 79, 17–23.

Carlsson, G.E. (2006) Facts and fallacies: an evidence base for complete dentures. *Dental Update*, 33, 134–42.

Christensen, J. (1988) Domiciliary care for the elderly patient. *Dental Update*, 15, 284–90.

Douglass, C.W., Shih, A. & Ostry, L. (2002) Will there be a need for complete dentures in the United States in 2020? *Journal of Prosthetic Dentistry*, 87, 5–8.

Drummond, J.R., Newton, J.P. & Yemm, R. (1988) Dentistry for the elderly: a review and an assessment of the future. *Journal of Dentistry*, 16, 47–54.

Feine, J.S., Carlsson, G.E., Awad, M.A., Chehade, A., Duncan, W.J., Gizani, S., Head, T., Heydecke, G., Lund, J.P., MacEntee, M., Mericske-Stern, R., Mojon, P., Morais, J.A., Naert, I., Payne, A.G., Penrod, J., Stoker, G.T., Tawse-Smith, A., Taylor, T.D., Thomason, J.M., Thomson, W.M. & Wismeijer, D. (2002) The McGill consensus statement on overdentures. Mandibular two-implant overdentures as first choice standard of care for edentulous patients. *Journal of Prosthetic Dentistry*, 88, 123–4.

Fiske, J., Dougall, A. & Lewis, D. (2009) *A Clinical Guide to Special Care Dentistry*. British Dental Association, London.

Fiske, J., Gelbier, G. & Watson, R.M. (1990) The benefit of dental care to an elderly population assessed using a sociodental measure of oral handicap. *British Dental Journal*, 168, 153–6.

Fiske, J., Griffiths, J., Jamieson, R. & Manger, D. (2000) Guidelines for oral health care for long-stay patients and residents. *Gerodontology*, 17, 55–64.

Fiske, J. & Lewis, D. (2000) The development of standards for domiciliary dental care services: guidelines and recommendations. *Gerodontology*, 17, 119–22.

Grabowski, M. & Bertram, U. (1975) Oral health status and need of dental treatment in the elderly Danish population. *Community Dentistry and Oral Epidemiology*, 3, 108–14.

Hamilton, F.A., Sarll, D.W., Grant, A.A. & Worthington, H.V. (1990) Dental care for elderly people by general dental practitioners. *British Dental Journal*, 168, 108–12.

Haraldson, T., Karlsson, U. & Carlsson, G.E. (1979) Bite force and oral function in complete denture wearers. *Journal of Oral Rehabilitation*, 6, 41–8.

Harkins, K. (2002) Social gerodontology. In: *Elderly Medicine – A Training Guide* (eds G.S. Rai & G.P. Mulley), pp. 9–12. Martin Dunitz, London.

Heath, M.R. (1972) Dietary selection by elderly persons, related to dental state. *British Dental Journal*, 132, 145–8.

Hoad-Reddick, G., Grant, A.A. & Griffiths, C.S. (1987) Knowledge of dental services provided: investigations in an elderly population. *Community Dentistry and Oral Epidemiology*, 15, 137–40.

Holm-Pedersen, P. & Loe, H. (1986) *Geriatric Dentistry*. Munksgaard, Copenhagen.

MacEntee, M.I. (1985) The prevalence of edentulism and diseases related to dentures – a literature review. *Journal of Oral Rehabilitation*, 12, 195–207.

MacEntee, M.I., Dowell, T.B. & Scully, C. (1988) Oral health concerns of an elderly population in England. *Community Dentistry and Oral Epidemiology*, 16, 72–4.

MacMahon, D.G. & Battle, M. (2002) Developing and planning services. In: *Elderly Medicine – A Training Guide* (eds G.S. Rai & G.P. Mulley), pp. 19–28. Martin Dunitz, London.

Mojon, P., Thomason, J.M. & Walls, A.W. (2004) The impact of falling rates of edentulism. *International Journal of Prosthodontics*, 17, 434–40.

Moynihan, P.J., Butler, T.J., Thomason, J.M. & Jepson, N.J.J. (2000) Nutrient intake in partially dentate patients: the effect of prosthetic rehabilitation. *Journal of Dentistry*, 28, 557–63.

Murphy, W.M., Morris, R.A. & O'Sullivan, D.C. (1974) Effect of oral prostheses upon texture perception of food. *British Dental Journal*, 137, 245–9.

Newton, J.P., Yemm, R. & Abel, R.W. (1993) Changes in human jaw muscles with age and dental state. *Gerodontology*, 10, 16–22.

O'Mullane, D. & Whelton, H. (1992) *Oral Health of Irish Adults 1989–1990*. The Stationery Office, Dublin.

Österberg, T., Carlsson, G.E. & Sundh, V. (2000) Trends and prognoses of dental status in the Swedish population: analysis based on interviews in 1975 to 1997 by Statistics Sweden. *Acta Odontologica Scandinavica*, 58, 177–82

Öwall, B., Kayser, A.F. & Carlsson, G.E. (1996) *Prosthodontics – Principles and Management Strategies*. Mosby-Wolfe, London.

Rai, G.S. & Mulley, G.P. (2002) *Elderly Medicine – A Training Guide*. Martin Dunitz, London.

Seymour, R. A. (1988) Dental pharmacology problems in the elderly. *Dental Update*, 15, 375–81.

Shapiro, S., Bomberg, T.J. & Hamby, C.L. (1985) Postmenopausal osteoporosis: dental patients at risk. *Gerodontics*, 1, 220–5.

Smith, J.M. & Sheiham, A. (1979) How dental conditions handicap the elderly. *Community Dentistry and Oral Epidemiology*, 7, 305–10.

Steele, J.G., Sheiham, A., Marcenes, W. & Walls, A.W.G. (1998) National Diet and Nutrition Survey: People aged 65 years and over. Vol. 2, Report of the oral health survey. The Stationery Office, London.

Steele, J.G., Treasure, E., Pitts, N.B., Morris, J. & Bradnock, G. (2000) Total tooth loss in the United Kingdom in 1998 and its implications for the future. *British Dental Journal*, 189, 598–603.

Strayer, M.S., DiAngelis, A.J. & Loupe, M.J. (1986) Dentists' knowledge of aging in relation to perceived elderly patient behavior. *Gerodontics*, 2, 223–7.

Thomason, J.M, Feine, J., Exley, C., Moynihan, P., Müller, F., Naert I., Ellis, J.S., Barclay, C., Butterworth, C., Scott B., Lynch, C., Stewardson, D., Smith, P., Welfare, R., Hyde, P., McAndrew, R., Fenlon, M., Barclay, S. & Barker, D. (2009) Mandibular two implant-supported overdentures as the first choice standard of care for edentulous patients – the York Consensus Statement. *British Dental Journal*, 207, 185–6.

Thomason, J.M., Lund, J.P., Chehade, A. & Feine, J.S. (2003) Patient satisfaction with mandibular implant overdentures and conventional dentures 6 months after delivery. *International Journal of Prosthodontics*, 16, 467–73.

Walker, A. & Cooper, I. (2000) *Adult Dental Health Survey. Oral Health in the United Kingdom 1998*. The Stationery Office, London.

Walls, A.W.G. & Barnes, I.E. (1988) Gerodontology: the problem? *Dental Update*, 15, 186–91.

Walsh, K., Roberts, J. & Bennett, G. (1999) Mobility in old age. *Gerodontology*, 16, 69–74.

WHO (1982) *Introductory Document: Demographic Considerations*. World Assembly on Aging, Vienna.

WHO (1992) *Country Profiles on Oral Health in Europe 1991*. WHO, Regional Office for Europe, Copenhagen.

Wright, S.M. (1997) Denture treatment for the stroke patient. *British Dental Journal*, 183, 179–84.

Xie, Q., Ainamo, A. & Tilvis, R. (1997a) Association of residual ridge resorption with systemic factors in home-living elderly subjects. *Acta Odontologica Scandinavica*, 55, 299–305.

Xie, Q., Närhi, T.O., Nevalainen, J.M., Wolf, J. & Ainamo, A. (1997b) Oral status and prosthetic factors related to residual ridge resorption in elderly subjects. *Acta Odontologica Scandinavica*, 55, 306–13.

Factors Influencing the Outcome of Prosthetic Treatment

2

The successful outcome of prosthetic treatment depends upon the combined efforts of three people:

- *The clinician* – who makes a diagnosis, prepares a treatment plan and undertakes the clinical work.
- *The dental technician* – who constructs the various items, which culminate in the finished dentures.
- *The patient* – who is faced with coming to terms with the loss of all the natural teeth, having to adapt to the dentures and accepting and accommodating their limitations.

This chapter will:

- focus on the patient's contribution to the success of complete denture treatment,
- review the information on the success rate of this treatment, and
- consider whether it is possible to predict treatment outcome.

The patient's contribution

The patient needs to know, with the clinician's help, what to expect when new dentures are provided and to be motivated to wear them long enough for adaptation to take place. This willingness, even determination, of the patient to persevere with new prostheses in the face of initial difficulties – so that adaptation can occur – is vital to success for two main reasons:

- There is nothing 'normal' about having to wear conventional complete dentures. The change to the oral environment when two large foreign bodies are inserted into the mouth is so great that a substantial positive effort has to be made to come to terms with it.
- The wearing of these foreign bodies is under the complete control of the patient. When difficulties are experienced with the new dentures they can be removed from the mouth, considered, discussed, compared and even set aside. If this is the patient's main response to the feeling of strangeness

Prosthetic Treatment of the Edentulous Patient, Fifth Edition, © R.M. Basker, J.C. Davenport and J.M. Thomason
Published 2011 by Blackwell Publishing Ltd.

then adaptation will not occur and the treatment is likely to fail.

To cope with the drastic change within the oral cavity, the patient must:

- be able to come to terms with the loss of the natural teeth and their artificial replacement,
- become accustomed to the sensation of the dentures, a process known as habituation,
- learn to control the dentures, and
- accept and hopefully appreciate the new appearance.

The psychological effects of tooth loss

Chapter 1 discussed the effect that tooth loss had on the residual ridges. Whereas a lot of research work has been undertaken on that topic, it is only in more recent years that investigations have been carried out to discover the effect of tooth loss on people's feelings (Fiske et al. 1998; Davis et al. 2000; Hyland et al. 2009).

In an investigation of patients receiving prosthetic treatment, most having lost their remaining natural teeth several years previously and seeking replacement dentures, 45% admitted to having found it difficult to accept the loss (Davis et al. 2000).

Many of those who had difficulties took longer than a year to get over the loss, and more than one-third had still not accepted it by that time. They expressed feelings of sadness, anger and depression and many felt that these last extractions had made them feel prematurely old and that they had lost a part of themselves. There was loss of confidence, a restriction in choice of food and a lowered enjoyment of that food. Relationships with others were affected and many patients avoided looking at themselves without their dentures in place. The impact of the limitations of complete dentures imposed on edentulous patients was also highlighted in a qualitative study comparing patients treated with either conventional complete dentures or implant-supported

overdentures (Hyland et al. 2009). The findings again demonstrated that the functional limitations of complete dentures often impose significant restrictions on edentulous patients, particularly in terms of limiting social participation with family and friends and in the choice of foods, especially when eating with others.

The disturbing picture for edentulous patients painted by these studies was reinforced by findings from a national survey of adult dental health (Walker & Cooper 2000), which revealed that 61% of those who still retained their natural teeth found the idea of complete dentures a very upsetting one. More women were upset than men and those people who attended their clinicians on a regular basis were more likely to be troubled than those who did not. Interestingly, the older the dentate person the more likely they were to find the idea of complete dentures very upsetting. It is as if the longer a person has been able to put off the evil day the more troubled they will be if, in spite of every effort, they succumb.

From the above account, it may be concluded that total tooth loss has a profound effect on a significant proportion of the edentulous population and may well introduce added complications to the process of successful rehabilitation. The following points clearly emerge from the research work:

- Prevent total tooth loss if possible.
- If total loss is inevitable, plan the transition from the remains of the natural dentition to the artificial dentition with great care (see Chapter 3).
- Ensure that the patient is properly prepared for treatment and that everything possible is done to reduce the inevitable feeling of anxiety.
- Remember that many wearers of complete dentures are still likely to have profound worries some considerable time after becoming edentulous, and that if these worries are addressed in a sympathetic and encouraging manner, there will be a greater chance of the course of treatment being successful.

Habituation

Habituation has been defined as follows: 'A gradual diminution of responses to continued or repeated stimuli.'

When new dentures are placed in the mouth, they stimulate mechanoreceptors in the oral mucosa. Impulses arising from these receptors, which record touch and pressure, are transmitted to the sensory cortex with the result that the patient can 'feel' the dentures. For the first-time denture wearer this bombardment of the sensory nervous system almost inevitably results in pronounced salivation which, fortunately, only lasts for a few hours. The continuing stimulation of these receptors does not result in a corresponding continuous stream of impulses. The receptors adapt to this stimulation and as a consequence the patient begins to lose conscious awareness of the new shapes in the mouth. Of course, if replacement dentures are constructed whose shape is dissimilar to existing ones, a new set of stimuli will be evoked and the process of habituation starts all over again. This concept is one of the main reasons for copying dentures, using a method such as that described in Chapter 8.

In addition to the mechanoreceptors in the oral mucosa being stimulated by the shape of the new dentures, further stimulation arises as a result of contact between the occlusal surfaces during function. The forces generated by contraction of the muscles of mastication are transmitted through the dentures to the underlying tissues, resulting in a pattern of stimulation of the mechanoreceptors which enables the patient to recognise the presence or absence of occlusal harmony. This is dealt with in greater detail in Chapter 14.

Control of the dentures

A discussion of the behaviour of sensory receptors is equally relevant when considering the patient's ability to control dentures. This is because the successful manipulation of dentures depends upon purposeful and effective muscular activity, which in turn is dependent on adequate sensory feedback. When sensory nerve endings in the oral cavity are anaesthetised, the retention of complete lower dentures is reduced. In other words, loss of sensory input results in a lower level of purposeful muscle activity directed at keeping the dentures in place.

The patient's ability to control dentures involves a learning process that, initially, is a conscious endeavour. The first few faltering steps of the inexperienced denture wearer are often discouraging both to the patient and to the clinician. However, it is comforting to realise that the vast majority of these patients return to the surgery after a few days showing few signs of their initial difficulty. The learning process has come to the rescue. As a result of repetition, new reflex arcs have been set up in the central nervous system and the conscious effort has been replaced by a subconscious behaviour pattern. Constant repetition of impulses lowers the synaptic resistance and facilitates the formation of conditioned reflexes. At the same time, however, it must be realised that the synaptic resistance will be increased in the absence of these repeated stimuli. In other words, practice makes perfect whilst idleness leads to decay.

The observation that the first few faltering steps are usually quickly overcome does not provide a license to ignore a more staged transition to the edentulous state through both partial dentures and more particularly overdentures as outlined in Chapter 3.

Appearance

The patient's perception

'Beauty is in the eye of the beholder', and in the prosthetic context one is concerned with the patient assessing the appearance of the new dentures in a mirror. Because a pleasing appearance is a subjective evaluation, there is obviously room for the clinician and patient to have differing opinions. However, open disagreement does not predispose to successful treatment and so it is vitally important that the clinician should take careful notice of a patient's views on appearance. However, this does not mean that the clinician should blindly follow the patient's requests if they are likely to lead to a poor aesthetic result. Indeed, advice and particularly demonstration may well succeed in convincing the patient that a more pleasing appearance can be obtained by introducing features such as slight irregularities in the positioning of the anterior teeth and a more natural shade. However, if demonstration of such modifications fails to convince the patient of their merits then it is likely that the patient's mind is made up and that success will be obtained only if an appearance is produced which conforms to the original request.

The clinician's judgement

Although the patient clearly has the final word on the appearance of the dentures, there are some situations in which clinical judgement is particularly important. Examples of these are as follows:

- The patient may be tolerating an upper denture whose tooth position has been placed too near the crest of the resorbed ridge. It is often possible to improve the appearance of replacement dentures by a judicious expansion of the upper dental arch. However, if the dental arch is expanded too far, the increased lip pressure on the labial face of the upper denture can lead to instability.
- Patients may request that new dentures are designed to 'iron out' creases around the mouth or generally to provide more facial support. Occasionally under such circumstances, it is possible to reduce the creases and so improve the appearance by expansion of the upper dental arch or by thickening the denture border as mentioned above. In both these situations, if it has proved pos-

sible to expand the upper arch the possibility of placing the mandibular denture teeth further buccally and/or labially arises and so avoids, or reduces, the dangers of 'tongue cramping'.

- The clinician may recognize that there would be an advantage in constructing replacement dentures with a lower occlusal plane so that the tongue, by resting on the occlusal surface of the mandibular denture, can be more effective in stabilising it. However, this lowering of the occlusal plane will alter the appearance and may lead to objections from the patient.

On occasions such as those described above, it is advisable for the clinician to explain, test and demonstrate the possible denture changes to the patient. This demonstration can be carried out on the patient's old dentures at the first appointment; wax additions can be made to simulate the possible changes to see if the alterations are likely to achieve the hoped-for benefits, or whether they are likely to have any detrimental effects such as instability. An example of success is shown in Fig. 8.8, whilst Fig. 2.1 is an example where the patient's wishes could not be met.

The value of compromise

On all these occasions where it is necessary to seek a compromise between function and appearance, the ability of the patient to accept the modified appearance will depend just as much on the persuasiveness of the clinician's explanation as on the deeds. Having said this, one must always be aware of the occasional patient who will not accept advice. In this case, the clinician has the choice of refusing to undertake a form of treatment that is unlikely to satisfy the patient's objectives of both appearance and function, or of making the dentures conform to the patient's request after warning the patient of the possible outcome and ensuring that he or she accepts responsibility for the design.

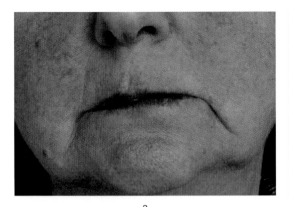
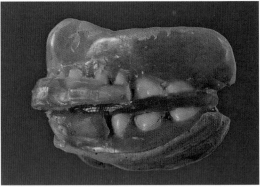

a   b

Figure 2.1   (a) The patient requested that replacement dentures be made to eliminate marked creasing at the angles of the mouth. (b) Possible alterations in design were demonstrated by addition of wax to the existing dentures; the dental arches were expanded and the occlusal vertical dimension increased. With the modified dentures in the mouth, it was possible to show the patient that her request could not be met and that the creases were, in fact, an age change.

Occasionally, it may be possible to satisfy the demanding patient by constructing two sets of dentures, one set with which to eat and one set in which to be seen! Needless to say it is vitally important that the eventual decision and reasons for that decision are noted in the patient's treatment record.

One further aspect of appearance is worthy of consideration. It is not uncommon for patients to seek replacement dentures in circumstances where the existing set has deteriorated to such an extent that a great deal of occlusal vertical dimension and lip support has been lost. In such circumstances, the patients commonly seek treatment to improve appearance. Replacement dentures that correct the aesthetic faults in the old dentures will undoubtedly make a dramatic change in appearance – a change hopefully appreciated by the patient. However, there is the risk that the change in appearance is so marked that it will be noticed by the patient's friends and relatives. The patient's initial enthusiasm for the new image is likely to be dampened if people stare rather pointedly, or even ask somewhat tactless questions about the new dentures. Such unwelcome comments can undermine the patient's confidence because they indicate that the friend recognises that the patient is a denture wearer. When obvious but necessary changes in appearance are being made, it is, therefore, a wise policy to warn the patient in advance of possible reactions from friends so that he or she is mentally prepared for them, and therefore, less likely to be discouraged.

Success rate of treatment

The discussion so far has ranged around the concept of the patient adapting to new dentures. The degree of success with which patients cope with the inevitable limitations of an artificial replacement varies enormously. Fortunately, the majority of patients have surprisingly little difficulty in adapting to an artificial dentition. However, it has been reported that about 15% of patients are dissatisfied with their new dentures (van Waas 1990a; Al Quran et al. 2001) and that this level may rise to 20% where treatment is being provided for patients who have had persistent problems (Lechner et al. 1995). It has also been shown that even if very high levels of satisfaction are recorded immediately after new dentures have been fitted, a significant deterioration occurs after 1 year (Berg 1988; Mersel et al. 1995). Most of the recurring dissatisfaction is blamed on the fit and comfort of the lower denture and the inability to eat effectively. This comment emphasises the importance of recalling patients and maintaining the dentures (Chapter 15). For example, relining or replacing dentures can readily restore chewing ability and the level of enjoyment when eating (Garrett et al. 1996). In addition, many patients simply accept a range of limitations as inevitable and 'learn to live with them' even though their general satisfaction and quality of life is adversely affected. In spite of these difficulties, such patients may not admit to them unless the relevant questions are put directly to them in a sympathetic manner (Hyland et al. 2009). Some patients present very considerable difficulties that can in fact be treated successfully by using special techniques. However, there remain a few patients who never become successful denture wearers. Can they be identified before treatment commences? The next section attempts to answer this question.

Predicting treatment outcome

How can one predict the outcome of complete denture treatment? Various attempts have been made to select various factors which, over the years, have been thought, either individually or collectively, to influence the eventual outcome of treatment. These factors include the following:

- Age of the patient
- Quality of care provided and previous complete denture experience
- The patient's expectations and attitude towards dentures
- Opinion of a third party
- General health

A review of the literature has led to the conclusion that there are still no reliable methods to predict the outcome of complete denture treatment (Carlsson 1998) and that satisfaction with dentures for most patients is individually determined, and for clinician and patient, is often unpredictable (van Waas 1990a). Nevertheless, the research offers some helpful pointers, and just as importantly, debunks some cherished beliefs.

The various factors will now be considered briefly.

Age of the patient

Age has not been found to be an accurate predictor of success or failure to adapt to new dentures (Beck et al. 1993). In general, as patients grow older, it takes longer for them to adapt successfully to new dentures for the reasons already discussed in Chapter 1. As the rate of ageing varies greatly between individuals, the actual age of a patient may be an unreliable guide to adaptive potential. A better basis for this assessment is the biological age, which may be estimated by judging how old the patient looks. It is not uncommon for the biological and actual ages to differ markedly. For example, when comparing the two people in Fig. 2.2, one would not expect the woman to have greater difficulty in adapting to the dentures in spite of the fact that she is 23 years older than the man. Increasing age should be looked at as offering a particular advantage in that the patient is likely to be able to draw upon previous denture experience, which, if favourable, can play an extremely valuable part in achieving ultimate success.

At this point, there should be a word of warning. Little is yet known about the ability of elderly people to adapt to the change from what remains of the natural dentition to a totally artificial one. With advances in preventive dentistry and an increased expectancy of life, one can foresee the possibility of people being faced with their first set of complete dentures

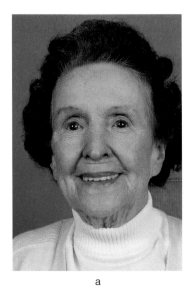 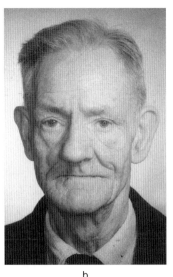

a   b

Figure 2.2 Variation of biological age with actual age. The woman, aged 89, is 23 years older than the man.

much later in life. The problems of adaptation with which prosthetic dentistry will be faced could well increase in the future for reasons mentioned earlier in this chapter.

The quality of care and previous denture experience

A survey of the literature shows inconsistency in identifying a positive association between patient satisfaction and denture quality. Whereas some researchers have reported no correlation (Vervoorn et al. 1988; de Baat et al. 1997), others have reported moderate correlation (van Waas, 1990a,b; Garrett et al. 1996) and still others have shown positive association with patient satisfaction (Reeve et al. 1984; Smith & Hughes 1988; Beck et al. 1993; Lamb et al. 1994; Fenlon et al. 2000; Fenlon & Sherriff 2008).

We conclude that of all the predictors of success which have been investigated, the quality of the prosthetic care provided stands out as the factor which is most strongly linked with patient satisfaction. This conclusion should not really be surprising and it highlights the fun-

damental importance of routinely adopting the best possible clinical and technical practices and of continually seeking to enhance the quality of care. These points are emphasised throughout this book.

The significance of the past dental history, its link with quality and with adaptability, can be illustrated by considering two common yet contrasting situations. There are those patients who seek new dentures to replace existing ones that have been worn for very many years. So often it is apparent that the old dentures are now ill-fitting and the occlusion is no longer balanced, and yet the patient has tolerated an increasing inadequacy for some time. Although this state of affairs may well indicate initial high denture quality and a well-marked ability to adapt to dentures and to overcome difficulties, such a level of perseverance can be dangerous, as it can result in accelerated resorption of the underlying bone and may induce pathological changes in the mucosa. This picture of stoicism is in marked contrast to the second group, made up of patients who have been provided with several sets of dentures in a short period of time. Such a story of repeated failure may at first sight indicate a patient who is unable or unwilling to accept complete dentures. However, there is another potent reason for repeated failure of prosthetic treatment and this may become apparent during examination of the various old dentures as obvious errors in design and construction are identified in each of them. If patients receive inadequate treatment on one or more occasions and are told that the problems experienced are due to them, confidence in prosthetic treatment is lost rapidly and a mental barrier is built up against dentures.

At first thought, it might seem common sense that there would be an obvious relationship between patient satisfaction and the quality of the denture-bearing tissues. In other words, it is easier to achieve success for a patient who has well-formed ridges on which to place dentures and vice versa. However, not all the investigations support such a relationship – perhaps because those patients who have poor ridges have learned to accept the inevitable limitations and have adapted particularly well to the handicap (van Waas 1990a; de Baat et al. 1997).

Nevertheless, in the cases where examination of the mouth indicates that the prognosis for dentures is poor, it is essential for the clinician to warn the patient in advance of the difficulties and to describe the steps that will be taken to minimise them. If a patient is not advised of the limited prognosis in the particular circumstances, any shortcomings in performance may be blamed on the dentures and the patient becomes discouraged prematurely.

It should also be remembered, as stated at the beginning of the chapter, that there is nothing 'normal' about having to wear conventional complete dentures. As such we should not be surprised that patients have difficulties accommodating to them and that this accommodation may only be partial. Thus, the possibility of other treatment alternatives, such as the use of dental implants for denture support, should be actively considered as a means of enhancing the possible success rates.

The patient's expectations and attitude towards dentures

Patients requesting replacement dentures generally do so for reasons of function and appearance; function includes fit and comfort of the dentures as well as the ability to eat effectively. As mentioned earlier, a satisfactory outcome to treatment is generally related to the level of function achieved and to the technical quality of the dentures (Fenlon & Sherriff 2008). It is of interest to note that concern over appearance seems to be under-reported, both before and after treatment. If functional requirements have been satisfied by the new dentures, patients may be inclined to look more closely at appearance. If they are unhappy with what they see, there is occasionally a reluctance to complain directly. Instead, patients may resort to making complaints about function to draw the clinician's attention to their real concern in a somewhat roundabout way. Functional complaints that seem to have no logical cause should always be considered in this particular light.

One study (van Waas 1990b) has pointed out that a patient's attitude to dentures can be a useful predictor of satisfaction or dissatisfaction. Agreement or disagreement to the following statements might be obtained from a patient before commencing treatment:

- I expect to have problems with my new dentures.
- I think I'll soon get used to my new dentures.
- I think it is difficult to make good dentures for me.
- I think they'll manage to make good dentures for me.
- I did not receive dentures that like me.

The 'wrong' answers should at least make one aware of the possibility of an unsatisfactory outcome.

Nevertheless, it should also be noted that the patient's expectations of what conventional complete dentures are capable of may not actually be realizable and that implant-supported dentures may be a more reliable way of satisfying the patients' wishes. One recent study has suggested that post-treatment satisfaction with conventional complete dentures was significantly lower than the patients' pre-treatment expectations, whereas the pre-treatment expectations of implant-supported overdenture were largely met (Heydecke et al. 2008). It may be the initial unrealistic expectation of what can be achieved with conventional complete dentures that ultimately leads to some patients' dissatisfaction with dentures even though constructed to a high standard.

The opinion of a third party

Earlier in the chapter, we drew attention to potential complications which might arise following critical comments about the new dentures from friends and relations. It has been shown that such comments, which are mostly centred on appearance, show a highly significant correlation with acceptance of the dentures by the patient (Berg et al. 1985). Negative comments can cause disappointment and rejection of the prostheses, whilst positive comments can promote cheerful acceptance of the treatment.

Health of the patient

Significant impairment of general bodily or mental health may affect the learning process adversely, with the result that the patient becomes discouraged because of major difficulties in mastering new dentures. In this respect, it should be remembered that the chances of impairment of health increase as people grow older. Therefore, when assessing a patient, it is very important to note details of the medical history, such as a chronic debilitating illness, which may reduce the patient's stamina to such an extent that there is little left to cope with the demands of new dentures. For example, patients suffering from any form of arthritis may

be persistently troubled with pain to the extent that it becomes a depressing and overwhelming part of life. The ability to manipulate dentures may be reduced severely by various neurological disorders, such as the muscle tremor and reduced muscular power of Parkinson's disease, and the muscle weakness of myasthenia gravis or bulbar palsy.

It has long been believed that any set of circumstances which impairs mental health may create a situation whereby anxiety, depression or other neurotic states may result in the patient being unable or unwilling to tolerate new dentures. Clues that such adverse psychological factors exist may be supplied by the medical history; for example, the patient may be taking tranquillisers or sedatives. To assist clinicians in recognising behavioural problems, various questionnaires have been designed to measure characteristics of personality and the levels of anxiety or depression.

The results of studies in this area are equivocal, whereas some point towards a link between, for example, neuroticism and dissatisfaction with the outcome of prosthetic treatment, others do not (Beck et al. 1993; Al Quran et al. 2001). At the beginning of the chapter, attention was drawn to the negative feelings shared by many people who had lost their remaining natural teeth. When coming across a patient who has had persistent dissatisfaction with complete dentures, it would seem sensible, at the very least, to discover their feelings and attitudes to prosthetic treatment, to offer advice or seek help from a dental or medical colleague as appropriate.

Readers may reasonably conclude at the end of this chapter that the pre-treatment assessment of a patient with respect to the level of ultimate success is far from being an exact science. They would be correct.

Clinical prosthetic experience is littered with pleasant surprises and with disappointments. Our review of current knowledge leads us to conclude that as long as a high standard of treatment is provided the disappointments, though inevitable, will at least be kept to a minimum.

References and additional reading

Al Quran, F., Clifford, T., Cooper, C. & Lamey, P.-J. (2001) Influence of psychological factors on the acceptance of complete dentures. *Gerodontology*, 18, 35–40.

Beck, C.B., Bates, J.F., Basker, R.M., Gutteridge, D.L. & Harrison, A. (1993) A survey of the dissatisfied denture patient. *European Journal of Prosthodontics and Restorative Dentistry*, 2, 73–8.

Berg, E. (1984) The influence of some anamnestic, demographic, and clinical variables on patient acceptance of new complete dentures. *Acta Odontologica Scandinavica*, 42, 119–27.

Berg, E. (1988) A 2-year follow-up study of patient satisfaction with new complete dentures. *Journal of Dentistry*, 16, 160–5.

Berg, E., Backer Johnsen, T. & Ingebretsen, R. (1984) Patient motives and fulfillment of motives in renewal of complete dentures. *Acta Odontologica Scandinavica*, 42, 235–40.

Berg, E., Backer Johnsen, T. & Ingebretsen, R. (1985) Social variables and patient acceptance of complete dentures. *Acta Odontologica Scandinavica*, 43, 199–203.

Berry, D.C. & Mahood, M. (1966) Oral stereognosis and oral ability in relation to prosthetic treatment. *British Dental Journal*, 120, 179–85.

Brill, N., Tryde, G. & Schübeler, S. (1959) The role of exteroceptors in denture retention. *Journal of Prosthetic Dentistry*, 9, 761–8.

Brill, N., Tryde, G. & Schübeler, S. (1960) The role of learning in denture retention. *Journal of Prosthetic Dentistry*, 10, 468–75.

Carlsson, G.E. (1998) Clinical morbidity and sequelae of treatment with complete dentures. *Journal of Prosthetic Dentistry*, 79, 17–23.

Crum, R.J. & Loiselle, R.J. (1972) Oral perception and proprioception: a review of the literature and its significance to prosthodontics. *Journal of Prosthetic Dentistry*, 28, 215–30.

Davis, D.M., Fiske, J., Scott, B. & Radford, D.R. (2000) The emotional effects of tooth loss: a preliminary quantitative study. *British Dental Journal*, 188, 503–6.

de Baat, C., van Aken, A.A., Mulder, J. & Kalk, W. (1997) 'Prosthetic condition' and patients' judgement of complete dentures. *Journal of Prosthetic Dentistry*, 78, 472–8.

Fenlon, M.R. & Sherrif, M. (2008) An investigation of factors influencing patients' satisfaction with new complete dentures using structural equation modeling. *Journal of Dentistry*, 36, 427–34.

Fenlon, M.R., Sherrif, M. & Walter, J.D. (2000) An investigation of factors influencing patients' use of new complete dentures using structural equation modelling techniques. *Community Dentistry and Oral Epidemiology*, 28, 133–40.

Fish, S.F. (1969) Adaptation and habituation to full dentures. *British Dental Journal*, 127, 19–26.

Fiske, J., Davis, D.M., Frances, C. & Gelbier, S. (1998) The emotional effects of tooth loss in edentulous people. *British Dental Journal*, 184, 90–3.

Garrett, N.R., Kapur, K.K. & Perez, P. (1996) Effects of improvements of poorly fitting dentures and new dentures on patient satisfaction. *Journal of Prosthetic Dentistry*, 76, 403–13.

Heydecke, G., Thomason, J.M., Awad, M.A., Lund, J.P. & Feine, J.S. (2008) Do mandibular implant overdentures and conventional complete dentures meet the expectations of edentulous patients? *Quintessence International*, 39, 803–9.

Hyland, R., Ellis, J., Thomason, M., El-Feky, A. & Moynihan, P. (2009) A qualitative study on patient perspectives of how conventional and implant-supported dentures affect eating. *Journal of Dentistry*, 37, 718–23.

Lamb, D.J., Ellis, B. & Kent, G. (1994) Measurement of changes in complete mandibular denture security using visual analogue scales. *International Journal of Prosthodontics*, 7, 30–4.

Lechner, S.K., Champion, H. & Tong, T.K. (1995) Complete denture problem solving: a survey. *Australian Dental Journal*, 40, 377–80.

Mersel, A., Babayof, I., Berkey, D. & Mann, J. (1995) Variables affecting denture satisfaction in Israeli elderly: a one year follow-up. *Gerodontology*, 12, 89–94.

Reeve, P.E., Watson, C.J. & Stafford, G.D. (1984) The role of personality in the management of complete denture patients. *British Dental Journal*, 156, 356–62.

Smith, J.P. & Hughes, D. (1988) A survey of referred patients experiencing problems with complete dentures. *Journal of Prosthetic Dentistry*, 60, 583–6.

van Waas, M.A.J. (1990a) Determinants of dissatisfaction with dentures: a multiple regression analysis. *Journal of Prosthetic Dentistry*, 63, 569–72.

van Waas, M.A.J. (1990b). The influence of clinical variables on patients' satisfaction with complete dentures. *Journal of Prosthetic Dentistry*, 63, 307–10.

van Waas, M.A.J. (1990c). The influence of psychologic factors on patient satisfaction with complete dentures. *Journal of Prosthetic Dentistry*, 63, 545–8.

Vervoorn, J.M., Duinkerke, A.S., Luteijn, F. & van de Poel, A.C. (1988) Assessment of denture satisfaction. *Community Dentistry and Oral Epidemiology*, 16, 364–7.

Walker, A. & Cooper, I. (eds) (2000) *Adult Dental Health Survey. Oral Health in the United Kingdom 1998*. The Stationery Office, London.

Weinstein, W., Schuchman, J., Lieberman, J. & Rosen, P. (1988) Age and denture experience as determinants in patient denture satisfaction. *Journal of Prosthetic Dentistry*, 59, 327–9.

Zigmond, A.S. & Snaith, R.P. (1983) The Hospital Anxiety and Depression Scale. *Acta Psychiatrica Scandinavica*, 67, 361–70.

Transition from the Natural to the Artificial Dentition

The loss of the remaining natural teeth and provision of an artificial dentition is a major and irreversible procedure for the patient. The enormity of the change raises the question – why is it not more common to use overdentures over natural tooth remnants, at least as a staging post, in the transition to the edentulous state? This is particularly the case as such overdentures may last for so long that the patient is able to continue having the denture supported by these natural abutments for the rest of his or her life. The question as to why this transition is not more frequently used is brought into sharp focus when one considers the improvements seen in patient satisfaction and quality of life provided by implant-supported overdentures when compared with conventional dentures (Thomason 2007). Before discussing the various ways of making the transition, it is helpful to consider just how common is the sudden, complete transition to the edentulous state and the typical reaction that patients have to the prospect.

Regular national surveys of the dental health of adults enable us to examine the changing state of dentitions and the attitudes of people to their dental status (Todd & Lader 1991; Walker & Cooper 2000). The general improvement in oral health has already been described in Chapter 1. With respect to the transition, there have been parallel improvements with the loss of natural teeth becoming an increasingly gradual process. For example, whereas in 1978 two-thirds of those who had lost the remainder of their teeth had 12 or more teeth extracted at the final stage, this proportion was reduced to nearly half in the next decade and to a quarter in the 1990s.

The level of anxiety with which people face the prospect of losing all their teeth and having to rely on complete dentures can be seen in Fig. 3.1. Nearly two-thirds of those people who did not wear dentures of any kind found the thought of having to wear complete dentures very upsetting. The concern was felt more by women than by men and more by those people who were regular attenders for dental treatment. It is important that the clinician appreciates that the transition can be a cause of great concern to the patient and

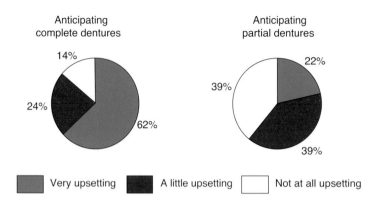

Figure 3.1 The attitude of adults (%) with only natural teeth to the thought of having complete dentures or a removable partial denture. (From Todd & Lader, 1991.)

takes the opportunity not only to manage this transition with understanding but also to offer alternatives to simply rendering the patient edentulous.

It can also be seen in Fig 3.1 that the concern about having complete dentures is much greater than that about partial dentures. Another important point to make is that this attitude had become more widespread over a 10-year period between surveys to the extent that the proportion of those who viewed the thought of having complete dentures as a very upsetting experience had gone up by 10%.

The level of concern felt by the general public can be examined in another way (Fig. 3.2). Here the level of anxiety was gauged amongst those who thought they were likely to need complete dentures within 5 years, those who would need complete dentures at sometime in the future and those who felt they would never require complete dentures. As expected, the proportion of those who were very upset about

the prospect of having complete dentures increased as their expectations of keeping their natural teeth increased. But even amongst those who thought they would need complete dentures in the next 5 years, one in five viewed the prospect as a very upsetting experience.

What is quite apparent is that a significant proportion of people who may have to have their remaining teeth extracted and complete dentures provided view the prospect with a great deal of concern and anxiety, thus making their acceptance of treatment much harder (see Chapter 2). The aim of this chapter is to outline the principles of treatment contributing to a successful transition either when forced to remove all the remaining tooth elements, or better still when at least some roots can be retained as overdenture abutments. The use of implants in place of tooth roots to support and stabilise the lower denture is also considered. Details of clinical techniques are, in the main, omitted.

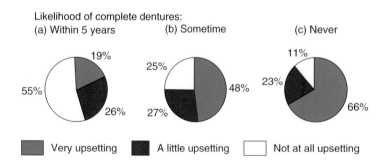

Figure 3.2 The attitude of adults (%) with only natural teeth to the thought of having complete dentures by the likelihood that they will need them. (From Todd & Lader, 1991.)

Methods of transition

The various methods of making the transition from natural to artificial dentition may be considered under the following headings.

Transitional partial dentures

Transitional partial dentures restore existing edentulous areas. They may be worn for a short period of time before the remaining natural teeth are extracted and the dentures are converted accordingly.

Overdentures

Overdentures are fitted over retained roots and derive some of their support and, if appropriately contoured, some stability from that coverage. Special attachments may be fixed to the root faces to provide mechanical retention for the denture which will further increase the denture stability. If, in due course, the roots have to be extracted, the overdenture can be converted into a mucosally-supported complete denture. In addition, overdentures can be supported and retained by implants.

Immediate dentures

Immediate dentures are constructed before the extraction of the natural teeth and are inserted immediately after removal of those teeth. An immediate denture can be either a conventional complete denture without support from the tooth roots, or a complete immediate overdenture.

Clearance of remaining natural teeth before making dentures

This approach differs from all those mentioned previously in that, after the extractions, time is allowed for initial healing and alveolar bone resorption to occur before providing complete dentures.

Factors influencing the decision of whether to extract all the remaining teeth or to retain some teeth or tooth roots

When the patient's dentition has reached the stage where it appears that complete dentures will be necessary in the foreseeable future, the clinician must consider carefully the timing of extraction of the remaining teeth and if it would be possible to retain some tooth roots, even if only in the short term. The following considerations will influence the decision.

The condition of the teeth and supporting tissues

The prognosis for each remaining tooth should be assessed carefully. Useful teeth can be retained if:

- it is feasible to undertake appropriate treatment to eliminate any disease present;
- if there is confidence in the patient's ability to maintain good, or even reasonable, oral health.

The presence of gross caries or advanced periodontal disease, coupled with an inability of the patient to maintain an acceptable level of oral hygiene, makes the decision of whether or not to extract the teeth a much simpler one; early extraction in such circumstances is probably advisable. Such a decision is perhaps especially important in the case of advanced periodontal disease where any undue delay will result in further destruction of what will become the bony denture foundation. Nevertheless, many patients who would be unwilling or unable to manage reasonable oral hygiene around multiple teeth, can often manage to clean two simple overdenture abutments, or at least to clean them well enough to delay significant short-term bone loss.

The position of the teeth

Natural teeth opposing an edentulous ridge

The situation in which one arch only is rendered edentulous can lead to major prosthetic complications. The combination most commonly found is a complete upper denture opposed by a number of lower natural teeth. A most unfavourable situation can develop in which the natural teeth generate high occlusal loads and excessive displacement of the denture, which may result in:

- rapid destruction of the denture-bearing bone;
- the production of a flabby ridge (see Chapter 16);
- complaints of a loose denture;
- a deteriorating appearance as the denture sinks into the tissues;
- fracture of the denture base.

The problems are accentuated in the lower jaw because the denture-bearing area is smaller.

Serious consideration must be given to preventing these problems from developing. The first step is to warn the patient of the possible consequences and arrange for regular inspection and maintenance to reduce the possibility of rapid, damaging resorption. If sufficient thought has been given to the problem in advance, it may be possible to utilise selected teeth as overdenture abutments so as to improve the loading on the underlying bone. It would be very rare for the clinician to consider trying to reduce the occlusal loads by extracting sound teeth in the opposing arch.

Over-eruption of the teeth

Extraction of over-erupted teeth may be required because they:

- excessively reduce the vertical space available for the opposing prosthesis;
- have a poor appearance.

In appropriate cases, endodontic therapy followed by decoronation of over-erupted teeth (so that they can be used as overdenture abutments) might be the preferred alternative approach. This also has the marked advantage that decoronating the tooth markedly improves its crown–root ratio and, therefore, creates a more favourable loading, usually resulting in a considerable reduction in mobility.

Age and health of the patient

As mentioned in Chapter 2, advancing years, frequently coupled by worsening health, may reduce the patient's ability to adapt successfully to complete dentures. This places the clinician on the horns of a dilemma when planning the timing of the extraction of teeth that have an uncertain prognosis:

- *Extract the remaining teeth earlier?* On the one hand, the teeth may be expected to have a few more years of useful life, but delaying extractions until they are unavoidable may postpone the patient's first experience of complete dentures to a time when ageing has seriously reduced adaptive capability. As a result, the patient may find it difficult, or even impossible, to cope with complete dentures when they are eventually fitted. It may therefore be argued that the best approach under such circumstances is to extract the teeth sooner rather than later so that the patient stands a better chance of adapting successfully to complete dentures. Better still, though, would be a planned progression through transitional partial dentures, the undertaking of endodontics on selected teeth for later overdenture support and eventually the conversion of the partial denture to a simple complete overdenture.
- *Extract the remaining teeth later?* As the rate of biological ageing and reduction in adaptive capability vary greatly from one patient to another, it is not possible to identify accurately a cut-off point in years at which

extractions should be carried out for the reason outlined above. It is true that early extractions may reduce problems of adaptation to dentures, but this advantage must be balanced against the immediate probability of reduced oral function and comfort in a patient who may be happy with a few remaining natural teeth and, perhaps, a partial denture.

The correct way out of the dilemma of whether or not to take the irrevocable step of a dental clearance may be determined by delaying the decision and placing the patient on a programme of regular review appointments. At each appointment, an assessment can be made of the rate of deterioration of the patient's dentition, and thus a clearer picture will emerge of the probable life of the teeth and their value to the patient. A somewhat crude judgement is to assess the health of the patient and the teeth and try to answer the question, 'Is the patient likely to outlive the remaining useful natural teeth, or is the reverse more likely to occur?' When it seems probable that the patient will outlive the remaining teeth in their current form, the first step should be the consideration of a staged transition, from partial dentures through to overdentures and, only if necessary, to conventional complete dentures. This way any decision to take action can be moderated by the patient's response to each phase of treatment.

It is important to remember that in the very elderly patient any elective alteration of oral status must be made only when absolutely necessary. On balance, extractions should probably be carried out only when they are unavoidable, not as an elective procedure in the hope that this will reduce adaptive difficulties later. In fact, those difficulties are likely to be present already.

To this end, there is a strong argument that every effort should be made to retain useful, strategic teeth which may either help to stabilise a partial denture or be converted into overdenture abutments. The argument may be extended by saying that if these last remaining teeth are extracted, and the patient experiences enormous problems with the complete dentures, the only way of minimising these problems is to provide an implant-retained overdenture. Such treatment is more costly. Thus, retaining these few natural teeth may well save the patient considerable trouble and expense and the clinician no little heartache.

The patient's wishes

The patient will often have views about whether or not the remaining teeth should be extracted and these views must of course be given high priority. If the views coincide with the clinician's judgement all is well. However, the following two scenarios occur occasionally and might cause the clinician some difficulty.

Hopeless teeth that the patient wants to retain

The clinician should carefully explain to the patient about the condition of the teeth and the possible harmful consequences of retaining them. If in spite of this the patient persists in wanting to retain the teeth, the clinician can do little apart from carefully noting the situation in the patient's record. A decision may still have to be made on whether to proceed with an alternative treatment plan, such as the provision of transitional partial dentures or an overdenture, or whether to withdraw from treatment.

Sound, useful teeth that the patient wants extracted

Again, the clinician's primary responsibility is to explain to the patient the nature of the clinical situation and to emphasise the harm that unnecessary extraction of the remaining teeth would cause. If this is done with care, the majority of patients will be persuaded of the value of keeping the teeth, or the tooth roots where this would be more appropriate. Judging from the relatively small number of tooth-supported overdentures it would appear that this is an area that the dental profession has probably not promoted sufficiently in the past. However, even after careful explanation a few patients will not accept the case for retaining the teeth; the appropriate action by the clinician is most likely to be withdrawal from the case, as to extract the teeth without clinical justification would be unethical.

Transitional partial dentures

Transitional partial dentures are of particular value in those cases where problems of adaptation to, or tolerance of, complete dentures are anticipated. Wearing a transitional partial denture provides:

- an opportunity to complete any denture adjustments found necessary to provide comfort and adequate function, before the remaining teeth are extracted or decoronated;
- a training period that allows the patient to develop some denture control and tolerance under circumstances made less demanding by the stabilising effect of the remaining teeth.

However true this may be, a study of unsuccessful and successful complete denture wearers did not conclude that a history of wearing a partial denture had any influence on the eventual outcome (Beck et al. 1993).

The chance of success of a transitional partial denture is influenced to a large extent by the particular teeth that remain in the mouth. For example, stability of a lower denture will be increased if an anterior saddle is present because the existence of the labial flange and contacts with the mesial surfaces of the abutment teeth will resist posterior displacement. Also, if the denture carries anterior teeth, the patient will be better motivated by the wish to retain a good dental appearance to persevere with the denture in the face of any initial difficulties. Success is also more likely if the denture design in-

corporates clasps (and preferably rests) to maximise retention and support. Although transitional partial dentures are a potentially valuable means of smoothing the passage from the partially dentate to the edentulous state, they can compound the difficulties of subsequent complete dentures unless they are correctly designed and adequately maintained. A partial denture that is under-extended, poorly fitting or which has an incorrect occlusion is likely to be unstable and uncomfortable, thus undermining the patient's confidence in denture wearing. Also, if the patient perseveres heroically with the partial denture in spite of the difficulties, destruction of the denture-bearing tissues is likely to occur, creating a more unfavourable foundation for subsequent complete dentures. Whilst traditionally these transitional partial dentures have been supported only by the soft tissues (so called tissue-borne) there is no reason why this should be the case. The important advantage of a transitional denture is that it can be added to when teeth need to be extracted; this usually means that the connector needs to be constructed from acrylic resin. It should be remembered that the transitional partial denture is the type of prosthesis usually provided for a patient whose dental awareness is highly suspect. In this situation, increased plaque formation and lack of adequate support can combine to cause severe tissue destruction in a relatively short time (Fig. 3.3). In such a

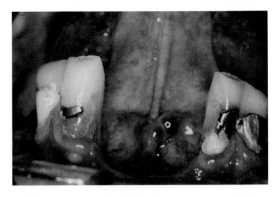

Figure 3.3 Severe tissue destruction caused by a tissue-borne partial denture.

case, a high-risk denture is provided for a high-risk patient.

Tooth-supported overdentures

In the transitional dentition the overdenture, like the partial denture, can be used to provide a training period, allowing the patient to prepare for the more demanding task imposed by future conventional complete dentures. If the life of the teeth is limited, treatment should normally be kept as simple as possible. However, even the simplest overdenture treatment usually entails root filling and decoronating two or three abutment teeth. As the loading of the teeth is more advantageous once they are decoronated, the simple overdenture may well extend the life of these remaining abutments. Therefore with tolerably acceptable oral hygiene, the tooth supported complete overdenture can be a long-term treatment option for many patients.

Advantages of tooth-supported overdentures

Preservation of the ridge form

Retaining the roots and periodontal tissues of the abutment teeth reduces resorption of the surrounding bone. This is the most important advantage of overdentures, particularly for the lower jaw where it has been shown that preserving the canine roots can reduce the rate of resorption in that region by a factor of 8. This preservation of alveolar bone has obvious benefits in providing support and promoting stability of dentures. If the retained roots are in the anterior region, the preservation of bone will also help to maintain support of the lips and thus will contribute to facial appearance.

Minimising horizontal forces on the abutment teeth

The reduction in crown length of the abutment teeth and the production of a domed shape to the root face reduces the mechanical advantage of potentially damaging horizontal forces. As mentioned above, the life of the abutment teeth may therefore actually be prolonged, and teeth that were very mobile before treatment commonly become firmer. This change in mobility is partly due to the improvement in the crown–root ratio. In addition, the absence of teeth on either side of these overdenture abutments facilitates oral hygiene measures which can be especially helpful for those who have found this a challenge in the past.

Proprioception

It has been suggested that while the roots and their periodontal ligaments remain, periodontal mechanoreceptors allow a finer discrimination of food texture, tooth contacts and levels of functional loading. A better appreciation of food and a more precise control of mandibular movements may therefore be possible than is provided for by receptors in the denture-bearing mucosa of edentulous patients. In theory this may mean that natural tooth roots may serve better in this regard than dental implants which are devoid of periodontal mechanoreceptors.

Correction of occlusion and aesthetics

Overdentures have a particular advantage over partial dentures in those cases where the crowns of the remaining few teeth are not ideal either in terms of occlusion or appearance. Removal of the offending crowns and covering of the roots with an overdenture provide the freedom in artificial tooth arrangement necessary to correct the undesirable features.

Denture retention

As mentioned earlier, more positive retention of the denture to the root faces may be obtained by means of precision attachments (Fig. 3.4). However, in many instances, such additional retention seems not to be needed. Indeed whilst precision attachments may make a positive

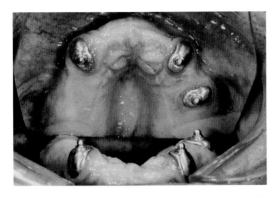

Figure 3.4   Stud attachments on the abutment teeth are engaged by spring clips within the overdenture to provide positive retention.

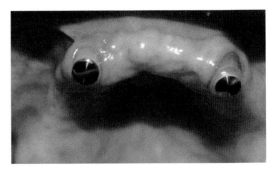

Figure 3.5   Keepers have been placed in the abutment teeth. The rare earth magnets are located within the overdenture.

contribution to retention on roots with good bone support, they are contraindicated for overdentures provided as a transitional stage of limited duration en route to conventional complete dentures for the following reasons:

- The increased height of the abutment arising from the precision attachment will adversely affect the crown–root ratio of the tooth. As a result, the tooth root will be subjected to larger horizontal forces.
- Attachments are relatively expensive and, therefore, may not be cost-effective if used on abutment teeth with a poor prognosis.
- The retention achieved with attachments can be too good, thus inhibiting the development of the patient's neuromuscular skills that will be required to control the future conventional complete dentures when the loss of these roots is inevitable.

An alternative method of augmenting retention is to use rare earth magnets located in the overdenture with the keepers incorporated into the abutment teeth (Fig. 3.5). These devices are less expensive than many precision attachments and provide effective retention. As a magnet applies less lateral force to the abutment tooth than does a precision attachment, it

can be used in situations where more advanced periodontal destruction has occurred.

The disadvantage of early designs of rare earth magnets is that they corroded in the oral environment. There has been significant improvement in this regard over the last decade with magnets now encased in a relatively inert capsule of titanium or stainless steel. In spite of this, corrosion can still be an occasional problem with some magnets when the oral fluids diffuse through the epoxy seal of the capsule (Riley et al. 1999). Longevity is improved if the magnet is enclosed in a laser-welded stainless steel casing (Thean et al. 2001).

Psychological benefits

The complete, irrevocable loss of all teeth can be a serious blow to a patient's morale as it signals, perhaps, that a major milestone in life has been reached. The retention of remnants of the natural dentition in the form of overdenture abutments can soften the blow and allow a period of mental adjustment before the edentulous state is reached. The patient's attitude to treatment and to conventional complete dentures may thus be more favourable. This particular benefit is not, in the authors' opinion, a common one. However, when it does arise, it can be of considerable value to both patient and clinician.

Disadvantages of tooth-supported overdentures

Root canal therapy

The preservation of roots as overdenture abutments usually necessitates endodontic treatment, thus extending the course of treatment and increasing its cost. The technical difficulty of achieving a satisfactory root filling may be increased because of partial obliteration of the root canal by secondary dentine due to ageing or in response to excessive loss of tooth substance. On the other hand, the same obliteration of the root canal may mean that the tooth may be shortened sufficiently without the need for endodontic treatment.

Caries

Covering root faces with an overdenture increases the risk of carious attack on these surfaces. The conclusions from a number of surveys reveal a caries prevalence ranging from 15% to 36%. Therefore, preventive measures are of great importance and comprise the following:

- Oral and denture hygiene instruction.
- Dietary advice.
- Careful smoothing and polishing of the domed root face to facilitate plaque removal.
- Sealing the root canal coronally with a glass-ionomer cement, as this material releases fluoride.
- Regular topical applications of fluoride using a fluoride varnish in the surgery and a fluoride toothpaste at home.
- Use of dentine bonding agents (Fenton 1998).

Periodontal disease

Covering the gum margins of abutment teeth with an overdenture has the potential for initiating periodontal disease or aggravating any existing disease process. There have been reports of gingival bleeding around all abutment teeth after 4 years and of obvious inflammation around 12% of abutment teeth after 3 years. The reduced number of teeth and their simple shaping may well mean that patients who found adequate home care a significant challenge may now be able to accomplish sufficient plaque removal to reduce the risk of these problems.

Budtz-Jørgensen (1995) has demonstrated that it is possible to maintain overdenture abutment teeth in older people who initially had poor periodontal and caries status by initial intensive treatment followed by four to five recall visits per year.

Technique for tooth-supported overdentures

The summary that follows outlines a simple technique appropriate for the construction of a complete overdenture.

Selection of abutments

As the mandibular residual ridge provides a less favourable foundation for a complete denture than the maxillary ridge and hard palate, the indications for retaining roots as overdenture abutments are greater in the lower jaw. Although any tooth amenable to root canal therapy may be retained as an overdenture abutment, single-rooted teeth are preferable on the grounds of simplicity. Teeth such as the canines, lower first premolars and upper central incisors are thus particularly suitable. Lower incisors and upper lateral incisors are not ideal abutments because of their smaller periodontal ligament area. Extraction of these teeth may, in fact, facilitate the task of cleaning adjacent abutments. Such extractions will usually be carried out at the appointment for fitting the overdenture.

Clinical and laboratory stages

After endodontic treatment of the abutment teeth has been carried out, the production of an overdenture follows the stages of conventional partial denture technique until the try-in stage has been completed.

Modifying the cast

The working cast is then modified by cutting off the crowns of the chosen abutment teeth and under-trimming the root faces to produce a domed preparation slightly larger and more supragingival than is intended for the actual root faces. It is useful to measure the height from the top of the dome to a fixed point at the gingival margin with dividers and to note this measurement in order to guide the preparation of the natural tooth at the next clinical visit. The crowns of any teeth to be extracted at the time of fitting the denture are also cut off the cast and the gingival contour modified to simulate any collapse likely to occur following tooth extraction. The denture is then processed in the normal way.

Fitting the denture

At the appointment for fitting the denture, the crowns of the teeth selected as overdenture abutments are removed and the root faces are domed, using the measurement made on the working cast. The openings of the root canals are then sealed with glass-ionomer cement or possibly amalgam, although the latter material does not have the advantage of caries inhibition resulting from fluoride release. The other teeth are extracted and the immediate overdenture is fitted.

Relining the denture

When the denture is checked at the next appointment, the restorations and the root faces are polished and fluoride varnish is applied to the dentine. An accurate fit of the denture to the root faces is achieved by using a cold-curing denture relining material based on acrylic resin within the recesses in the impression surface corresponding to the roots. Correct seating of the denture under occlusal pressure is facilitated by drilling a hole from each of the recesses

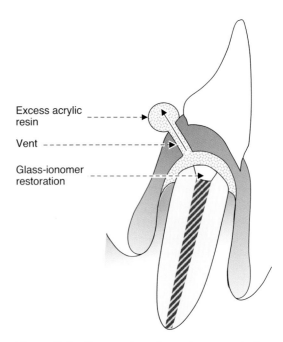

Figure 3.6 Cross-section of overdenture and abutment tooth showing correction of fit by addition of cold-curing acrylic resin.

to the polished surface to allow escape of any excess acrylic resin (Fig. 3.6).

Maintenance of tooth-supported overdentures

It is important to arrange a programme of review appointments to allow proper maintenance of the overdenture. This will involve maintaining oral and denture hygiene and reinforcing when necessary. Regular applications of topical fluoride should be made to the abutments. Temporary or permanent relining procedures will be required to compensate for alveolar resorption in regions where extractions were carried out at the time of fitting the denture. If caries of the root faces poses a problem in spite of topical fluoride applications, gold copings can be considered as a secondary procedure. If the patient is unable to control the denture as well as had been anticipated, magnets or stud attachments may be placed on the abutments to enhance retention. In one long-term study it was reported that treatment needs were greatest after 6 years. By that time, 36% of lower overdentures had lost stability but as few as 6% of upper and lower dentures had to be remade (Ettinger & Jakobsen 1997).

Implant-supported overdentures

Osseointegrated implant-supported overdentures are not generally an appropriate option for the short-term transition from the dentate state to that of complete denture wearing. Nevertheless, it is relevant to consider osseointegrated implants in this section of the book as both tooth roots and implants provide similar potential benefits for the enhanced support and retention of complete dentures.

Development of osseointegrated implants

Osseointegrated implants were developed in the second part of the twentieth century by Professor Per-Ingvar Brånemark. He was working in the early 1950s, using titanium-viewing chambers to examine blood flow in the bone of rabbits. When it became time to remove the chambers at the end of the experiment, the bone was firmly attached to the chamber. The phenomenon was termed osseointegration and describes the direct connection between vital bone and the implant without the presence of intervening connective tissue. It was later defined as 'direct structural and functional connection between ordered, living bone and the surface of a load carrying implant'.

Design

The vast majority of dental implants placed today are osseointegrated root-form titanium implants. These implants come in a wide variety

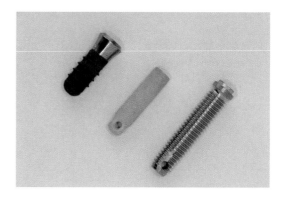

Figure 3.7 Examples of different types of implant design.

of designs (Fig. 3.7), but they all have certain basic components in common. These are:

- A submerged portion (usually referred to as the fixture) to which the bone integrates.
- A supra-bony portion that emerges through the mucosa into the mouth (the transmucosal element) to which various attachments can be added to support and retain the subsequent prosthesis (Fig. 3.8).

Success rates

Osseointegrated implants provide a successful and predictable way of replacing missing teeth which achieves a long-term survival, especially in the anterior part of the mandible where it is in excess of 98% after 20 years (Ekelund et al. 2003). Even so, the complications associated with such long-term restorations are probably greater than for the restoration of natural teeth (Pjetursson et al. 2007). The success of implant treatment has been followed by an explosion in the number of implant manufacturers each with their own specific designs.

Through the decades of development of osseointegrated prostheses for edentulous patients, the fixed restoration has been regarded as the 'gold standard of treatment'. The removable option tended to be considered only

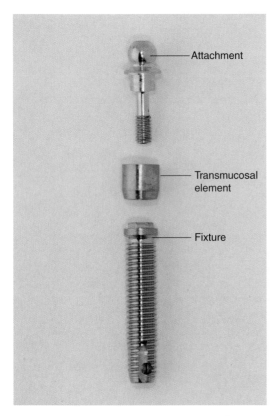

Attachment

Transmucosal element

Fixture

Figure 3.8 The three component parts of an implant.

where there were anatomical or financial restraints that excluded the fixed option. Nevertheless, work by various research groups has convincingly shown that even the provision of just two implants placed in the mandible can provide marked improvement both in patient satisfaction with a removable prosthesis and in oral health-related quality of life. These data have been summarised by Thomason et al. (2007).

There is an increasing body of research which provides support for the argument that an implant-supported mandibular overdenture should be offered as the preferred treatment option to edentulous patients. This view has gained momentum and is the key outcome statement from both the McGill Consensus statement (Feine et al. 2002) and the York Consensus statement (Thomason et al. 2009).

Barriers to implant treatment

It is difficult to overestimate the potential for improved treatment that dental implants offer. This potential has only been partially fulfilled however because of the low rates of uptake on a global basis, the greatest barriers being those of cost and training. The number of edentulous patients worldwide who have received implant treatment is probably less than 1% (Carlsson 2009) and for the majority of the world's edentulous patients the cost will continue to be an insurmountable barrier for the foreseeable future. Interestingly, even when offered implants 'free of charge', a significant proportion of patients have chosen to refuse the option for a variety of reasons (Walton & MacEntee 2005; Allen et al. 2006).

Implant placement

Traditionally, implants are inserted as a two-stage procedure. The first stage involves placing the implant, or fixture, within the alveolar and basal bone. A site for the implant is prepared in the bone with sets of graded drills so that it carefully matches the dimensions of the fixture. Great care must be taken to avoid increasing the temperature of the bone to a point that would cause necrosis and so prevent osseointegration. The fixtures are then placed into the prepared site and covered with the soft tissues. After a period for osseointegration, which is typically 3 months in the mandible and 6 months in the maxilla, the fixture is surgically exposed and the second stage or transmucosal element is attached to the fixture. After a short healing period the implants are restored with a fixed or removable prosthesis. More recently, the usual practice for simple overdentures has been to use a one-stage rather than a two-stage procedure and to attach the transmucosal element at the time of implant placement (Fig. 3.9).

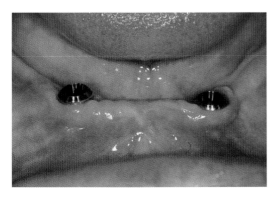

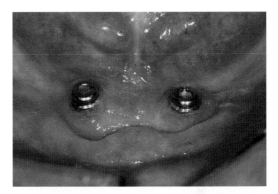

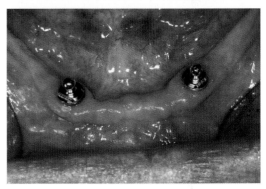

Figure 3.9 Non-submerged osseointegrated implants inserted as a single-stage procedure for the support and retention of a mandibular overdenture.

An attachment is subsequently added to the implant to provide support and retention for the overdenture (Fig. 3.10). There is a wide variety of attachments available and the number of designs continues to increase (Fig. 3.11). The attachments on each implant can be kept separate, or the implants can be linked together with a bar (Figs. 3.12a and 3.12b).

Impressions

It is critical for implant-supported dentures that the position of the implant abutments is recorded with great precision. This usually in-

Figure 3.11 The photographs show two different types of abutments widely used for implant-supported mandibular overdentures.

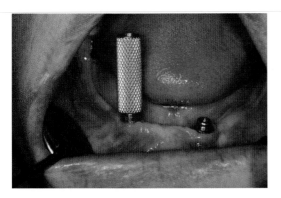

Figure 3.10 The attachment driver (patient's right) is used to carry the abutment to the fixture and secure it in place as seen on the patient's left.

volves some form of transfer impression which allows abutment-analogues (which are replicas of the abutment, or 'dummies') to be incorporated into the stone models on which the dentures will be constructed (Fig. 3.15). This can be achieved by taking an impression in a heavy bodied elastic impression material which includes the attachments on the implants. Then, when the impression is removed from the mouth, the abutment analogues can be inserted into the impressions of the attachments before the stone model is poured. Alternatively, transfer copings can be placed on the implants in the mouth (Fig. 3.13) which are then 'picked up' in the impression. Abutment replicas are placed onto the copings in the impression (Fig. 3.14) so that they will be incorporated into the master model (Fig. 3.15) on which the

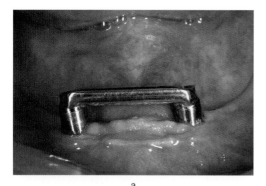

a

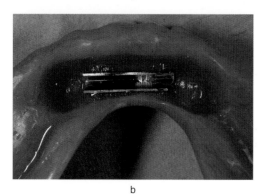

b

Figure 3.12   (a) shows two implants linked with a gold bar. (b) shows a retainer within the denture base which clips onto the bar.

denture is constructed allowing accurate positioning of the retainer within the denture base (Fig. 3.16).

Training

Whilst the placement of implants remains the province of those with appropriate additional training, the actual construction of overdentures supported by two implants is a straightforward procedure comparable to providing dentures supported by two tooth roots. Initial reports suggest that newly qualified clinicians with little implant experience can achieve very favourable results when restoring implants with overdentures (Esfandiari et al. 2006). As

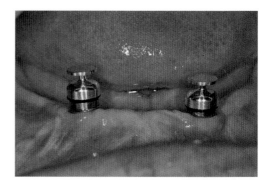

Figure 3.13   Two transfer copings have been placed on the implant abutments prior to impression-taking. The extension of the copings occlusally will be enveloped by the impression material so that when the impression is removed from the mouth the copings will be removed with it.

a result, there is an inevitable pressure to bring an understanding of the placement of implants and even clinical experience of the restoration and management of implant prostheses into the undergraduate curriculum (McAndrew 2010).

Immediate dentures

If the provision of overdentures is not possible, then providing a patient with a conventional

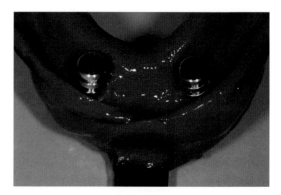

Figure 3.14   Abutment replicas have been inserted into transfer copings "picked up" in the impression of the denture bearing area.

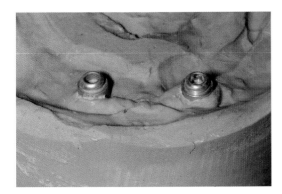

Figure 3.15 Abutment replicas incorporated into the master model on which the denture will be constructed.

immediate denture is the most effective way of making the transition from the natural to the artificial dentition (Jonkman et al. 1997). It was once said that this method was the appropriate treatment for those in the professions where they could not do without teeth for any length of time. The typical list would usually include vicars, doctors and business people – dentists were never mentioned! Thankfully, times and outlooks have changed and today the preservation of appearance is an almost universal wish.

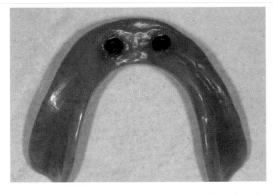

Figure 3.16 Retainers located accurately within the denture base.

Advantages of immediate dentures

Related to the patient

- Maintenance of dental appearance and facial contour.
- Minimising disturbances of mastication and speech.
- Facilitating adaptation to dentures. Difficulties with adaptation occur more commonly if the patient experiences an edentulous period of several months before dentures are fitted.
- Maintenance of the patient's physical and mental well-being.
- Provides a 'protective bandage' for the surgically traumatised area.

Related to the clinician

- *Transfer of the jaw relationship.* If the jaw relationship determined by the occlusion of the remaining natural teeth is acceptable in both horizontal and vertical planes, it can be transferred to the immediate dentures with reasonable accuracy. This obviates the need for the inspired guesswork of rest position estimation that is required if the patient is edentulous.
- *Achieving a good appearance.* The form and arrangement of the natural teeth can be reproduced in the immediate denture if the patient likes their appearance. When the appearance of the natural teeth is poor, or when their positions are likely to cause instability of the denture, planned improvements relative to the existing natural anterior tooth arrangement can be carried out. However, when such changes are anticipated, it is important to avoid radical changes in incisal relationship which may result in the undesirable consequences, as described in Chapter 12.
- *Reduction in ridge resorption.* It has been suggested that the rate of ridge resorption

following extractions is less if immediate dentures are worn than if no dentures are fitted. However, the evidence for this is inconclusive.

- *Haemostasis.* An immediate denture covers the sockets as a "protective bandage" and thus encourages haemostasis. It also supports and protects the clot during the immediate post-extraction period, reducing the chance of its mechanical dislodgement, for example, by food particles.

Disadvantages of immediate dentures

It is extremely important for the clinician to fully explain to the patient the following limitations of immediate dentures (Seals et al. 1996). Treatment should not normally be started unless the patient fully appreciates and accepts these limitations. Failure to achieve such an understanding is a common cause of complaint by patients against clinicians and can also result in failure of treatment:

- *Inability to complete a comprehensive trial stage.* As the trial stage is carried out while the remaining natural teeth are still present the try-in prosthesis consists of a partial denture restoring the existing edentulous spaces only. Therefore, artificial teeth that will eventually replace the natural teeth cannot be assessed. This is a particular disadvantage when anterior teeth are being replaced because neither the patient nor the clinician can make a full evaluation of the appearance of the dentures in situ.
- *Increased maintenance.* A number of visits are required after extraction of the teeth to allow for maintenance of the immediate dentures. Such maintenance may include:
  - relining with soft or hard materials;
  - occlusal adjustment;
  - addition of a labial flange to an open-face denture. If the dentures are not properly maintained, it usually results in exten-

sive destruction of the denture-bearing tissues.
- *Short service life.* An immediate denture will not normally last as long as a conventional complete denture. After 6–12 months of the adjustments outlined above, together with morphological changes in the oral environment, an immediate denture will commonly need replacing. Therefore, patients are likely to have to face the financial and time commitments associated with the provision of a replacement denture sooner than they would normally expect.

In spite of the disadvantages listed above, the advantages of conventional immediate dentures are normally overwhelming compared with tooth extraction and delayed denture fabrication after healing. This form of treatment should therefore be offered to the vast majority of patients for whom the transition from natural to artificial dentition must be made and where overdentures are not a possibility. With this caveat, there are relatively few circumstances in which the immediate denture is contraindicated.

Types of immediate complete denture

There are basically two types of immediate complete denture (Fig. 3.17).

Flanged
This design can be subdivided into:

- Complete flange – labial flange fully extended to the depth of the sulcus.
- Partial flange – labial flange usually finished with the border extended about 1 mm beyond the maximum bulbosity of the ridge.

Open-faced
There is no labial flange and the anterior teeth extend a few millimetres into the labial aspect of the sockets of their natural predecessors.

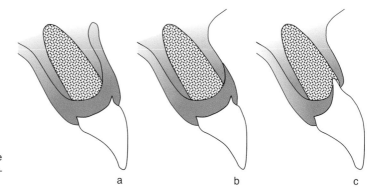

Figure 3.17 Types of immediate denture: (a) complete flange; (b) partial flange; (c) open face.

a   b   c

Comparison of flanged and open-face dentures

Appearance

- The appearance of a flanged denture does not alter after fitting whereas the appearance of an open-face denture, although good initially, can deteriorate rapidly as resorption creates a gap between the necks of the teeth and the ridge.
- The flange design allows considerable freedom in positioning the anterior teeth for optimum effect, whereas the anterior teeth on the open-face denture have to be positioned with their necks in the sockets of their natural predecessors.

Stability

A flange on an upper denture creates a more effective border seal, and therefore better retention, than is achieved with an open-face design. In the lower denture a border seal is not normally so significant. However, stability is of the greatest importance and this is improved by a labial flange because it helps to resist posterior displacement of the denture.

Strength

- The presence of a labial flange produces a stronger denture, which is less likely to fracture as a result of accidental impacts or high occlusal loads.

- A labial flange will also make the denture stiffer so that the likelihood of a midline fatigue fracture caused by repeated flexing across the midline is reduced.

Maintenance

- As the bone resorbs following extraction of the teeth, the immediate denture becomes loose and a reline is required. The presence of a labial flange makes it easier to add either a short-term soft lining material or a cold-curing polybutylmethacrylate relining material as a chairside procedure.
- As the colour of some of the chairside reline materials is not always ideal, they may be visible and unsightly when used with an open-face denture, but discreetly concealed by a flange.

Haemostasis

- The flanged denture covers the clots completely and protects them more effectively than does an open-face denture.
- The flanged denture also exerts pressure on both lingual and labial gingivae, reducing the likelihood of post-extraction haemorrhage.

Remodeling of the ridge

There is always the danger that the patient will fail to attend for a maintenance appointment. The consequent wearing of an ill-fitting

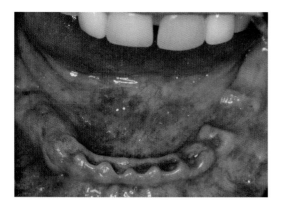

Figure 3.18 Tissue damage produced by an open-face lower immediate denture.

denture can, if it is open-faced, produce a scalloped ridge in the region of the extracted teeth (Fig. 3.18). This danger is avoided in the case of a flanged denture, which also has the advantage of distributing the functional loads more favourably to the underlying ridge, thus minimising bone resorption. For this reason alone, the authors would discourage the use of an open-faced denture in the upper arch and do not advocate its use in the lower arch at all.

Tolerance of replacement dentures

A significant clinical problem can be the difficulty that patients commonly experience in accepting a labial flange on a replacement denture when they have got used to an open-face immediate denture. Although a correctly designed flange only replaces bone that has resorbed, its presence in the richly innervated oral cavity frequently promotes a complaint of 'fullness' of the upper lip. If a flanged denture has been worn from the very beginning, this problem does not occur.

For the reasons listed above, the flange design is usually preferable; however, it is essential that the flange is kept thin and positioned correctly against the labial surface of the ridge, otherwise over-distension of the lip will result in poor facial appearance. In this context, selection of the correct path of insertion of the denture is essential (Fig. 3.19).

Where the ridge morphology produces a deeply undercut area, it may not be possible to fit a full labial flange unless there is surgical reduction of that undercut. Under such circumstances, a partial flange may be acceptable unless the patient has a smile line high enough to reveal the edge of the flange.

An outline of relevant clinical and technical procedures

The essential steps in the construction of immediate dentures follow the same sequence as those for conventional partial dentures until

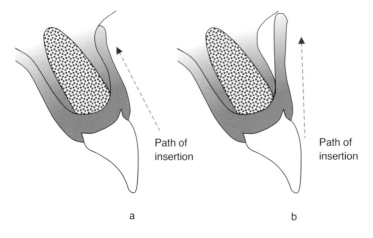

Path of insertion

Path of insertion

a

b

Figure 3.19 Diagram of a flanged immediate denture showing the effect of the path of insertion on the placement of the flange: (a) path of insertion parallel to the labial surface of the ridge – flange position favourable; (b) path of insertion at right angles to the occlusal plane – flange position unfavourable.

after the try-in stage. The subsequent conversion of the try-in to the complete denture requires modification of the cast in the laboratory.

Impressions for immediate dentures can be problematic if the remaining teeth are particularly mobile as a result of terminal periodontal disease. Under such circumstances, a conventional alginate impression can even act as an instrument of extraction with some or all of the remaining teeth coming out in the impression. The risk of such an undesirable and potentially upsetting accident can be minimised by either:

- *Loosening the 'grip' of the impression on the loose teeth.* One way that this can be achieved if there are several teeth adjacent to each other is by moulding soft red carding wax into the sub-contact point spaces and around the necks of the teeth so that the alginate is prevented from locking into the undercuts. Solitary teeth can be protected by placing a loose-fitting copper band over them before taking the impression.
- *Temporarily strengthening the attachment of the vulnerable teeth.* A stronger attachment of the loose teeth can be produced by splinting them to adjacent teeth with composite resin.

The nature of the modification depends upon whether the denture is to be flanged or open-face. The extent of the adjustment will be influenced by clinical assessment of the bone levels around the teeth to be extracted and on the amount of surgical reshaping of the ridge that is required. Therefore, as a general rule it is highly desirable for the cast to be modified by the clinician rather than by the dental technician.

Flanged dentures

Extraction without alveolar surgery
If the arrangement of the natural anterior teeth is to be reproduced in the denture, a record of

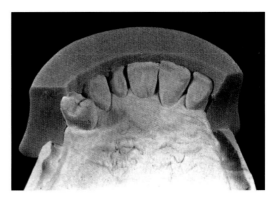

Figure 3.20 Position of the anterior teeth recorded by a silicone putty index.

their position must be obtained in one of the following ways:

(i) Produce a labial index of the natural teeth before they are cut off the cast. The index can be produced quite simply by moulding silicone putty against the labial surface of the teeth and ridge on the cast (Fig. 3.20). The artificial teeth are then set into the index while it is held against the cast.
(ii) Remove teeth singly from the cast and immediately wax an artificial tooth into position so that the adjacent teeth serve as a guide to the position of the artificial replacement.
(iii) Scribe guidelines on the cast recording the position, angulation and incisal level of the natural teeth (Fig. 3.21).

Once the artificial teeth have been positioned, the flange is added in wax before the denture is processed.

Alveolotomy following interseptal alveolectomy
This procedure is intended to eliminate moderate labial alveolar undercuts so that a flanged denture can be used without that flange distorting the upper lip unduly.

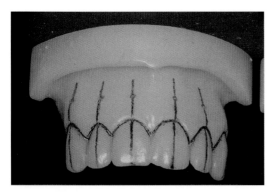

Figure 3.21 Long axes of the teeth marked on the cast to assist in placing the artificial teeth in similar positions. The location of incisal edges can be determined by direct measurement with dividers.

The denture is constructed on a working cast which is trimmed to the anticipated contour of the ridge after surgery as follows:

(i) The gingival margins are marked and the teeth removed.
(ii) Guidelines are drawn on the cast (Fig. 3.22).
  • A line is drawn on the crest of the ridge, passing across the centre of the sockets of the incisors and through the junction of the labial third and palatal two-thirds of the canine sockets.

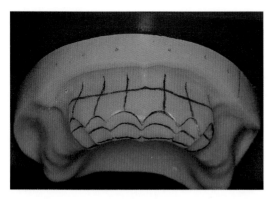

Figure 3.22 Alveolotomy following interseptal alveolectomy: lines drawn on the cast to guide model trimming (see text for details).

• A second line is drawn horizontally along the labial aspect of the ridge; it is placed approximately two-thirds down the length of the shortest root, usually the lateral incisor, and is continuous around all the teeth at that level.
(iii) All that part of the cast contained within these two lines is trimmed away and the edges are rounded over.
(iv) A clear acrylic template is processed on a duplicate of this cast and is used as a guide to control the amount of bone removal at operation.

The surgical procedure involves the following:

(i) Extraction of the teeth.
(ii) Removal of the associated interseptal bone.
(iii) Collapse of the labial cortical plate of bone and mucoperiostium, back into the resulting 'gutter'.
(iv) Insertion of the clear acrylic template to check if bone removal has been sufficient. Blanching of the mucosa is clearly seen beneath the template in any area where there is excessive pressure.
(v) Further bone removal, if necessary, until re-insertion of the template ceases to cause blanching.
(vi) Suturing of the sockets and insertion of the immediate denture.

Alveolectomy

The most common indication for an alveolectomy in association with the fitting of immediate dentures is the reduction of a prominent premaxilla to allow a more favourable placing of anterior teeth on the dentures.

A clear acrylic template is processed on a duplicate of the working cast trimmed to produce the desired ridge form. The template is used as a guide to bone removal during surgery in the same way as described for an alveolotomy following interseptal alveolectomy.

Open-face dentures

The purpose of extending the labial aspect of the necks of the denture teeth into the sockets, just enough to compensate for the gingival retraction that occurs immediately after extractions, is to maintain an acceptable appearance in the immediate post-extraction period. Without this, an unsightly gap would soon appear between tooth and mucosa. The amount of gingival retraction will depend on the degree of pocketing and bone loss that is present around the natural teeth. These aspects should therefore be assessed before deciding whether the necks of the denture teeth should be placed sub-gingivally to a depth of 2 mm, or whether a greater anticipated gingival collapse indicates that they should be placed more deeply. When this decision has been taken, the teeth are cut off the cast and a recess of the required depth is cut in the labial aspects of the sockets. No recessing of the palatal aspects of the sockets is undertaken. The artificial teeth are carefully positioned in the prepared recesses and the denture is processed.

Contraindications to immediate dentures

Patients at risk from a bacteraemia

Some clinicians believe that movement of an immediate denture can disturb the clots and surrounding tissues sufficiently to precipitate a bacteraemia. They are therefore opposed to the provision of immediate dentures for patients where such a bacteraemia may be perceived as a danger. Nevertheless, it can be argued that the potential for clot disturbance in the absence of a baseplate covering the wounds may be even greater.

Patients with a genuine history of post-extraction haemorrhage

As multiple extractions of anterior teeth are generally required when immediate dentures are fitted, such treatment is inappropriate when there is a proven history of post-extraction haemorrhage that has been difficult to control. A more cautious approach is indicated, involving the extraction of a few teeth at a time followed by suturing the sockets. Dentures are then fitted at a later date when the initial healing is complete.

The presence of gross oral sepsis

Although it is possible to provide immediate dentures for a neglected mouth, it is generally unwise to do so. The anterior teeth are often unsightly because of surface deposits, caries, gingival inflammation or recession; therefore, their retention for aesthetic reasons is unjustified. Furthermore, a patient who has neglected the mouth in this way may be less concerned about appearance anyway. The benefits of an immediate denture are therefore reduced significantly.

Clearance of teeth without immediate provision of dentures

When a decision is taken to extract the remaining teeth before denture construction, it is a common practice to allow a period of several months for healing and initial alveolar modelling. This delay before taking impressions will produce more stable supporting areas for the dentures, although resorption will continue indefinitely but at a slower rate. The main advantage of this method, that the dentures retain their fit for a longer period, is outweighed by the following disadvantages:

- Loss of masticatory function and appearance during the healing period.
- The undesirable mental and physical effects that the absence of teeth creates on a patient.
- Tongue and cheeks may invade the future denture space, making adaptation to subsequent dentures more difficult.

- Difficulty in assessing vertical and horizontal jaw relationships when constructing new dentures.
- The difficulty in restoring appearance if all information on the natural dentition has been lost.

It is surprising, in view of the disadvantages listed above, that the more efficient alternative method of making the transition from the natural to the artificial dentition via immediate dentures is not used routinely unless definite contraindications exist. The authors would strongly advocate that, where possible, long-term planning should encompass transition through partial dentures and then overdentures, thus avoiding the very abrupt "leap" from the dentate to the edentulous state. An additional benefit of this step-by-step approach is that it provides flexibility in the long-term treatment plan, allowing it to be modified appropriately in response to changes in clinical circumstances.

Postscript

A well-managed transition from what remains of the natural dentition to the totally artificial dentition carries a good level of success. With regard to the more problematic lower denture, studies have shown that, after 1 year, 85% of patients were satisfied both with complete immediate conventional dentures and with complete immediate overdentures (Jonkman et al. 1995; van Wass et al. 1997). This result was the consequence of careful clinical and technical procedures and a considerable amount of interim care.

Implant supported overdentures, as an alternative to conventional complete dentures, are becoming much more widely accepted as they now provide a realistic option for edentulous patients (Thomason et al. 2009). The available data convincingly show that patients are more satisfied with implant-supported mandibular overdentures than conventional dentures – typically by some 30%. There is also strong evidence that oral health-related quality of life can be significantly improved by this treatment (Thomason et al. 2007). However, whilst high satisfaction ratings have been reported for maxillary implant prostheses, the overall ratings given to them have not been shown to be any greater than for maxillary conventional dentures. Despite the positive improvements provided by mandibular implant overdentures the overall uptake of this treatment remains low, even in affluent countries and in the UK in particular (see above and Chapter 1). For many years to come, the most common treatment alternative for edentulous individuals worldwide will be conventional complete dentures (Carlsson 2006). This is in no small part due to the additional expense involved in implant treatment – even though this is relatively modest for two-implant overdentures, particularly when spread over the life of the patient (Heydecke et al. 2005). The relatively slow uptake of implant treatment is also a consequence of a need for further training of the dental workforce, both for implant placement and for rehabilitation. Fortunately, for the latter, the principles of implant-supported complete denture construction and conventional complete denture construction are similar. Therefore, those well trained in conventional denture provision are also well prepared for the provision of implant supported complete dentures.

References and additional reading

Allen, P.F., Thomason, J.M., Jepson, N.J., Nohl, F., Smith, D.G. & Ellis, J. (2006) A randomized controlled trial of implant-retained mandibular overdentures. *Journal of Dental Research*, 85, 547–51.

Basker, R.M., Harrison, A., Ralph, J.P. & Watson, C.J. (1993) *Overdentures in general dental practice*, 3rd edn. British Dental Association, London.

Beck, C.B., Bates, J.F., Basker, R.M., Gutteridge, D.L. & Harrison, A. (1993) A survey of the dissatisfied denture patient. *European Journal of Prosthodontics and Restorative Dentistry*, 2, 73–8.

Budtz-Jørgensen, E. (1995) Prognosis of overdenture abutments in elderly patients with controlled oral hygiene. A 5 year study. *Journal of Oral Rehabilitation*, 22, 3–8.

Carlsson, G.E. (2006) Facts and fallacies: an evidence base for complete dentures. *Dental Update*, 33, 134–42.

Carlsson, G.E. (2009) Critical review of some dogmas in prosthodontics. *Journal of Prosthodontic Research*, 53, 3–10.

Ekelund, J.A., Lindquist, L.W., Carlsson, G.E. & Jemt, T. (2003) Implant treatment in the edentulous mandible: a prospective study on Brånemark system implants over more than 20 years. *International Journal of Prosthodontics*, 16, 602–8.

Esfandiari, S., Lund, J.P., Thomason, J.M., Dufresne, E., Kobayashi, T., Dubois, M. & Feine, J.S. (2006) Can general dentists produce successful implant overdentures with minimal training? *Journal of Dentistry*, 34, 796–801.

Ettinger, R.L. & Jakobsen, J. (1997) Denture treatment needs of an overdenture population. *International Journal of Prosthodontics*, 10, 355–65.

Feine, J.S. & Carlsson, G.E. (eds) (2003) *Implant Overdentures: The Standard of Care for Edentulous Patients.* Quintessence Publishing, Chicago.

Feine, J.S., Carlsson, G.E., Awad, M.A., Chehade, A., Duncan, W.J., Gizani, S., Head, T., Heydecke, G., Lund, J.P., MacEntee, M., Mericske-Stern, R., Mojon, P., Morais, J.A., Naert, I., Payne, A.G., Penrod, J., Stoker, G.T., Tawse-Smith, A., Taylor, T.D., Thomason, J.M., Thomson, W.M. & Wismeijer, D. (2002) The McGill consensus statement on overdentures. Mandibular two-implant overdentures as first choice standard of care for edentulous patients. *Journal of Prosthetic Dentistry*, 88, 123–4.

Fenton, A.H. (1998) The decade of overdentures: 1970–1980. *Journal of Prosthetic Dentistry*, 79, 31–6.

Heydecke, G., Penrod, J.R., Takanashi, Y., Lund, J.P., Feine, J.S. & Thomason, J.M. (2005) Cost-effectiveness of mandibular two-implant overdentures and conventional dentures in the edentulous elderly. *Journal of Dental Research* 84, 794–9.

Johnson, K. (1977) A study of the dimensional changes occurring in the maxilla following open-face immediate denture treatment. *Australian Dental Journal*, 22, 451–4.

Johnson, K. (1978) Immediate denture treatment for patients with class II malocclusions. *Australian Dental Journal*, 23, 383–8.

Jonkman, R.E., van Waas, M.A., van't Hof, M.A. & Kalk, W. (1997) An analysis of satisfaction with complete immediate (over)dentures. *Journal of Dentistry*, 25, 107–11.

Jonkman, R.E.G., van Wass, M.A.J. & Kalk, W. (1995) Satisfaction with complete immediate dentures and complete immediate overdentures. A 1 year survey. *Journal of Oral Rehabilitation*, 22, 791–6.

McAndrew, R., Ellis, J., Lynch, C.D. & Thomason, M. (2010) Embedding implants in undergraduate dental education. *British Dental Journal* 2010, 208, 9–10.

Murphy, W.M., Huggett, R., Handley, R.W. & Brooks, S.G. (1986) Rigid cold curing systems for direct use in the oral cavity. *British Dental Journal*, 160, 391–4.

Mushimoto, E. (1981) The role in masseter muscle activities of functionally elicited periodontal afferents from abutment teeth under overdentures. *Journal of Oral Rehabilitation*, 8, 441–55.

Nairn, R.I. & Cutress, T.W. (1967) Changes in mandibular position following removal of the remaining teeth and insertion of immediate complete dentures. *British Dental Journal*, 122, 303–6.

Pjetursson, B.E., Bräggur, U., Lang, N.P. & Zwalen, M. (2007) Comparison of survival and complication rates of tooth-supported fixed dental prostheses (FDPs) and implant-supported FDPs and single crowns (SCs). *Clinical Oral Implants Research*, 3, 97–113.

Preiskel, H.W. (1996) *Overdentures Made Easy*, Quintessence Publishing, London.

Quinn, D.M., Yemm, R., Ianetta, R.V., Lyon, F.F. & McTear, J. (1986) A practical form of pre-extraction records for construction of complete dentures. *British Dental Journal*, 160, 166–8.

Ralph, J.P. & Basker, R.M. (1989) The role of overdentures in gerodontics. *Dental Update*, 16, 353–60.

Riley, M.A., Williams, A.J., Speight, J.D., Walmsley, A.D. & Harris, I.R. (1999) Investigations into the failure of dental magnets. *International Journal of Prosthodontics*, 12, 249–54.

Seals, R.R., Kuebker, W.A. & Stewart K.L. (1996) Immediate complete dentures. *Dental Clinics of North America*, 40, 151–67.

Tallgren, A., Lang, B.R., Walker, G.F. & Ash, M.M. (1980) Roentgen cephalometric analysis of ridge resorption and changes in jaw and occlusal relationships in immediate complete denture wearers. *Journal of Oral Rehabilitation*, 7, 77–94.

Thean, H.P.Y., Khor, S.K.L. & Loh, P.-L. (2001) Viability of magnetic denture retainers: a 3-year case report. *Quintessence International*, 32, 517–20.

Thomason, J.M, Feine, J., Exley, C., Moynihan, P., Müller, F., Naert I., Ellis, J.S., Barclay, C., Butterworth, C., Scott B., Lynch, C., Stewardson,

D., Smith, P., Welfare, R., Hyde, P., McAndrew, R., Fenlon, M., Barclay, S. & Barker, D. (2009) Mandibular two implant-supported overdentures as the first choice standard of care for edentulous patients – the York Consensus Statement. *British Dental Journal*, 207, 185–6.

Thomason, J.M., Heydecke, G., Feine, J.S. & Ellis, J.S. (2007) How do patients perceive the benefit of reconstructive dentistry with regard to oral health related quality of life and patient satisfaction? *Clinical Oral Implants Research*, 18, 168–88.

Todd, J.E. & Lader, D. (1991) *Adult Dental Health 1988 United Kingdom*. HMSO, London.

van Wass, M.E.J., Kalk, W., van Zetten, B.L. & van Os, J.H. (1997) Treatment results with immediate overdentures. An evaluation of 4.5 years. *Journal of Prosthetic Dentistry*, 76, 153–7.

Walker, A. & Cooper, I. (eds) (2000) *Adult Dental Health Survey Oral Health in the United Kingdom 1998*. The Stationery Office, London.

Walton, J.N. & MacEntee, M.I. (2005) Choosing or refusing oral implants: a prospective study of edentulous volunteers for a clinical trial. *International Journal of Prosthodontics*, 18, 483–8.

Stability of Dentures 4

A stable denture is one that moves little in relation to the underlying bone during function. It is perhaps surprising that what we now refer to as conventional dentures stay in place at all, as they simply rest on mucous membrane and lie within a very active muscular environment. They stay in place if the retentive forces acting on the dentures exceed the displacing forces and the dentures have adequate support. Clearly, when complete dentures are supported by implants, this balance between retentive and displacing forces is greatly tipped in favour of the denture staying in place. For conventional complete dentures, this support is determined by the form and consistency of the denture-bearing tissues and the accuracy of fit of the denture. The relationship of these factors is summarised in Fig. 4.1.

Retentive forces

Retentive forces offer resistance to vertical movement of a denture away from the underlying mucosa and act through the three surfaces of a denture. These surfaces may be defined as follows:

(1) *Occlusal surface*: that portion of the surface of a denture which makes contact or near contact with the corresponding surface of the opposing denture or dentition.
(2) *Polished surface*: that portion of the surface of a denture which extends in an occlusal direction from the border of the denture and which includes the palatal surface. It is that part of the denture base which is usually polished, includes the buccal and lingual surfaces of the teeth, and is in contact with the lips, cheeks and tongue.
(3) *Impression surface*: that portion of the surface of a denture that had its shape determined by the impression. It includes the borders of the denture and extends to the polished surface.

The retentive forces that act upon each of these surfaces (Fig. 4.2) are of two main types, muscular forces and physical forces:

Prosthetic Treatment of the Edentulous Patient, Fifth Edition, © R.M. Basker, J.C. Davenport and J.M. Thomason
Published 2011 by Blackwell Publishing Ltd.

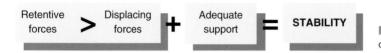

Figure 4.1 Relationship of factors contributing to denture stability.

1. *Muscular forces*. These forces are exerted by the muscles of the lips, cheeks and tongue upon the polished surface of the denture and by the muscles of mastication indirectly through the occlusal surface.
2. *Physical forces*. These rely on the presence of an intact film of saliva between the denture and mucosa. They act primarily between the impression surface of the denture and the underlying mucosa, and are to a large extent dependent on the maintenance of a seal between the mucosa and the border regions of the denture and upon the accuracy of fit.

Muscular forces

Patients who wear their dentures successfully do so primarily because they have learnt to control them with the muscles of their lips, cheeks and tongue. This skill may be developed to such a high degree that a denture which appears loose to the clinician may be perfectly sat-isfactory from the patient's point of view. There are even instances of patients who can eat without difficulty in spite of the fact that the denture has broken into two or more pieces.

Cineradiographic studies show that many complete dentures move several millimetres in relation to the underlying tissues during mastication. Consequently loss of physical retention occurs frequently during mastication, as movement of this extent breaks the border seal upon which physical retention depends. Muscular control is therefore extremely important, particularly in the case of the lower denture where the reduced area of the impression surface and the difficulty of obtaining a border seal reduce the influence of physical retention.

The successful muscular control of dentures depends on two factors:

1. The design of the dentures.
2. The ability of the patient to acquire the necessary skill.

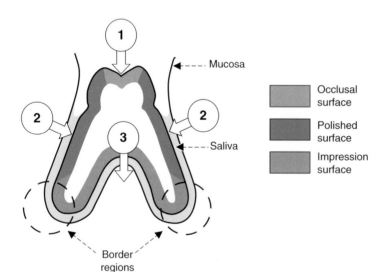

Figure 4.2 Retaining forces acting on a denture: (1) force of the muscles of mastication acting through the occlusal surface; (2) muscular forces of lips, cheeks and tongue acting through the polished surface; (3) physical forces acting through the impression surface.

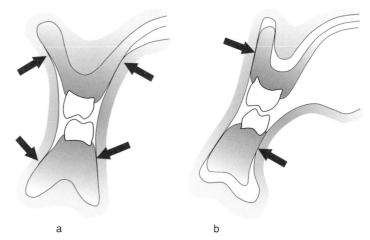

Figure 4.3 Influence of soft tissue forces on dentures: (a) seating the dentures when the polished surfaces are correctly shaped; (b) displacing the dentures when the polished surfaces are incorrectly shaped.

a

b

Design of dentures

During mastication the muscles of the cheeks, lips and tongue control the bolus of food, move it around the oral cavity and place it between the occlusal surfaces of the teeth. In doing so, they press against the polished surfaces of the dentures. If these surfaces are correctly shaped with the buccal and lingual surfaces converging in an occlusal direction, this muscular force will seat the dentures on the underlying mucosa (Fig. 4.3a). In addition to this active muscular fixation of the dentures during function, there will be a certain amount of passive fixation when the muscles are at rest, as the relaxed soft tissues 'sit' on the dentures, thereby maintaining them in position. Conversely an incorrectly shaped denture results in the muscular force dislodging that denture (Fig. 4.3b). In short, the muscles can either help or hinder denture stability.

Patient's skill

The patient's ability to acquire the necessary skills to control new dentures tends to be related to biological age. In general, the older the patient, the longer the learning period. In the extreme case, the older or senile patient may not be able to acquire this skill at all and so new dentures may fail even though they are technically satisfactory. It is for this reason that replacement dentures for an older patient should normally be constructed in such a way that the patient's skill in controlling the previous denture shapes can be transferred directly to the replacements. This is achieved by copying the old dentures as closely as possible, ideally using a technique such as that described in Chapter 8.

A specific example of the muscular control of dentures is seen when a patient incises (Fig. 4.4). The forces tend to tip the upper denture, causing the posterior border to drop. This movement is normally resisted by the dorsum of the tongue, which presses against the denture and reseats it. Patients who complain of difficulty when incising with dentures, which otherwise appear to be satisfactory, should be examined very carefully to establish whether or not tongue control is present. If it is not, it is essential for the clinician to draw the patient's attention to the problem and to institute appropriate training (Basker & Watson 1991). This takes the form of explaining the central role of the tongue, lips and cheeks in controlling the denture and giving specific advice – such as supporting the posterior border of the upper denture with the tongue when incising.

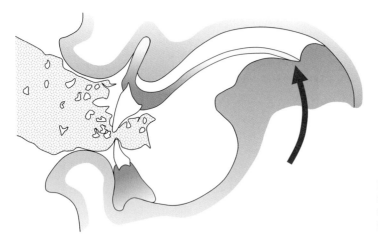

Figure 4.4 As the patient incises, the upper denture is controlled by the tongue pressing against the posterior border.

A reduction in displacing forces to bring them within the ability of the patient to control the dentures can be achieved by offering advice, for example, cutting food into smaller pieces before inserting them into the mouth, chewing on both sides of the dental arch simultaneously and starting with softer 'easier' foods before progressing to more challenging morsels. Unless purposeful muscular activity is learnt, replacement dentures will fail to overcome the patient's complaint.

When dentures are first fitted, muscular control takes some time to develop and is therefore likely to be inefficient in the early stages. Thus, it is during this initial learning period that the physical forces of retention are particularly important. The stronger these forces are, the smaller will be the demand on the patient's skill in controlling the dentures. If the prospects for physical retention are poor, the resulting looseness of the dentures may lead to their rejection by the patient. In difficult cases it may be helpful to advise the use of a denture fixative, as improved retention and stability will give the patient confidence during the period of adaptation (Grasso et al. 1994). There are real physical limitations of conventional complete dentures, particularly the lower denture, and as

such it is not surprising that some patients are unhappy with their function despite apparently seeming to have learned to control them well. As an example, such a patient may be aware of movements of the dentures during function although these movements are undetectable to the observer. This may lead to dissatisfaction and concerns for the patient which may ultimately impact on their interaction with other people (Thomason et al. 2009).

As alveolar resorption progresses, the fit of the dentures deteriorates with a consequent reduction in physical retention. However, this will not necessarily result in a reduction in the overall retention, as there will have been a compensating increase in the level of muscular control. Nevertheless, the fit may eventually become so poor that complete compensation is no longer possible and movement of the dentures begins to increase. The degree of denture mobility that elicits a complaint of looseness will vary considerably between individuals; some patients are quite happy with dentures which perform 'acrobatics' in the mouth while others complain bitterly about dentures which hardly move at all.

The topic of the patient's skill is considered further in Chapter 2.

Physical forces

The contribution of physical forces to the retention of a denture is heavily dependent upon the presence of a continuous thin film of saliva between denture and mucosa, which wets both surfaces. The forces of adhesion and cohesion play a part in achieving this condition.

Adhesion

Adhesion is the force of attraction between dissimilar molecules such as saliva and acrylic resin or saliva and mucosa, which promotes the wetting of the denture and mucosal surfaces.

Cohesion

Cohesion is the force of attraction between like molecules, which maintains the integrity of the saliva film. These intermolecular forces of adhesion and cohesion may be thought of as forming a chain between the denture and the mucosa (Fig. 4.5).

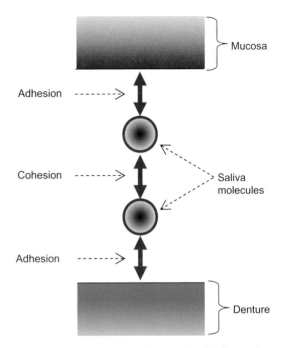

Figure 4.5 The chain of intermolecular forces between the denture and the mucosa contributing to retention.

Surface tension

Surface tension is the result of cohesive forces acting at the surface of a fluid. It has been suggested that in the case of saliva these cohesive forces result in the formation of a concave meniscus at the surface of the saliva in the border region of the denture. When a fluid film is bounded by a concave meniscus, the pressure within the fluid is less than that of the surrounding medium; thus, in the intra-oral situation a pressure differential will exist between the saliva film and the air (Fig. 4.6). The size of this pressure differential is inversely related to the diameter of the meniscus, i.e. the closer the fit of the denture to the tissues the stronger the retentive force attributable to surface tension. This is discussed further in the section below, 'Obtaining optimum physical retention'.

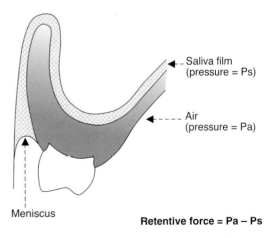

Retentive force = Pa – Ps

Figure 4.6 Retention due to the pressure differential between the saliva film and the air.

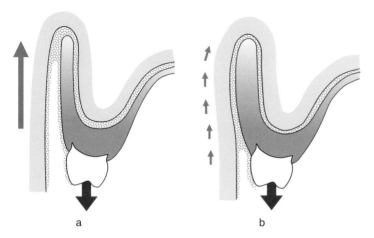

a   b

Figure 4.7 Relationship between the width of the buccal channel and resistance to flow of saliva: (a) wide channel, rapid flow, poor retention; and (b) narrow channel, slow flow, good retention.

Viscosity

As a denture is pulled away from the tissues, saliva is drawn into the space being created beneath the denture. A retentive force is generated by a resistance to this flow of saliva, resulting from the viscous properties of the saliva and the dimensions of the channel through which it flows (Fig. 4.7). It follows that the narrower the channel and the greater the viscosity of the saliva, the more effective should be the retention. This certainly holds true clinically for the dimensions of the channel, but it appears that very viscous saliva is associated with relatively poor retention. It may be that retention is low in this instance because the excessive viscosity of the saliva results in a thick and discontinuous film between the denture and the mucosa. Any discontinuities, such as air bubbles, in the saliva film reduce retention dramatically because air flows infinitely more readily than saliva and therefore offers very little resistance to denture displacement.

It is important to appreciate that the walls of the buccal channel through which the saliva flows differ from each other. The denture flange is rigid while the soft tissues of the cheeks or lips are movable. If the denture is displaced, the pressure within the saliva film drops and the mucosa is drawn tightly against the denture surface so that the channel between the two becomes very narrow indeed. This causes a greatly increased resistance to the flow of saliva and a corresponding increase in retention (Fig. 4.8). Incidentally, this will also increase retention due to surface tension, because narrowing of the channel between denture and mucosa will reduce the diameter of the meniscus

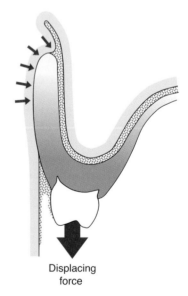

Displacing
force

Figure 4.8 Drop in pressure of the saliva film beneath the denture causing impaction of the buccal mucosa and greatly increased retention.

and therefore increase the pressure differential between the saliva film and air. If, however, the denture is constructed with flanges which are too thin, resulting in a wide buccal channel (Fig. 4.7a), impaction of the buccal mucosa will not occur, and saliva and air will be rapidly drawn towards the impression surface as the denture is displaced. Retention in this instance will be poor.

The retentive mechanism resulting from the viscosity of the saliva and the valve-like action of the soft tissues is best able to resist large displacing forces of short duration. Small forces acting over an extended period of time, such as the influence of gravity on the upper denture, result in a much smaller pressure differential between the saliva film and the air because they allow saliva to be drawn gradually into the space being created beneath the prosthesis. If the effect of gravity is unopposed, a progressive downwards movement of the upper denture is likely to occur until eventually all retention is lost and the denture drops. However, in this situation, occlusal forces are important in restoring the denture to its former position. Whenever the patient occludes (e.g. during swallowing), excess saliva which has accumulated beneath the denture is squeezed out again, the denture is re-seated and retention is re-established.

Obtaining optimum physical retention

The aspects of complete dentures that influence the amount of physical retention obtained are:

- Border seal
- Area of impression surface
- Accuracy of fit

Border seal

For optimum retention, the denture border should be shaped so that the channel between it and the sulcus tissues is as small as possible.

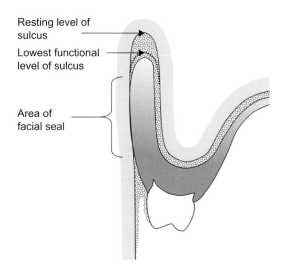

Figure 4.9 Lateral extension of the buccal flange to produce a facial seal.

It is not possible to maintain a close approximation between the border of a denture and the mucosal reflection in the sulcus at all times because the depth of the sulcus varies during function. The denture has to be constructed so that the border conforms to the shallowest point that the sulcus reflection reaches during normal function. This means that for some of the time when the patient is at rest the denture will be slightly under-extended. If the denture were extended further in an attempt to produce a more consistent seal in this area, displacement might occur when the sulcus tissues move during function. The problem of achieving a constant border seal is overcome by extending the flanges of the denture laterally so that they contact and slightly displace the buccal and labial mucosa to produce a facial seal (Fig. 4.9).

It is not possible to produce a facial seal along the posterior border of the upper denture as it crosses the palate. In this area, the solution to achieving the smallest possible space between denture and mucosa is to create a post-dam – a raised lip along the posterior border which becomes embedded a little way into the palatal mucosa. One way of producing this is to cut a groove into the working cast where the posterior border of the denture is to be located which is normally at the vibrating line (Figs. 10.1 and 10.3).

Alternatively, the post-dam may be developed during the first stage of the master impression by using a mucocompressive impression material along the posterior border of the impression tray to displace the mucosa locally in the post-dam area (p. 145).

However, although an enhanced posterior seal is achieved with a post-dam it differs from the facial seal against the flanges in that, even a small downwards movement of the posterior border of the denture is likely to break the seal with a resultant loss of retention. If the post-dam has width as well as depth, the basic retention of the denture will be improved.

Area of impression surface

The degree of physical retention is proportional to the area of the impression surface. It is important therefore to ensure maximum extension of the dentures so that the optimum retention for a particular patient may be obtained.

The denture on the right side in Fig. 4.10 was poorly retained because the thin flanges failed to create a facial seal, and the palatal coverage did not make the most of the area available. The replacement denture on the left corrected these errors and as a result had excellent retention.

Accuracy of fit

The thinner the saliva film between the denture and underlying mucosa, the greater the forces of retention; therefore, it is important that the fit of the dentures is as accurate as possible. A poor fit will increase the thickness of the saliva film and increase the likelihood of air bubbles occurring within the film. These bubbles will further reduce the retention of the denture. In addition, as the pressure of the saliva film drops due to displacing forces acting on the denture, the air bubbles will expand and may extend to the border area, resulting in a breaking of the border seal.

Other factors

Bony undercuts

If bony undercuts exist, retention may be enhanced by designing a denture that utilises these undercut areas. In order to achieve this without traumatising the mucosa on insertion and removal of the denture, special care is

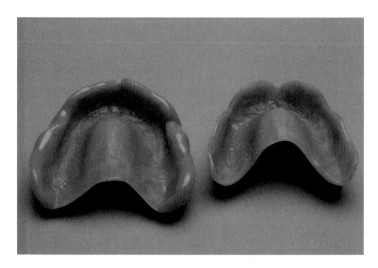

Figure 4.10 Right: denture poorly retained because the thin flanges failed to create a facial seal and the palatal coverage did not make the most of the area available. Left: the replacement denture corrected these errors and as a result had excellent retention.

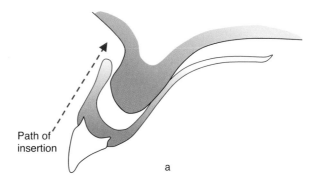

Path of
insertion

a

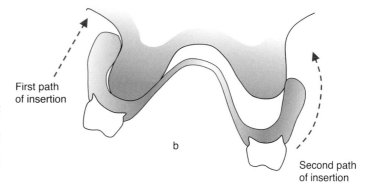

First path
of insertion

b

Second path
of insertion

Figure 4.11 Selection of path of insertion to improve retention by utilising undercuts: (a) single path of insertion to engage labial undercut; (b) dual path of insertion to engage unilateral undercut.

required in planning the path of insertion (Fig. 4.11).

Retention aids

In exceptional cases, such as surgical or congenital defects of the hard palate, it may not be possible to obtain the required retention by routine clinical techniques. In such circumstances, the use of denture fixatives, long-term soft liners, springs or implants may be of value.

Denture fixative

A denture fixative can be an invaluable aid to retention, particularly under difficult anatomical circumstances. Fixatives come in powder, paste or sheet form, the latter having the advantage of staying longest between the denture and mucosa. The more adhesive that can be incorporated in the sheet of material, the better the retention (Uysal et al. 1998). It should be noted that there is a potential health risk associated with long-term, excessive use of zinc-containing denture adhesives; high levels of zinc in the body have been associated with symptoms such as numbness or tingling in the arms and legs, difficulties with walking and balance, and anaemia. As a result these products have been currently withdrawn from the market.

Long-term soft liners

Soft liners enable free, flexible margins to extend into the anatomical defect and engage tissue undercuts. The liner can be constructed as an integral part of the denture base or as a separate obturator section retained on the denture base by rare earth magnets. Long-term soft lining materials are considered further in Chapter 16.

Denture springs

Denture springs are usually of coil type and are attached by pivots to the buccal flanges of upper and lower dentures in the premolar region. The springs are often partially covered by acrylic flanges, or 'hooded', to stabilise the springs and reduce irritation of the buccal mucosa. The springs exert a force which acts to separate the dentures and thus helps to maintain the dentures in contact with the supporting tissues. These devices are rarely used but can occasionally be of value when the anatomical circumstances are exceptionally unfavourable as can be the case in a patient who has undergone a maxillectomy.

Implants

It was proposed in the McGill Consensus Statement (Feine et al. 2002) and again in the York Consensus statement (Thomason et al. 2009) that 2-implant supported overdentures should be the minimum offered to edentulous patients as the first choice of treatment. Available data strongly support this suggestion in terms of patient satisfaction and Quality of Life outcomes (Thomason et al. 2007). The available evidence has resulted in this form of treatment being recognised and provided under private and state administered insurance schemes in a number of different countries over the last few years. The situation currently in the UK remains with almost all implant provision occurring privately or to a limited extent in the secondary care environment.

Displacing forces

Acting through the occlusal surface

Occlusal imbalance

If, when the dentures occlude, tooth contact on one side of the dental arch is not balanced by

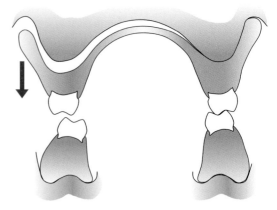

Figure 4.12 Tipping of the denture due to an unbalanced occlusal contact.

contact on the other side the dentures will tip, causing the border seal to break, with consequent loss of retention (Fig. 4.12). When the mandible moves into lateral or protrusive occlusal positions, interference between opposing teeth resulting from interlocking cusps or an excessively deep overbite can cause horizontal displacement and tipping of the dentures. This type of instability can be minimised by reducing or eliminating the occlusal interferences (pp. 167–171). It should be borne in mind that occlusal displacing forces can be dramatically increased in patients exhibiting parafunctional activity such as bruxism.

Mastication

Forces related to the posterior teeth

During mastication, pressure exerted by the food on the teeth tends to displace the denture. This problem may influence the positioning of artificial posterior teeth. For example, stability of the lower denture can be improved by careful consideration of the posterior extension of the occlusal table. If that table extends to the steeply sloping part of the ridge posteriorly, pressure from the bolus will tend to make the denture slide forwards (Fig. 4.13). Therefore the occlusal table should terminate on the

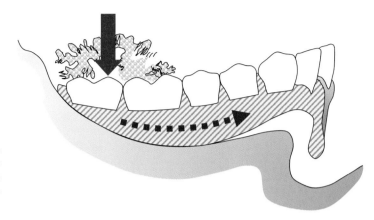

Figure 4.13 Pressure from the bolus on the posterior part of the lower occlusal table, which overlies a sloping part of the ridge, causes the lower denture to slide forwards.

relatively horizontal part of the ridge where effective support is available and displacement prevented. It may be necessary to reduce the number of posterior teeth to achieve this aim.

Forces related to the anterior teeth

Occasionally, the problem of occlusal displacement can create a conflict of interests between the requirements of optimum appearance and denture stability. This is illustrated by the example of the experienced denture wearer who expresses a strong preference for having upper anterior teeth placed close to the crest of the ridge where strong incising forces can be applied with minimal leverage effects, despite the fact that lip support and appearance would be compromised. In the face of such a clearly stated preference it is usually wise for the clinician to comply with the patient's request. But it is important that the likely aesthetic penalty is explained to, and accepted by, the patient before treatment is started.

During the opening phase of the masticatory cycle, when the teeth begin to separate after penetrating a bolus of food, the adhesive properties of the food generate a displacing force in an occlusal direction. Sticky foods therefore tend to move the dentures away from the mucosa.

Acting through the polished surface

The muscles of the lips, cheeks and tongue, in addition to being of fundamental importance in the retention of dentures, are also capable of causing denture instability. Displacement will occur, as mentioned earlier, if the polished surfaces have an unfavourable slope (Fig. 4.3b) and also if the denture interferes with the habitual posture and functional activity of the surrounding musculature. For example, distal movement of a lower denture may be produced by the lower lip if the anterior teeth are placed too far labially (Fig. 4.14). The teeth should therefore be placed just far enough lingually to prevent this displacement but not so far as to allow excessive tongue pressure to develop.

It is not uncommon to see lower dentures that are unstable because the posterior teeth have been placed too far lingually; under such conditions of restricted tongue space, movement of the tongue during function will tend to lift the denture. There is an area between the tongue on the one side and the cheeks and lips on the other where the muscular displacing forces acting on a denture are least. This area is known as the neutral zone or zone of minimal conflict. Positioning a prosthesis within this zone is most important for the lower denture as the physical retentive forces are normally

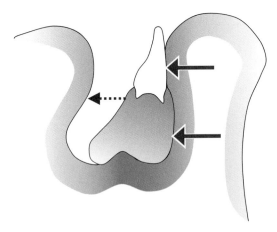

Figure 4.14 Distal displacement of the lower denture caused by placing teeth too far labially.

small and can do little to resist muscular displacement.

Post-extraction changes may lead to a gradual shifting of the neutral zone. For example, it is common for posterior teeth to be extracted some considerable time before the anterior teeth. If a partial denture is not fitted, the tongue spreads laterally into the edentulous space. This, in effect, moves the neutral zone laterally as well as reducing its bucco-lingual dimension so that there is a reduced space in which to place a denture. This space might be re-established, at least in part, when a new complete denture is fitted. However, the modification in tongue posture and behaviour required to achieve this, increases the demand on the patient's ability to adapt. Some patients may find it difficult or even impossible to meet this challenge and so the denture could fail.

Changes in the neutral zone also occur between the lower lip and the tongue as a result of post-extraction changes affecting the mentalis muscle. Resorption of the alveolar bone leads to the superior fibres of the origin of the mentalis muscle lying on top of the residual ridge and a lingual migration of the neutral zone. Certainly, in these circumstances, it is no longer possible to position the artificial teeth where once the natural ones were situated.

A further disturbance of muscle balance can arise as a consequence of incorrect tongue posture. If the tongue takes up a 'defensive posture' towards the back of the mouth a lower denture, of whatever design, will be unstable. It is necessary to explain matters to the patient and train the tongue to touch the lingual surfaces of the lower incisors in order to restore the lingual balancing force and, thus, stability (Likeman 1997).

Gravity

The effect of gravity on an upper denture has been described on p. 61. In order to minimise this effect, it is important that the upper denture is of light construction. Heavy denture base materials, such as cobalt-chromium alloy, should be avoided unless other requirements, such as strength, are of overwhelming importance.

Support

This chapter has shown that stability of dentures can be obtained only if retentive forces exceed displacing forces. However, there is one more factor in the equation, that of adequate support for the dentures by the underlying tissues. A reduction in support promotes instability, as indicated in the following examples:

- Instability of an upper denture follows resorption of the supporting bone. This resorption is largely confined to the region of the alveolar ridges, as there is remarkably little resorption of bone in the centre of the palate. Thus, after a period of time, the denture will be well supported by the hard palate, but there will be limited contact between the impression surface of the denture and the alveolar ridges. In these circumstances, occlusal contact readily produces tipping, with the denture pivoting about the mid-line of the palate.
- Support will be inadequate if the ridges are small because resistance to lateral displacing forces will be poor.

- Support will be reduced if the ridges are flabby (p. 242). The denture will move considerably during function even though the retention may be good and contact with the mucosal surface is maintained.

References and additional reading

Basker, R.M. & Watson, C.J. (1991) Tongue control of upper complete dentures – a clinical hint. *British Dental Journal*, 170, 449–50.

Brill, N. (1967) Factors in the mechanism of full denture retention – a discussion of selected papers. *Dental Practitioner and Dental Record*, 18, 9–19.

Culver, P.A.J. & Watt, I. (1973) Denture movements and control – a preliminary study. *British Dental Journal*, 135, 111–16.

Darvell, B.W. & Clark, R.K.F. (2000) The physical mechanisms of complete denture retention. *British Dental Journal*, 189, 248–52.

Davenport, J.C. (1984) Clinical and laboratory procedures for the production of a retentive silicone rubber obturator for the maxillectomy patient. *British Journal of Oral and Maxillofacial Surgery*, 22, 378–86.

Feine, J.S., Carlsson, G.E., Awad, M.A., Chehade, A., Duncan, W.J., Gizani, S., Head, T., Heydecke, G., Lund, J.P., MacEntee, M., Mericske-Stern, R., Mojon, P., Morais, J.A., Naert, I., Payne, A.G., Penrod, J., Stoker, G.T., Tawse-Smith, A., Taylor, T.D., Thomason, J.M., Thomson, W.M. & Wismeijer, D. (2002) The McGill consensus statement on overdentures. Mandibular two-implant overdentures as first choice standard of care for edentulous patients. *Journal of Prosthetic Dentistry*, 88, 123–4.

Grasso, J.E., Rendell, J. & Gay, T. (1994) Effect of denture adhesive on the retention and stability of maxillary dentures. *Journal of Prosthetic Dentistry*, 72, 399–405.

Jagger, D.C. & Harrison, A. (1996) Denture fixatives – an update for general dental practice. *British Dental Journal*, 180, 311–13.

Kelsey, C.C., Lang, B.R. & Wang, R.F. (1997) Examining patients' responses to the effectiveness of five denture adhesive pastes. *Journal of the American Dental Association*, 128, 1532–8.

Likeman, P.R. (1997) Tongue control of lower complete dentures: a clinical hint. *British Dental Journal*, 182, 229–30.

Lindstrom, R.E., Pawelchak, J., Heyd, A. & Tarbet, W.J. (1979) Physical–chemical aspects of denture retention and stability. A review of the literature. *Journal of Prosthetic Dentistry*, 42, 371–5.

Sheppard, I.M. (1963) Denture base dislodgement during function. *Journal of Prosthetic Dentistry*, 13, 462–8.

Slaughter, A., Katz, R.V. & Grasso, J.E. (1999) Professional attitudes toward denture adhesives. *Journal of Prosthetic Dentistry*, 15, 159–65.

Thomason, J.M, Feine, J., Exley, C., Moynihan, P., Müller, F., Naert I., Ellis, J.S., Barclay, C., Butterworth, C., Scott B., Lynch, C., Stewardson, D., Smith, P., Welfare, R., Hyde, P., McAndrew, R., Fenlon, M., Barclay, S. & Barker, D. (2009) Mandibular two implant-supported overdentures as the first choice standard of care for edentulous patients-the York Consensus Statement. *British Dental Journal*, 207, 185–6.

Thomason, J.M., Heydecke, G., Feine, J.S. & Ellis, J.S. (2007) How do patients perceive the benefit of reconstructive dentistry with regard to oral health related quality of life and patient satisfaction? *Clinical Oral Implants Research*, 18, 168–88.

Tyson, K.W. (1967) Physical factors in retention of complete upper dentures. *Journal of Prosthetic Dentistry*, 18, 90–7.

Uysal, H, Altay, O.T., Alparslan, N. & Bilge, A. (1998) Comparison of four different denture cushion adhesives – a subjective study. *Journal of Oral Rehabilitation*, 25, 209–13.

Jaw Relations – Theoretical Considerations 5

The clinical procedure of recording the jaw relationship enables the clinician to provide the dental technician with the following information:

- An appropriate vertical and horizontal relationship of the mandible to the maxilla.
- The required shape of the dentures.

This information is given to the dental technician in the form of wax record rims, which have been adjusted by the clinician, to enable the casts to be mounted on an articulator. The shape of the record rims provides the dental technician with a blueprint on which to base the design of the trial dentures.

This chapter is devoted to a discussion of the theoretical background to occlusion. The points arising from the discussion are used to justify the clinical techniques described in Chapter 11.

Basic mandibular positions

- *Rest position.* The rest position can be defined as the vertical and horizontal position the mandible assumes when the mandibular musculature is relaxed and the patient is upright. When the mandible is in the rest position there is a space between the occlusal surfaces of the teeth which is known as the freeway space or interocclusal rest space. This space is wedge-shaped, being larger anteriorly where the separation between the teeth is most commonly within the range 2–4 mm, although there can be considerable variation between individuals and within an individual depending on the particular circumstances operating at the time.
- *Muscular position.* The muscular position is the vertical and horizontal position of the mandible produced by balanced muscle activity raising the mandible from the rest position into initial tooth contact.
- *Intercuspal position.* The intercuspal position is the vertical and horizontal position of the mandible in which maximum occlusal contact occurs. In the denture wearer, the intercuspal and muscular positions should coincide.

Prosthetic Treatment of the Edentulous Patient, Fifth Edition, © R.M. Basker, J.C. Davenport and J.M. Thomason
Published 2011 by Blackwell Publishing Ltd.

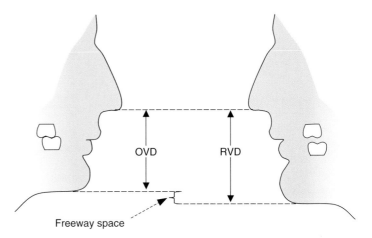

Figure 5.1 The difference between the rest vertical dimension (RVD) and the occlusal vertical dimension (OVD) is the freeway space.

The distance between two selected points, one related to the maxilla and one related to the mandible, when the upper and lower teeth are in contact is known as the *occlusal vertical dimension*. When the mandible is in its resting position, this distance is the *rest vertical dimension* (Fig. 5.1). The difference between the measurements is the *freeway space*.

- *Retruded contact position.* With light tooth contact maintained, movement of the mandible in a posterior direction from the intercuspal position is usually possible. This posterior position is known as the retruded contact position and is separated from the intercuspal position by approximately 1 mm. Further retrusion of the mandible is prevented by the lateral ligaments of the temporomandibular joints.

With the condyles maintained in the retruded position, the movement of the mandible as it opens is hinge-like until jaw separation in the incisal region is approximately 2 cm. The path taken by the mandible up to this point is known as the retruded arc of closure. Further opening of the mandible results in a forwards and downwards translation of the condyles.

The interrelationship of the mandibular positions is shown in Fig. 5.2.

In the past, there has been confusion with regard to the associated nomenclature. The terms used in this book, together with the alternatives commonly used elsewhere in the dental literature, are shown in Table 5.1.

The rest position
Clinical significance

- *Constructing or assessing dentures.* The rest position is used as a reference position when determining the appropriate occlusal vertical dimension for new complete dentures or checking the occlusal vertical dimension of existing dentures. The clinical procedure is to measure the rest vertical dimension and the occlusal vertical dimension and then calculate the freeway space.
- *Relaxation of the masticatory apparatus.* When the mandible is in the rest position and the teeth are out of contact, the tissues which support the dentures are not loaded, there is no strain on the temporomandibular joint capsules and only minimal, if any, activity in the elevator and depressor muscles of the mandible.

If new dentures have no freeway space, the denture-bearing tissues are subjected to excessive loading, the elevator muscles are unable to

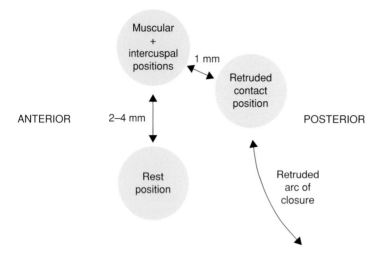

Figure 5.2 Diagrammatic representation of the basic positions of the mandible in the sagittal plane.

return to their normal resting length, and the continuous muscular activity results in an accumulation of metabolites and subsequent pain in the affected muscles.

If, on the other hand, an excessive freeway space is provided, the load on the tissues is of course reduced. However, there is a reduction in masticatory efficiency and the patient's appearance is usually adversely affected.

Table 5.1   Nomenclature for basic mandibular positions.

Terms used in this book	Alternative terms
Rest position	Physiologic rest position
Muscular position	Habitual position
Intercuspal position	Centric occlusion Maximum intercuspation Tooth position
Retruded contact position	Centric occlusion Centric relation Ligamentous position Posterior border position
Freeway space	Inter-occlusal rest space

Control of the rest position

The rest position of the mandible at any one time is the result of a balance of forces as shown in Fig. 5.3. Both passive and active forces are described. The relative importance of active and passive forces in determining the rest position is a controversial issue. One school of thought maintains that active forces are the major factor, another that passive forces alone are responsible for the true rest position, while yet a third school suggests that the rest position is the product of both active and passive forces in combination.

Passive forces

Passive forces are derived from the following:

- *Muscles attached to the mandible.* Passive forces arising from the muscles attached to the mandible result from the elastic nature of the muscle fibres and of the connective tissue elements. Although it has been suggested that, in the truly relaxed state, the passive forces inherent in the muscles are able to maintain the rest position, this state is rarely evident and variables such as change in posture or emotional state affect the

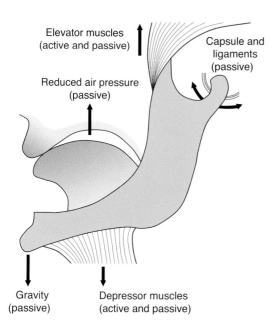

Elevator muscles (active and passive)

Capsule and ligaments (passive)

Reduced air pressure (passive)

Gravity (passive)

Depressor muscles (active and passive)

Figure 5.3 Forces which determine the rest position of the mandible.

equilibrium, resulting in the introduction of active forces.

- *The elastic properties of the capsules and ligaments of the temporomandibular joints.* The elastic properties of the capsules and ligaments of the temporomandibular joints exert forces on the condyles that tend to return them to a central position within the glenoid fossae. Thus, these passive forces will encourage the mandible to adopt the rest position.
- *Reduced intra-oral air pressure.* A contribution to the balance of forces acting on the mandible in the rest position may come from a reduction in intra-oral air pressure.

When the mandible is in the rest position, the lips are together and the patient is breathing through the nose, the oral cavity is a closed 'box' sealed anteriorly by the lips and posteriorly by contact between the soft palate and the posterior surface of the tongue. There is a tendency for the space inside this closed box, between the dorsum

of the tongue and the hard palate, to be increased by the weight of the mandible pulling downwards. It has been suggested that the pressure in this closed space is thus reduced and that the resulting differential between the intra-oral pressure and atmospheric pressure helps to support the mandible in the rest position.

- *Gravity.* The force of gravity is a constant factor. However, its influence on the balance of forces acting on the mandible varies with the position of the head in the gravitational field and with the mass of the mandible. Thus, the gravitational effect is reduced when the patient is supine, when lower teeth are extracted or when a lower denture is removed from the mouth.

Active forces

Active forces influencing the rest position are generated by continuous low-grade motor unit activity in the muscles attached to the mandible. This activity is seen predominantly in the elevator muscles and is influenced by the following factors:

- *Mass of the mandible.* Activation of the stretch reflex increases motor unit activity. If the mass of the mandible is increased by the insertion of a lower denture or record block, the mandible will tend to drop and the elevator muscles will be stretched. Muscle spindles within the stretched muscles are activated and initiate impulses which increase motor unit activity in the same muscles and inhibit activity in the depressor muscles. This activity acts to oppose the displacing effect of the lower denture and returns the mandible towards its original rest position.
- *Changes in position of the mandible.* Other mechanoreceptors which may play a part in influencing the rest position following changes in position of the mandible, or of the head as a whole, are to be found in the temporomandibular joint, the middle ear and the cervical spine.

- *Pain, drugs and emotional stress.* External factors are able to facilitate or inhibit motor unit activity via the reticular system. For example, the amount of jaw separation at rest is reduced by pain, drugs such as adrenalin and caffeine, and emotional stress. Emotional stress itself may be caused by factors in the patient's own domestic environment, or by disturbing visual, auditory or olfactory stimuli in the dental surgery. Jaw separation is increased during sleep or by drugs such as tranquillisers and sedatives.

An alternative explanation

The rest position of the mandible has been considered from an entirely different viewpoint – its association with the function of respiration (Fish 1964). When a patient is at rest, respiration is the primary function affecting the oral region. It has been suggested that the rest position of the mandible is determined by the demands of the tongue in performing its respiratory function of completing the anterior wall of the pharyngeal part of the respiratory tract (Fig. 5.4a). Following extraction of teeth and resorption of the alveolar bone, the tongue spreads laterally into the edentulous space. When the resorption of bone is extensive, the tongue spreads to such a degree that the posterior oral seal cannot be maintained (Fig. 5.4b). The response of the mandible in this situation is to rise, thus allowing the posterior oral seal to be re-established (Fig. 5.4c). A lower denture replaces the natural teeth and alveolar bone and, when inserted into the mouth, controls the lateral tongue spread and allows the mandible to return to a lower resting position while still maintaining the posterior seal.

Variation in the rest position

At one time, the rest position of the mandible was thought to be constant throughout life. From the foregoing discussion, it is apparent that this is not so. The rest position of the edentulous patient can be affected by the short-term

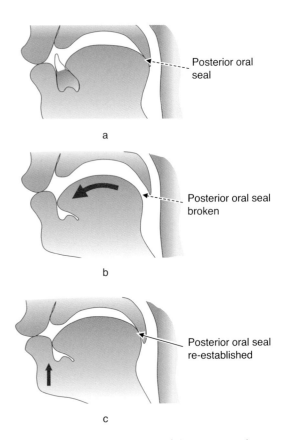

a

b

c

Figure 5.4   The association of the tongue with respiration and its influence on the rest position of the mandible: (a) posterior oral seal established between the soft palate and the tongue – lower denture in situ; (b) the tongue spreads into the area vacated by the denture; the posterior oral seal cannot be maintained; (c) the mandible is raised so that the posterior oral seal can be re-established (the rest vertical dimension when the denture is in the mouth is therefore larger than when it is removed) (Fish 1964).

variables listed in Table 5.2, and by long-term variables. However, these variables in no way reduce the value of the rest position as a reference point in establishing the occlusal vertical dimension.

Short-term variables

The short-term variables can reduce the reproducibility of the rest vertical dimension while

Table 5.2 Short-term variables that may affect the rest position of the edentulous patient.

Variable	Rest vertical dimension
Patient supine	Reduced
Head tilted back	Increased
Head tilted forwards	Reduced
Insertion of lower denture or record block	Increased
Stress	Reduced
Pain	Reduced
Drugs	Variable

the clinician is attempting to record it, but that influence can be minimised by careful clinical technique as discussed in Chapter 11.

Long-term variables

Prosthetic treatment has an important long-term influence on the rest position of the mandible. If the same dentures are worn for many years and are not maintained, a reduction in the occlusal vertical dimension occurs as a result of alveolar resorption and occlusal wear. The rest position of the mandible adapts to this change and takes up a position closer to the maxilla. Longitudinal studies of the change in the vertical dimension have been undertaken and it has been shown that an average 7-mm reduction in occlusal vertical dimension occurs in as many years (Fig. 5.5). The rest vertical dimension responds in a similar manner, although to a lesser degree. As a result, the freeway space becomes larger. Where these changes have taken place in young patients, it is often possible to recover much of the lost vertical dimension when new dentures are constructed. However, with the older patient, any attempt to restore the occlusal vertical dimension to its original level may be met with problems that are discussed more fully in Chapter 8. The long-term variables will not affect the reproducibility

of the rest vertical dimension during the period of a dental appointment, but their likely effect on the recorded rest vertical dimension needs to be recognised by the clinician and allowed for, if appropriate.

The muscular and intercuspal positions

The precise nature of the muscular and intercuspal positions in a dentate subject depends upon the arrangement of the natural teeth and the proprioceptive impulses arising from receptors in the periodontal ligaments and muscles of mastication. The muscular position is not constant and may be modified by sensory feedback resulting from changes in intercuspal position. For example, a protrusive relationship may be adopted following loss of posterior teeth and consequent restriction of mastication to the incisal region. A similar situation can develop where an edentulous patient has been wearing dentures whose pattern of occlusal contact has been altered through tooth wear and resorption of underlying bone. In this instance, altered sensory input from receptors in the denture-bearing mucosa and muscles encourages the mandible to adopt a protrusive position closer to the maxilla. The resulting clinical picture is one of uneven occlusal contact, reduction in the occlusal vertical dimension and protrusion of the mandible. Such a modification of the muscular position will complicate the provision of new dentures. Although the position will appear to be reproducible, it is unwise to set up the new dentures in relation to it because once they are fitted the muscular position is likely to change yet again in response to the new sensory feedback initiated by the improved occlusion. Muscular position and intercuspal position will then no longer be coincident. This is a highly undesirable situation because it increases the likelihood of damage to the denture-bearing tissues and discomfort in the muscles of mastication. The situation can be avoided by recording the retruded jaw relation

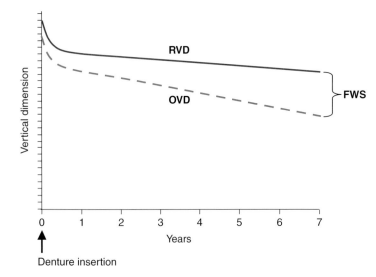

Figure 5.5 Average changes in occlusal and rest vertical dimensions after fitting complete dentures. (Modified after Tallgren (1966).)

rather than the muscular position, as discussed below.

The retruded jaw relation

This relation is determined by the lateral ligaments of the temporomandibular joints and does not depend upon the presence of teeth. Therefore, it does not alter when the natural teeth are extracted or when a new occlusal surface replaces an unsatisfactory one. It has been suggested that the retruded position has practical significance during normal functional movements, as tooth contact in this position is the termination of the heavy masticatory strokes needed to break up pieces of hard food.

Reference positions of the mandible to be used when recording the jaw relationship

When providing complete dentures, the relationship of the mandible to the maxilla in both horizontal and vertical planes must be determined.

In the vertical plane, it is of prime importance that the occlusal vertical dimension of the

dentures allows for an adequate freeway space. If existing dentures have been entirely satisfactory from this point of view their occlusal vertical dimension may be copied in the new prostheses. Otherwise the occlusal vertical dimension must be calculated with reference to the rest position.

The issue is perhaps less clear-cut with respect to the jaw relationship in the horizontal plane. Some authorities prefer to record the antero-posterior relationship of the mandible to the maxilla in the muscular position, while others describe techniques for obtaining the retruded position.

Evidence indicates that it is possible to record the retruded position with greater consistency than the muscular position. It has been shown that variation of the muscular position in the antero-posterior plane is especially affected by the posture of the patient, whereas the reproducibility of the retruded position remains high. In addition, it is quite possible that the muscular position may have been influenced by an abnormal occlusion and may alter once the new occlusal surface has been provided. Because the retruded jaw relationship is more consistent than the muscular position, and because the former is known to be close to an acceptable intercuspal position, the authors recommend using the retruded position as the point of reference in the horizontal plane. However, when positioning the artificial teeth, allowance must be made for the patient to adopt the muscular position. This concept is considered further on p. 170.

References and additional reading

Brill, N. & Tryde, G. (1974) Physiology of mandibular positions. *Frontiers of Oral Physiology*, 1, 199–237.

Brill, N., Lammie, G.A., Osborne, J. & Perry, H. (1959) Mandibular positions and mandibular movements. A review. *British Dental Journal*, 106, 391–400.

Crum, R.J. & Loiselle, R.J. (1972) Oral perception and proprioception: a review of the literature and its significance to prosthodontics. *Journal of Prosthetic Dentistry*, 28, 215–30.

Faigenblum, M.J. (1966) Negative oral pressures. A research report. *Dental Practitioner and Dental Record*, 16, 214–16.

Fish, S.F. (1961) The functional anatomy of the rest position of the mandible. *Dental Practitioner and Dental Record*, 2, 178–88.

Fish, S.F. (1964) The respiratory associations of the rest position of the mandible. *British Dental Journal*, 116, 149–59.

Helkimo, M., Ingervall, B. & Carlsson, G.E. (1971) Variation of retruded and muscular position of mandible under different recording conditions. *Acta Odontologica Scandinavica*, 29, 423–37.

Nairn, R.I. & Cutress, T.W. (1967) Changes in mandibular position following removal of the remaining teeth and insertion of immediate complete dentures. *British Dental Journal*, 122, 303–6.

Posselt, U. (1952) Studies in the mobility of the human mandible. *Acta Odontologica Scandinavica*, 10 (Suppl. 10).

Preiskel, H.W. (1965) Some observations on the postural position of the mandible. *Journal of Prosthetic Dentistry*, 15, 625–33.

Tallgren, A. (1957) Changes in adult face height due to ageing, wear and loss of teeth and prosthetic treatment. *Acta Odontologica Scandinavica*, 15 (Suppl. 24).

Tallgren, A. (1966) The reduction in face height of edentulous and partially edentulous subjects during long-term denture wear. *Acta Odontologica Scandinavica*, 24, 195–239.

Yemm, R. (1969) Variations in the electrical activity of the human masseter muscle occurring in association with emotional stress. *Archives of Oral Biology*, 14, 873–8.

Yemm, R. (1972) Stress-induced muscle activity: a possible etiologic factor in denture soreness. *Journal of Prosthetic Dentistry*, 28, 133–40.

Yemm, R. & Berry, D.C. (1969) Passive control in mandibular rest position. *Journal of Prosthetic Dentistry*, 22, 30–6.

Introductory Remarks to the Clinical Chapters 6

A preview of the clinical chapters

It is much more common for a dentist to have to provide complete dentures as replacements for existing dentures than to provide them for a patient who has not worn dentures before.

What is the reason for this pattern of treatment? Clearly, one of the main factors is that the average life expectancy of patients receiving complete dentures for the first time is considerably greater than the average life expectancy of the dentures themselves. This is, of course, particularly the case if the patient's first complete dentures were immediate restorations whose useful life is relatively short. Thus, dentures are likely to be replaced several times during the life of the patient.

The remaining chapters of this book are largely concerned with clinical procedures and, because of the pattern of demand mentioned above, the major emphasis is placed on the treatment of patients requiring replacement dentures.

Chapter 7 deals with the first stage of treatment, i.e. history, examination and treatment planning. Then in Chapter 8, the use of old dentures is discussed as their existence affects treatment from the outset. The next logical step is to consider the measures that may be required to prepare the oral tissues (Chapter 9) before continuing with the stages of denture construction (Chapters 10–15). The book concludes with a discussion of some clinical problems and their possible solutions (Chapter 16).

Of course, there are patients who require complete dentures, who have not had dentures before. In these cases the initial assessment is usually a less complicated procedure. After mouth preparation, the conventional clinical stages of treatment are followed, as described in the appropriate chapters.

Quality of treatment – its control and enhancement

In recent years much emphasis has been placed on measures designed to evaluate and improve

Prosthetic Treatment of the Edentulous Patient, Fifth Edition, © R.M. Basker, J.C. Davenport and J.M. Thomason
Published 2011 by Blackwell Publishing Ltd.

the quality of care. This has led to the active promotion of two concepts:

1. Clinical audit
2. Peer review

Clinical audit

Clinical audit has been defined as:

> the systematic, critical analysis of the quality of dental care, including the procedures and processes used for diagnosis, intervention and treatment, the use of resources and the resulting outcome and quality of life as assessed by both professionals and patients.
>
> (Clinical Audit and Peer Review in the General Dental Services, April 2001)

The aim of the concept is self-examination by the clinician. For example, criteria are established to judge the quality of outcome of a procedure, the actual outcome is measured against the criteria and, where the criteria have not been fully met, changes are made to improve the procedure and the audit cycle is repeated after a convenient time.

Peer review

Peer review

> provides an opportunity for groups of dentists to get together to review aspects of practice. The aim is to share experiences and identify areas in which changes can be made with the objective of improving the quality of service offered to patients.
>
> (Clinical Audit and Peer Review in The General Dental Services, April 2001)

We hope that this textbook will be seen as providing a useful foundation on which quality initiatives can be built. As a contribution to the thinking behind clinical audit and peer review we have included short sections in the clinical chapters entitled 'Quality control and enhancement' where we offer ideas on clinical topics which might be examined more closely within an audit cycle.

The clinician/dental technician interface

The quality of care provided for the edentulous patient is heavily dependent upon effective communication between the dental clinician and dental technician and a mutual understanding of the objectives for each clinical stage.

Previous studies have indicated that the standard of communication between a dental clinician and a dental technician can be very variable (Basker et al. 1993; Barsby et al. 1995). Even in those cases when the instructions from the dentist are clear they are not necessarily followed by the dental technician, as shown in the survey of quality of complete dentures by Barsby et al. (1995), where the actual position of the postdam on the finished dentures only coincided with the correct position which had been clearly marked previously by the clinician in 65 of the 101 instances.

The outcome of a study into the quality of copy dentures (Kippax et al. 1998) strongly suggested that the objectives behind the procedure were not fully understood by either clinician or dental technician with the result that the dentures produced were poor 'copies'.

To emphasise the importance of clear communication, we have included specific sections on the topic at the end of each appropriate chapter. We have not included such basic items as names and addresses of the patient and the dentist and the date when the next item of work is required. Rather, we have listed the minimum amount of information that the dental technician requires in order to provide what is really wanted by the clinician.

At this point it is worth noting that the accuracy of the clinician's prescription and the way it is acted upon by the dental technician are fruitful areas for clinical audit and peer review. A greater understanding of each other's role would foster this communication and may be best built on joint training and shared education (Clark et al. 2010).

The control of cross-infection

Much has been written about cross-infection control in the last decade. It is not appropriate in this book to go into any detail about techniques that should be used. Rather, we simply make the point that the reader will find up-to-date information provided by professional, governmental and statutory bodies as well as in the dental literature and in information provided by the manufacturers of dental products.

We restrict ourselves to a brief discussion on three points:

1. The surgery/laboratory interface
2. Impression materials
3. Avoiding contamination of stock materials

The surgery/laboratory interface

The dental technician is an integral member of the dental team, and the dental laboratory, wherever it is situated, is an integral part of the dental environment. Therefore, it is essential that cross-infection policies are fully discussed, understood and agreed on by both dental technician and clinician. Without this close cooperation, the chain upon which cross-infection control depends will be broken and the mutual protection lost.

Cross-infection within the dental laboratory can be a problem. One study attributed a high prevalence of eye infections among dental technicians to contaminated pumice. It was found that the pumice was heavily infected but that the bacterial count could be significantly reduced by mixing up the slurry with a solution of a commercially available disinfectant. It was concluded that untreated pumice slurries pre-

sented an unacceptable risk of cross-infection (Witt & Hart 1990).

The key to preventing transmission of infection between the two areas is a disinfectant 'barrier' through which all items must pass before being dispatched in either direction. The precise nature of this barrier will vary according to the item involved. Prior to dispatch of an item from the clinic to the laboratory the responsibility for disinfection lies solely with the clinician. It is a good practice to agree the protocol to be used with the laboratory and this would broadly consist of rinsing the item, immersing it in an ultrasonic bath if it is grossly contaminated, disinfecting it with an approved product and then rinsing again before packing. The package should be labelled to indicate its disinfection status. When items are being returned from the laboratory to the clinic, they should be similarly disinfected before dispatch (British Dental Association, 2009).

Impression materials

The basic point is that the dentist must choose a combination of impression material and disinfectant where the latter is not only effective but will not adversely affect the dimensional stability and surface accuracy of the impression.

Care needs to be taken not to breach cross-infection procedures when using impression compound. This material is commonly softened in a thermostatically controlled water-bath. However, these baths must be regarded as contaminated once the impression has been completed, and therefore must be emptied, cleaned and disinfected before being used for another patient – a cumbersome procedure. A better and simpler procedure is to use a bowl in which hot water is poured and which can be autoclaved after use.

Handling materials

When handling prosthetic materials, it is important to develop a regimen that avoids contamination of stocks and unacceptable levels of wastage. Careful advanced planning for each prosthetic appointment so that, as far as possible, all the required materials and instruments are placed ready, is the key to minimising the chance of contaminating stock. However, even then it is difficult to avoid the situation in which it is necessary to collect additional items during a procedure. This can be done only by changing the gloves, or by placing a barrier between the contaminated gloves of the clinician and the stock. This barrier may take the form of a 'clean' dental nurse to hand the item to the clinician, cheap vinyl over-gloves which are subsequently discarded, or sterile forceps. Rummaging through stocks with contaminated gloves clearly creates a breach in any cross-infection policy.

It is important for economic reasons to minimise wastage. Dispensing prosthetic materials (such as the various waxes) in portions appropriate for single use keeps the residue of unused materials to a level at which they can be discarded without incurring an unacceptable financial penalty.

References and additional reading

Barsby, M.J., Hellyer, P.H. & Schwarz, W.D. (1995) The qualitative assessment of complete dentures produced by commercial dental laboratories. *British Dental Journal*, 179, 51–7.

Basker, R.M., Ogden, A.R. & Ralph, J.P. (1993) Complete denture prescription – an audit of performance. *British Dental Journal*, 174, 278–84.

British Dental Association (2009) *Infection Control in Dentistry (England)*. Advice sheet A12. BDA, London.

Clark, R.K.F., Radford, D.R. & Juszczyk, A.S. (2010) Current trends in complete denture teaching in British Dental Schools. *British Dental Journal*, 208, 214-15.

Croser, D. & Chipping, J. (1989) *Cross-infection control in general dental practice – a practical guide for the whole dental team*. Quintessence, London.

Department of Health (2001) *Clinical Audit and Peer Review in the General Dental Services*. Department of Health, London.

Kippax, A., Watson, C.J., Basker, R.M. & Pentland, J.E. (1998) How well are complete dentures copied? *British Dental Journal*, 185, 129–33.

Witt, S. & Hart, P. (1990) Cross-infection hazards associated with the use of pumice in dental laboratories. *Journal of Dentistry*, 18, 281–3.

Assessment of the Patient

7

A thorough and systematic history and examination of the patient will ensure that all relevant details are recorded so that the clinician can determine the following:

- Diagnosis
- Treatment plan
- Prognosis

The purpose of this chapter is to describe a systematic approach to this all-important stage preceding treatment. The significance of the information obtained is discussed more fully in other chapters of the book.

History

Reason for attendance

After noting personal particulars such as name, address, age and occupation, the clinician should record the concern or complaint in the patient's own words. For example, if the patient says that the denture is loose, it may be positively misleading if the clinician records the comment as 'the denture lacks retention'. The denture may, in fact, exhibit excellent physical retention but is being displaced by an uneven occlusal contact.

History of the present complaint

It is essential to obtain full details of any complaint. If, for example, the complaint is of pain in relation to a denture, the location, character and timing of the pain should be determined; relieving and aggravating factors should also be recorded. It is important to ascertain the relationship of the time of onset of the symptoms with the time that the present set of dentures was fitted.

If a denture is loose, it is necessary to enquire when the looseness was first noticed. If the denture has been worn satisfactorily for several years before trouble developed, it indicates that the dentures were initially satisfactory and that subsequent changes such as resorption of the residual ridges or wear of the occlusal surfaces are responsible for the problem. In this situation, it is essential – in addition to identifying the cause of the complaint – to note the good features of the denture, as it is usually sensible to replicate these in the replacement dentures.

On the other hand, if the looseness was present from the time the denture was fitted, the cause may be attributed to a basic design fault in the denture, to unfavourable anatomical factors or perhaps to the inability of the patient to adapt to dentures. Until an examination is made, it is not possible to distinguish between these causes.

Dental history

When obtaining a patient's dental history, it is necessary to determine:

- when the natural teeth were extracted;
- the reasons for the extractions;
- the occurrence of any surgical complications;
- how many dentures have been worn subsequently;
- the degree of success or failure with the dentures.

This history can provide important information on the following:

- *The rate of bone resorption.* The history of tooth loss provides a basis on which to make an assessment of the current rate of bone resorption. If extractions were carried out in the previous few months, resorption will still be continuing at a rapid rate, so that if dentures are provided at this time they will soon become loose and require rebasing. The patient should therefore be warned of this likelihood. If, however, the teeth were extracted several years ago, the alveolar bone will have reached a relatively stable state and the life of a replacement denture will be considerably extended.
- *Retained roots.* If there is a history of difficult extractions, it is advisable to obtain radiographs in order to check for the presence and location of retained roots.

- *The adaptive capability of the patient.* Clues can be obtained as to the adaptive capability of the patient. For example, if three sets of dentures have been worn successfully over a period of 15 years, it may be assumed that adaptation has been satisfactory, whereas if the same number have been provided over the last 2 or 3 years – and each has been troublesome – the ability to adapt will be suspect. However, it is vitally important not to jump to conclusions and to put the blame on the patient until one is satisfied that the complaint cannot be related to defects in the design of previous dentures (see Chapter 2). It is thus a wise practice to ask the patient to bring all available sets of dentures when attending the initial assessment, as inspection of them can yield valuable clues and increase the accuracy of the diagnosis.

Medical history

Notes should be made of a patient's past and present medical history that is relevant to future dental treatment. Information should include particulars of drug therapy and the name of the patient's medical practitioner. A patient for whom sedatives and tranquillisers are being prescribed may have a reduced capacity in adapting to dentures, as may a person suffering from a protracted chronic disability. It should also be noted that many antidepressants and tranquillisers produce xerostomia. This condition may reduce the physical retention of a denture and may cause a generalised soreness of the denture-bearing mucosa. It has also been reported that certain antidepressants and tranquillisers may adversely affect the tonicity of the facial muscles and may produce facial grimacing and trismus or bizarre tongue movements.

It can be helpful when taking a medical history to work with a questionnaire to make certain that no significant aspect is overlooked.

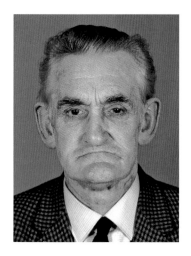 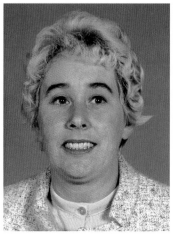

Figure 7.1 Both patients are wearing complete dentures which are in occlusion. The man shows obvious signs of a gross loss of occlusal vertical dimension; the freeway space is approximately 10 mm. On the other hand, the woman's facial appearance leads one to suspect that the occlusal vertical dimension of her dentures is excessive.

Social history

When entering into a discussion with some patients, it may be helpful to explain that one is not being 'nosy' but that there are important reasons for such an enquiry. For example:

- A history of domestic worries may well tie in with the medication that has been prescribed or with a parafunctional habit which is resulting in pain under an existing lower denture.
- If the patient has been widowed, preparing food and eating alone can well take all the enjoyment out of mealtimes and an unbalanced diet could lead to tissue changes in the oral cavity.
- Because the clinician has a responsibility for the health of the patient, it is important to obtain information on risk factors related to oral cancer such as smoking or chewing tobacco, a high alcohol consumption, a prior history of cancer, familial or genetic predisposition. Age on its own is not a risk factor but exposure to other risks clearly increases with age.

Examination

Examination of the patient

Extra-oral examination of the patient

Simply by talking to the patient, and making careful observations at the same time, the clinician may obtain important information that will help in treatment planning:

- *Discrepancy between actual and biological ages.* Any discrepancy between the actual age and biological age should be noted as this can be important in assessing the likely adaptive capability, an aspect discussed more fully in Chapter 2.
- *Skeletal relationship.* The skeletal relationship of the patient should be assessed because this will indicate the appropriate incisal relationship of the planned dentures (Chapter 12).
- *Occlusal vertical dimension.* The facial appearance provides valuable information about the occlusal vertical dimension of existing dentures (Fig. 7.1). If loss of occlusal vertical dimension is noted, correction may be required before the provision of new dentures is started (p. 93).

- *Dental appearance.* If the patient already has dentures, the dental appearance should be evaluated at this stage of the examination. It is particularly important that the appearance of the dentures is assessed during speaking and smiling. Features such as inadequate lip support or poor appearance of the anterior teeth should be noted. If the patient has a complaint regarding the appearance of the current dentures it is essential that the details are carefully recorded when obtaining the history of the complaint.
- *Extra-oral lesions.* Inflammation and fissuring at the corners of the mouth (angular stomatitis) may be present; the significance and treatment of this condition are described on p. 119.
- *Intolerance or other difficulties with the dentures.* While the patient is speaking it may be possible to detect any obvious looseness of dentures, or whether the patient is having difficulty in controlling the prostheses.

Intra-oral examination of the patient

The broad objectives of this part of the examination are to determine:

- whether there is any pathology in the mouth (Figs. 7.2a and 7.2b);
- what the prospects are for the new dentures providing a satisfactory level of comfort and function.

Detecting systemic disease

The mouth has been aptly described as a mirror which reflects the state of health of the individual. When systemic disease develops, the powerful combination of microorganisms, normal wear and tear, and moisture and warmth present in the mouth frequently result in visible changes in the oral tissues before signs of disease are evident elsewhere in the body. Investigation of these changes may allow an

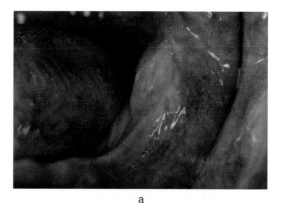

a

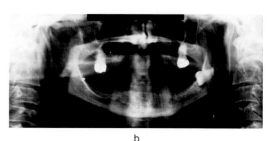

b

Figure 7.2 (a) The swelling in the left molar region should be reviewed for associated pathology. (b) A radiograph showed an unerupted third molar.

early diagnosis of the systemic condition to be made. For example, there may be a change in the population of papillae on the tongue; this change occurs first on the tip and sides, the areas of maximum trauma. The filiform papillae are progressively lost so that the fungiform papillae become more noticeable and produce the appearance of a 'pebbly' tongue; eventually, the fungiform papillae also disappear and the tongue becomes smooth (Fig. 7.3). These changes should lead the clinician to suspect deficiencies such as iron, vitamin B_{12} and folic acid. Diagnosis may be confirmed by the appropriate haematological investigations.

Screening for oral cancer

Clinicians, because of their training, experience and equipment, are uniquely qualified to examine the oral cavity thoroughly and to recognise

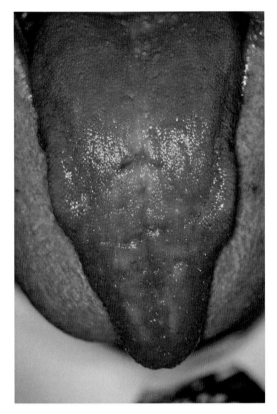

Figure 7.3 Reduction in population of filiform and fungiform papillae as a result of a folic acid deficiency.

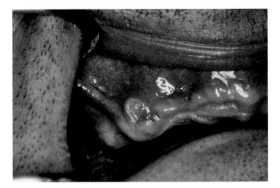

Figure 7.4 The ulcer in the upper right canine region has a raised, rolled margin; there was no history of trauma. Biopsy confirmed a malignant change.

any features which are outside the range of normal variation. Large numbers of people are examined dentally each year; the clinician therefore plays the central role in screening the population for oral manifestations of systemic disease. Of particular relevance in the older patient with complete dentures is the presence of oral malignancy. It has been reported that the oral cavity and pharynx combined, constitute the sixth commonest site for cancer and that oral cancer is increasing in a number of countries in both the developed and developing world. Although the overall prevalence of oral cancer is low, 95% of cases, excluding salivary gland tumours, occur in patients who are over 45 years of age. Early detection by the clinician increases the chance that treatment may affect

a cure. Any ulceration, change in character of the mucosa or swelling, whose presence cannot be readily explained, should be regarded with suspicion (Fig. 7.4). In all instances, appropriate steps such as radiographic examination, biopsy or immediate referral should be undertaken. There is widespread agreement that opportunistic screening for oral cancer should be part of every dental examination procedure (British Dental Association 2000; Conway et al. 2002). There is evidence that this is particularly effective in developing countries with a high incidence of the disease (Downer et al. 2006). However, there is a concern that the individuals who are at the highest risk tend not to be regular dental attenders and, therefore, additional strategies are needed to also allow screening of this group (Yusof et al. 2006).

Other assessments

If there are no signs of systemic disease, the findings of the intra-oral examination assume a primarily local significance by helping to diagnose the patient's dental complaint, to formulate a treatment plan and to determine a prognosis. Features of interest are:

- The shape and size of ridges and hard palate.
- The depth and width of the sulci, including the presence of prominent frena.

- The degree of compressibility of the denture-bearing mucosa determined by palpation.
- The size of the tongue.
- Any pathology such as mucosal inflammation, ulceration, hyperplasia, sinuses or swellings. If pathological conditions of the underlying bone are suspected, radiographs must be taken. These conditions, described in Chapter 9, should normally be treated before starting prosthetic treatment so that a stable and healthy denture foundation is produced.
- The quality and quantity of saliva. The relevance of such observations to the stability of complete dentures is discussed more fully in Chapters 4 and 16.

Examination of the dentures

Extra-oral examination of the dentures

The dentures are removed from the mouth and a detailed and systematic extra-oral examination is made of their impression, polished and occlusal surfaces. Any relevant findings are recorded.

Impression surface
- The presence or absence of a post-dam (p. 153) and palatal relief (p. 162).
- Width of borders.
- The amount and distribution of plaque, an important cause of denture stomatitis (Chapter 9). Painting disclosing solution on the impression surface will help to visualise the plaque (Fig. 14.10).
- Evidence of adjustments, relines or repairs.
- Surface roughness.

Polished surface
- Shape and inclination. In essence, is the shape such that it will allow the muscles to help rather than hinder the control of the denture?
- Condition and general cleanliness of the denture material.

Occlusal surface
- Amount of wear; presence of shiny facets.
- Teeth – size, shape and colour.

Intra-oral examination of the dentures

The first point to make in this section is that the clinicians' judgements of the quality of dentures often do not match the level of satisfaction reported by patients. For example, a denture border which is judged clinically to be under-extended, may not necessarily have led the patient to complain of looseness because the denture foundation is particularly favourable. Furthermore, the point needs to be made that clinicians may well vary in their judgements of quality.

This insecurity has prompted the development of an approach which judges the following important aspects of upper and lower dentures (Corrigan et al. 2002):

- Occlusal vertical dimension
- Occlusion
- Retention of upper denture
- Tongue control of upper denture
- Stability of upper denture
- Stability of lower denture

Occlusal vertical dimension
Every effort should be made to obtain an accurate estimation of the freeway space at this stage because the result will be of fundamental importance both in the diagnosis and in the formulation of a treatment plan; the clinical techniques for obtaining this information are described in Chapter 11. However, it should be remembered that an assessment of the freeway space at this stage may, in some instances, only be a rough estimate because it may be impossible to induce a relaxed state at the patient's first visit. Further estimations will be made when the occlusion is recorded and will serve to check on the accuracy of the original assessment.

Occlusion

Having asked the patient 'to close gently on the back teeth' several times from a relaxed and slightly open position, occlusal contact is judged to be either satisfactory (when there is even meeting of teeth and consistent return to an intercuspal position) or unsatisfactory (when there is uneven contact, an inconsistent return to the intercuspal position or a slide greater than 4 mm).

Retention of the upper denture

Tests of retention are usually only of value in assessing the upper denture as the physical retention of lower dentures is often minimal. Two functional tests are of particular value for the upper denture:

1. Seat the upper denture and attempt to dislodge it by pulling vertically downwards with the thumb and first finger on the buccal aspects of the right and left premolar teeth. Lack of resistance indicates poor retention.
2. Seat the upper denture and ask the patient to open the mouth until the incisal separation is about 2 cm. If this degree of opening causes the denture to drop, an error in either the impression or the polished surface should be suspected.

Tongue control of the upper denture

This is particularly important because, in its absence, a complaint of looseness when biting on a piece of food is unlikely to be cured (Culver & Watt 1973; Basker & Watson 1988). A cotton wool roll is inserted between the incisors and the patient is instructed to initially hold the roll gently and then, when instructed, to bite on it as if it were a piece of food. This test can be repeated three times and a check made on the last occasion as to whether or not the tongue has been raised to stabilise the posterior border of the denture (Fig. 7.5).

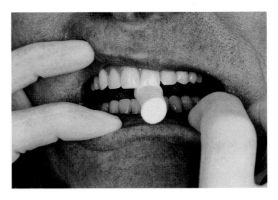

Figure 7.5   From this position the patient is asked to bite on the cotton wool roll. The clinician is in a position to judge whether or not the tongue has pushed itself against the back edge of the upper denture so as to stabilise it.

Stability of the upper denture

The upper denture is seated in the mouth and an attempt made to rotate it in the horizontal plane. Any resulting lateral movement of the midline is noted. Some movement is inevitable because of the compressibility of the mucosa, but a movement of 3 mm or more either side of the midline is an indication of loss of fit or the presence of a flabby ridge. A similar conclusion can be drawn if an attempt to rock the denture across the midline results in clearly detectable movement of the prosthesis with the centre of the hard palate acting as a fulcrum.

Stability of the lower denture

This can be judged in four ways:

1. With the upper denture in place to support the muscles of the cheeks, the patient is asked to open the mouth by about 2 cm. A judgement can then be made as to whether the denture stays on the tissues or has been noticeably displaced in an occlusal direction. This judgement can be made only if the tongue is brought forwards so that its tip lightly contacts the lingual surfaces of the anterior teeth (Fig. 7.6).

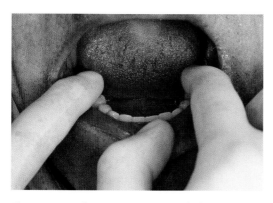

Figure 7.6 The tongue is in a retruded position and thus it is impossible to assess if the denture is in the neutral zone. The tip of the tongue should touch the lingual aspect of the anterior teeth before the judgement is made.

2. The stability of a lower denture can be further investigated by seeing if it stays seated on the ridge when the patient is instructed to move the tongue so that the tip rests gently at the angle of the mouth, first one side and then the other. Lack of tongue space within the arch of teeth will readily result in movement of the denture (Fig. 7.7).

3. The lower denture is held against the ridge by a finger and thumb in the incisor region and an attempt is made to move it in an antero-posterior direction. Pronounced

movement is highly suggestive of lack of extension of the denture base over the all-important pear-shaped pads and into the retromylohyoid fossa.

4. It is also advisable to assess the height of the occlusal plane of the lower denture and determine whether it is in such a position that the tongue is able to rest on the occlusal surface and thus play a part in stabilising the denture.

Border extension

Having completed the functional assessment of the dentures, there will usually be a need to focus on the border extension of the dentures so as to link functional concerns with design errors. Under-extension of the upper and lower denture buccally, labially and at the post-dam can be determined by direct vision. Over-extension is present if the denture moves occlusally when the muscles are gently pulled. Lingual extension is less easy to assess. Anteriorly a mouth mirror can help, and overextension can be inferred if the lower denture lifts when the tongue is raised. A fully border moulded alginate wash impression within the denture can be very informative, indicating either over- or under-extension. The correct extension of a denture base is described in Chapter 10.

Appearance

Having completed the functional assessment of the dentures, a further assessment of the appearance of the dentures should be made. The lips can be retracted and features such as orientation of the occlusal plane, and the colour, shape and arrangement of the anterior teeth can be noted. The findings at this stage will supplement those obtained during the extra-oral examination of the patient described previously.

Special tests

It may be necessary to take radiographs, organise blood tests, arrange for microbiological

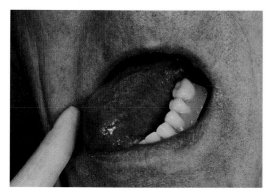

Figure 7.7 The tongue movement has produced marked instability of the denture. There is inadequate space for the tongue.

examination of swabs or smears, or to carry out diagnostic modifications of existing dentures. The reasons for undertaking any of these procedures are discussed in the relevant sections of the book.

Diagnosis

By correlating the findings of the examination and special tests with the patient's history, the cause or causes of the complaint should be identified and recorded. It is important to realise that, unless a diagnosis is made, there is little prospect of solving a patient's problems by providing new dentures, and in some cases, it is unwise to embark on such treatment.

Treatment plan

Following the diagnosis, a treatment plan is formulated. Possible treatment options include the following:

- No treatment
- Preparatory treatment such as denture adjustment or a short-term reline (Chapter 8)
- Definitive denture modifications such as reline, rebase (Chapter 15), repair or cleaning
- Replacement dentures

If replacement dentures are to be made, it can be of great value to write down a 'shopping list' in the patient's records that clearly identifies those features in the existing dentures which will be:

- Modified in the replacement dentures in order to overcome the patient's complaint. An indication of the nature of the modifications should also be included.
- Copied and incorporated in the replacement dentures because these features have proved successful previously. Such written comments serve as an invaluable reminder and checklist during subsequent clinical stages.

There are several approaches to designing and constructing complete dentures. The clinician should make a positive decision at the treatment plan stage as to which is appropriate for the patient:

- *Carving record rims.* The shape, or design, of the dentures may be determined by the clinician carving the record rims as described in Chapter 11.
- *Copy dentures.* Where dentures have provided satisfactory service for the patient in the past, it may be advisable to base the design of replacement dentures on the well-accepted features of the old ones. Although such an approach is particularly appropriate for the treatment of older patients who have a reduced ability to adapt, it can also be of value in a number of other clinical situations. A potentially accurate method of maintaining the well-accepted features of existing dentures is to use a copy technique (Chapter 8).
- *Biometric guides.* Another approach to design involves the use of biometric guides – measurements from certain anatomical landmarks which allow the denture teeth and base to be placed in positions similar to those formerly occupied by the natural teeth and alveolar bone. The desirability of so doing has been a source of controversy for many years but has received a considerable measure of support. Anatomical guidelines have now been researched which assist the clinician in trying to achieve this aim (Chapter 10).
- *Functional neutral zone impression.* When there are particular problems in achieving stability of a lower denture – for example, if there is abnormal muscular activity or intraoral anatomy – the clinician can record the neutral zone by getting the patient to mould a soft record rim into a position of stability between the tongue and cheeks and lips by means of swallowing and speaking. A lower denture is then produced whose shape

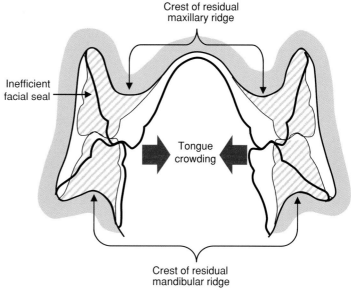

Crest of residual
maxillary ridge

Inefficient
facial seal

Tongue
crowding

Crest of residual
mandibular ridge

Figure 7.8 Pattern of resorption in the maxilla and mandible following loss of the natural teeth. A mechanistic upper denture (heavy outline) has been produced with teeth on the crest of the residual ridge. Occlusion with the lower denture has been achieved by producing a cross-bite on the patient's right and excessive lingual placement of the lower teeth on the left.

Position formerly occupied by the natural teeth and supporting bone

is derived from the neutral zone impression. This clinical technique has been shown to enhance the tongue's retentive ability over a conventional design (Miller et al. 1998). Details of this technique are described in Chapter 12.

All these approaches to complete denture design are based on sound clinical principles and require an adequate prescription to be sent by the clinician to the laboratory. In the absence of such a prescription, the technician may be tempted to produce a denture design which is essentially mechanistic with the teeth placed on the crest of the ridge. The greater the amount of resorption that has occurred, the greater the problem this approach can create. This is because the pattern of bone resorption of the residual ridges is not uniform. For example, in the maxilla the bone loss is predominantly from the buccal and labial aspects of the ridge, causing its crest to progressively migrate palatally. Setting the upper teeth on the crest of the ridge

as shown in Fig. 7.8 has the following undesirable consequences:

- Poor facial appearance due to inadequate lip and cheek support.
- Reduced physical retention associated with an inefficient or absent facial seal.
- Encroachment on tongue space, resulting in denture instability, tongue soreness and interference with tongue function during speech and food transport.
- Problems in achieving a satisfactory occlusal relationship with the lower denture. For example, in Fig. 7.8 the alternatives are to accept a posterior cross-bite or place the lower teeth so far lingually that instability of the lower denture is bound to result.

In view of these undesirable consequences, it can be argued that a mechanistic approach which results from the clinician failing to supply a design prescription to the laboratory is an avoidance of professional responsibilities by the clinician, who alone has the clinical information necessary to make an informed decision on the design.

Prognosis

The findings of the history and examination will enable the clinician to assess the degree of success the proposed line of treatment is likely to achieve. If problems are anticipated, they should be explained to the patient before treatment proceeds. The patient is then more likely to accept and to cope with the unavoidable limitations of the new dentures.

References and additional reading

Basker, R.M. & Watson, C.J. (1991) Tongue control of upper complete dentures. *British Dental Journal*, 170, 449–50.

Boyle, P., Macfarlane, G.J., Maisonneuve, P., Zheng, T., Scully, C. & Tedesco, B. (1990) Epidemiology of mouth cancer in 1989: a review. *Journal of the Royal Society of Medicine*, 83, 724–30.

British Dental Association (2000) *Opportunistic Oral Cancer Screening*. BDA, London.

Conway, D.I., Macpherson, L.M.D., Gibson, J. & Binnie, V.I. (2002) Oral cancer: prevention and detection in primary dental healthcare. *Primary Dental Care*, 9, 119–23.

Corrigan, P.J., Basker, R.M., Farrin, A.J. Mulley, G.P. & Heath, M.R. (2002) The development of a method for functional assessment of dentures. *Gerodontology*, 19, 41–5.

Culver, P.A.J. & Watt, I. (1973) Denture movements and control: a preliminary study. *British Dental Journal*, 135, 111–6.

Downer, M.C., Moles, D.R., Palmer, S. & Speight, P.M. (2006) A systematic review of measures of effectiveness in screening for oral cancer and precancer. *Oral Oncology*, 42, 129–31.

Duxbury, A.J., Leach, F.N. & Smart, T.E. (1982) Oral dyskinesia induced by Tryptizol. *Dental Update*, 9, 299–302.

Lamey, P.J. & Lewis, M.A.O. (1999) *A Clinical Guide to Oral Medicine*, 2nd edn. British Dental Journal, London.

Likeman, P.R & Watt, D.M. (1974) *Morphological changes in the maxillary denture bearing area*. British Dental Journal, 136, 500–3.

Miller, W.P., Monteith, B. & Heath, M.R. (1998) The effect of variation of the lingual shape of mandibular complete dentures on lingual resistance to lifting forces. *Gerodontology*, 15, 113–19.

Watt, D.M. (1977) Tooth positions on complete dentures. *Journal of Dentistry*, 6, 147–60.

Watt, D.M. & Likeman, P.R. (1974) Morphological changes in the denture bearing area following the extraction of maxillary teeth. *British Dental Journal*, 136, 225–35.

Yusof, Z.Y., Netuveli, G., Ramli, A.S. & Sheiham, A. (2006) Is opportunistic oral cancer screening by dentists feasible? An analysis of the patterns of dental attendance of a nationally representative sample over 10 years. *Oral Health and Preventive Dentistry*, 4, 165–71.

The Relevance of Existing Dentures

8

This chapter makes the following key points:

- Existing dentures are often invaluable for diagnosis and treatment planning. For this a thorough assessment of the dentures, as described in Chapter 7, is essential. Most existing dentures, whether or not they have been worn successfully, can provide important information for all stages of treatment. Therefore they should be referred to regularly as treatment proceeds.
- Existing dentures are often very useful when carrying out certain treatment procedures.
- Most complete denture provision is concerned with the construction of replacement, rather than first dentures.
- The copy technique is an effective way of transferring design information accurately from existing to replacement dentures.
- As with most prosthetic treatments, good clinician/dental technician teamwork is of the utmost importance in achieving a successful outcome.

To summarise, existing dentures can play an important part in the following:

- Diagnosis
- Treatment planning
- Preparation of the mouth
- Impression procedures
- Recording the jaw relationship
- Denture copying

Diagnosis

A thorough assessment of a patient's denture history and of the dentures themselves will provide key information which leads to a sound diagnosis and an effective treatment plan. Patients requesting replacement dentures fall into three broad categories.

Those wearing immediate dentures

Patients requesting replacement of their immediate dentures usually do so because the post-extraction resorption of bone has led to a loss of retention and stability. Apart from a desire for better fitting dentures, many of these patients are anxious that the appearance of the original dentures should be maintained. The clinician

Prosthetic Treatment of the Edentulous Patient, Fifth Edition, © R.M. Basker, J.C. Davenport and J.M. Thomason
Published 2011 by Blackwell Publishing Ltd.

needs to satisfy these demands if a successful outcome is to be achieved. Improving the fit is seldom a major problem, but considerable care is needed to maintain the other well-accepted characteristics, such as position and arrangement of the artificial teeth. This challenge may best be met by using a copying technique, as described later in this chapter.

Those whose most recent dentures have been worn successfully for a significant period of time

It is important when providing new dentures for those patients whose previous dentures have been satisfactory for a number of years that the features considered to have contributed to that success are incorporated into the new prostheses. Failure to conform to this principle, which is particularly relevant to the treatment of older patients, who may adapt to change very slowly or be unable to adapt, is likely to lead to the construction of dentures which are poorly tolerated. Such failures account for a proportion of patients in the third group, who have experienced persistent denture problems.

Those with dentures that have caused persistent problems from the very beginning

For those patients with chronic denture problems, it is again vitally important to establish an accurate diagnosis. This is best achieved by asking the patient to bring in all sets of dentures in their possession so that the previous attempts can be analysed.

Within each of the three groups described, clinical situations may occur in which the clinician observes a shortcoming in the denture design which has not troubled the patient. There is then the dilemma – should the shortcoming be corrected or not? This can be a very difficult question to answer and possible pitfalls are discussed more fully under 'Category (f)' on p. 103. It is impossible to be dogmatic about this, particularly when treating older patients. In all instances, the clinician should consider whether it is likely to be possible to make successful new dentures if the error is retained. If it is decided to make an alteration, then it is essential to explain the reasons for this to the patient.

Treatment plan

Having assessed the patient's dentures and related problems, the treatment plan is likely to fall into one of the following categories:

- Make temporary modifications to the existing dentures to test a diagnosis.
- Make permanent modifications to the existing dentures (e.g. rebase or modify the occlusion).
- Construct replacement dentures using conventional techniques.
- Construct replacement dentures using a copy technique for one or both dentures.
- No treatment, or referral for specialist advice. Such a decision may be made when the clinician assesses that new dentures will not overcome the patient's complaint or where a diagnosis cannot be established with confidence, and thus there is a real risk of new dentures being no more successful than any of the existing ones.

Preparation of the mouth

Before commencing any of the treatment plans listed above, it is often necessary to carry out preparatory treatment to improve the condition of the mouth so that it is in the optimum state to receive the new prostheses. The existing dentures are often of value in carrying out this preparatory treatment – for example, when treating inflammation of the denture-bearing mucosa or when modifying an unsatisfactory jaw relationship.

Treatment of inflammation of the denture-bearing mucosa

The commonest causes of this condition are trauma from an existing denture and the proliferation of microorganisms on the impression surface of the denture. Denture trauma may be the result of an ill-fitting denture, an unbalanced occlusion, or lack of freeway space.

It is important that the inflammation of the mucosa is resolved before final impressions for the new dentures are taken. If not, the better fitting and more hygienic new dentures are likely to affect some improvement in the condition. Then, as the inflammation resolves, the shape of the denture-bearing mucosa will change causing the fit of the new dentures to deteriorate, re-establishing one of the causative factors of the original inflammation. Although the simplest method of treatment is to ask the patient not to wear the old dentures, such advice is unacceptable to the majority of patients. In such cases the dentures need to be corrected before the definitive treatment is started.

The fit of a denture can be improved quickly and effectively by temporarily relining with a short-term soft lining material (p. 234).

Occlusal imbalance can be corrected either by adjusting the occlusal surface through selective grinding or by applying a layer of cold-curing acrylic to the posterior teeth, provided this addition leaves an adequate freeway space.

Methods of eliminating infection by microorganisms are described on p. 117.

Modification of an unsatisfactory jaw relationship

Some patients still believe that once complete dentures have been provided there is no need for further treatment. This is borne out by a national survey of adult dental health in the UK which included information on the age of dentures being worn by edentulous people (Walker & Cooper 2000). A total of 39% were wearing a denture provided at least 20 years ago.

Added to this was the fact that although 41% of complete denture wearers had some problem, only 13% were planning to visit a dentist. As a result, cases are seen where, through lack of maintenance, there have been considerable changes in occlusal vertical dimension and in the intercuspal position. Severe wear of the acrylic occlusal surface and resorption of alveolar bone leads to a situation where the freeway space may be 10 mm or more. Patients seeking new dentures at this advanced stage of occlusal derangement may make such statements as 'I can't chew my food so well', or 'My teeth don't show as much as they used to'. Little imagination is required on the part of the clinician to appreciate the basis of their complaints (Fig. 8.1).

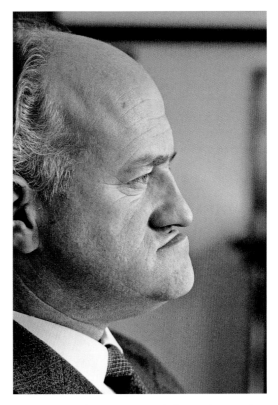

Figure 8.1 The patient is occluding on his complete dentures. Lack of maintenance has led to gross loss in occlusal vertical dimension and protrusion of the mandible.

However, patients are not usually aware of the problems produced in allowing the occlusion to deteriorate to such a degree.

There are two major uncertainties concerning the jaw relationship when providing replacement dentures:

1. *What increase in occlusal vertical dimension is likely to be tolerated?* If one attempts to reduce the freeway space to 3 mm in situations like those described above, the occlusal vertical dimension has to be increased by 7 mm or more. This may exceed a patient's ability to adapt. For example, such a magnitude of change can result in increased masticatory stress being transmitted to the denture-bearing mucosa which might have atrophied to the extent that it is no longer able to accept such stress. Furthermore, a patient possessing a generous freeway space has been able to eat large mouthfuls of food without having to open the mandible much beyond the rest position. If the same dietary habits continue once the new dentures are fitted, difficulties in eating are likely and the increased opening of the jaw to accommodate the large mouthfuls may well produce pain in the muscles of mastication.

2. *What is the correct jaw relationship in the horizontal plane?* The reduction in occlusal vertical dimension and the unbalanced occlusion result in protrusion of the mandible. This mandibular protrusion is partly anatomical and partly habitual and generally makes it difficult, sometimes impossible, to record the retruded position. A reduction in the apparent protrusion of the mandible is, to some degree, automatic on restoration of the occlusal vertical dimension, because the hinge-like nature of the temporomandibular joint causes the chin to move posteriorly as the occlusal vertical dimension is increased (Fig. 8.2). Correcting the habitual element is usually a more gradual process. If the protrusive habit is not corrected before constructing the

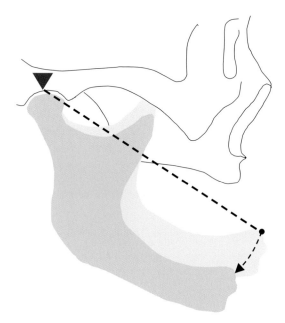

Figure 8.2   Movement of the chin posteriorly as the occlusal vertical dimension is increased.

new dentures the subsequent gradual reduction in the protrusive posture will result in a long programme of occlusal adjustment to these new dentures.

The uncertainties may be minimised by modifying the old dentures. The occlusal vertical dimension is increased by adding a layer of cold-curing acrylic resin to the occlusal surface of one of the dentures (Fig. 8.3). The new occlusal pattern initiates the breakdown of the habitual protrusion of the mandible as well as allowing an assessment of the patient's ability to accept the chosen increase in occlusal vertical dimension and the change in appearance. The temporary occlusal surface can be modified to accommodate the gradual change in the jaw relationship. New dentures can then be constructed when it becomes apparent that the planned increase in vertical dimension is acceptable and the protrusion of the mandible has been corrected.

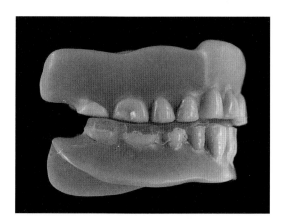

Figure 8.3 Occlusal vertical dimension corrected by the addition of a layer of cold-curing acrylic resin applied to the occlusal surface of the lower denture.

Impression procedures

Under certain circumstances an existing lower denture may be used as an impression tray to obtain the following types of master impression:

- Functional impression
- 'Wash' impression
- Copy of the existing impression surface of the old denture

Functional impression

A functional impression is one that is obtained by placing in the denture an impression material that exhibits plastic flow over a period of several hours. During this period the denture is worn and subjected to functional loads, e.g. during mastication. As a result the impression material records the shape of the denture-bearing tissues during function. This contrasts with the conventional impression techniques described in Chapter 10, which are in effect 'snapshots' of the shape of the denture-bearing tissues obtained at a single point in time. Such impressions are produced under conditions of loading applied by the clinician as the tray is

seated which bear little, if any, relationship to those occurring in normal function.

An additional advantage of the functional impression technique is that it allows an assessment of the patient's reaction to a new impression surface before proceeding with definitive treatment. For example, a patient may present with a history of persistent discomfort beneath a denture that has not responded to previous adjustments. If, after a careful evaluation of the situation, the clinician concludes that the problem is due to errors in the impression surface, it can be helpful to the clinician and reassuring to the patient to be able to test the hypothesis before being committed to definitive treatment. In the case described this can be achieved by correcting the fit of the denture with a short-term soft lining material. If the patient comments favourably on the result at the next visit, the operator has gained valuable evidence that the new impression surface is compatible with the comfortable, normal function and that a rebase or a replacement denture made to this new surface is likely to be equally well tolerated. If the patient does not comment favourably on the result the clinician can look for other possible causes of the complaint and, if necessary, remove the ineffective functional impression material. Using this approach, one is following the dictates of the saying, 'The proof of the pudding is in the eating'. It is very important, however, to sound a note of caution here. There are situations in which a patient has persistent problems with a number of dentures in which it may be very unwise to alter the existing dentures in any way. This is discussed further in the section 'Category (f)' on p. 103. The short-term soft lining materials used for functional impressions are discussed more fully in Chapter 16.

The 'wash' impression technique

In some instances an old denture can act as a very satisfactory special impression tray. This avoids the need for a separate appointment to take a preliminary impression in a stock tray

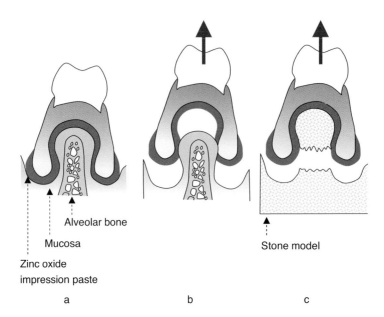

Figure 8.4   (a) Undercuts not removed from the impression surface. (b) Mucosal compressibility allows removal of the denture from the mouth. (c) Subsequent removal from the cast is impossible without damage.

in order to construct a special tray. However, it must be appreciated that corrections of any over- or under-extension of the old denture will be required before taking the master impression. If it is necessary to increase the extension of the border by more than 2 mm, it is advisable to use one of the rigid border-trimming materials which are discussed on p. 145.

It will be appreciated that if there are significant undercuts in the impression surface of the denture they have to be removed before taking the impression for the reason described in Fig. 8.4. In most cases it is unwise to tamper with such a denture in this way for fear of making it too loose or uncomfortable to wear. Fortunately, most of the dentures for which the technique might be considered appropriate will have been originally constructed on well-resorbed ridges where undercuts do not exist.

The impression surface of the denture should be dried thoroughly to ensure that the impression material adheres firmly to the denture. Either a low viscosity silicone impression material or a zinc oxide-eugenol impression

paste may be used to record the detail of the denture-bearing mucosa. Both materials are accurate when used in thin section but the former has the advantages of being tasteless, elastic and relatively clean to use. The denture is returned to the patient after the cast has been poured and the impression material has been removed.

Copying the existing impression surface of the lower denture

There are occasions when a new lower denture has been provided to replace an old ill-fitting one and the patient returns to the surgery with the comment that 'the old denture was much more comfortable'.

The impression surface of the old denture may only contact the mucosa along its borders (Fig. 8.5). However, the reactions of the patient and the appearance of the mucosa show that this state of affairs is perfectly acceptable. Why do the reactions of the patient differ from the evidence of the clinical examination? It is

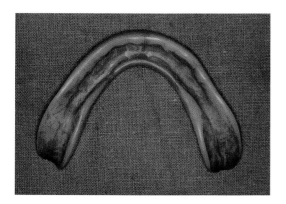

Figure 8.5 The impression surface of a lower denture which still provides comfort and stability after 10 years of wear. The border areas are well polished by continual contact with the border tissues. The middle of the impression surface is covered with calculus and is heavily stained, indicating that the denture no longer fits the tissues in that area.

because the denture-bearing tissues have gradually adapted to the progressive loss of fit of the old denture and the uneven distribution of load that is the result. It is also likely that the progressive loss of fit has been adequately compensated by the muscular control of the denture.

If a new denture is constructed with an accurate impression surface, the masticatory forces will be transmitted to tissues which have not been loaded for a long time. The mucosa overlying the ridge may no longer be able to accept the forces, so discomfort is experienced. Therefore, if one is faced with an old denture whose impression surface is well tolerated by the patient and which has not caused mucosal damage, an option which should be seriously considered is to pour dental stone directly into the impression surface and construct the new denture on the cast produced. In this way the comfortable fit of the old denture will be reproduced in the new one.

Recording jaw relations

If replacement dentures are being made by conventional techniques, reference to previ-

ous dentures is particularly rewarding when recording jaw relations. During this clinical stage, the clinician produces a blueprint, for example, by shaping the record rims so that the dental technician can construct dentures that faithfully follow the design concepts decided at the treatment planning stage. In the case of a patient requiring replacement dentures, the clinician has the advantage of a previous blueprint, the old dentures, which will yield valuable information on features to be copied or changed in the replacement dentures.

Assessing occlusal vertical dimension

Simply determining the occlusal vertical dimension by reference to the rest position alone can be rather imprecise. Thus, it is advisable to try to improve the reliability of this assessment by using several indicators. These include facial appearance, speech and the patient's experience with existing dentures.

If it is apparent from the patient's comments and the clinician's own observations that the existing dentures have an adequate freeway space, the occlusal vertical dimension can be recorded and copied in the new dentures.

On the other hand, if the patient complains of symptoms which signify a lack of freeway space and this is confirmed by clinical assessment, the clinician can still record the occlusal vertical dimension and then use the result for comparative purposes to ensure that the height of the record blocks is reduced by an amount sufficient to provide the required freeway space.

Where there is excessive freeway space, it may be advisable to correct this on the old dentures by adding a resin onlay, as described previously. Then, when the occlusal vertical dimension for the new dentures is determined, it is possible to refer directly to the successfully modified old dentures.

Shaping the upper record block

When replacing an existing upper denture which has provided several years of satisfactory wear, it is usually advantageous to carve the record block to a shape very similar to that of the denture so that the key details of design are passed on to the dental technician for incorporation into the new prosthesis. Particular attention should be paid to the following aspects.

Shape and width of the dental arch, together with its relationship to the underlying ridge

The shape and width of the dental arch determine the amount of tongue space within the confines of the upper denture. As the tongue is accustomed to functioning within a given space, a reduced space on the replacement denture is liable to induce speech difficulties, problems when manipulating a bolus of food, a sore tongue and a general difficulty in adapting to the new shape of the denture. The well-accepted shape of the old denture is conveniently reproduced by first assessing the overbite–overjet relationship of the buccal and labial segments on the old dentures. Then the upper record block is carved until, on occluding with the old lower denture in the mouth, the same relationship is produced. This procedure establishes the overall width of the dental arch. The palatal aspect of the record block is then adjusted to produce an occlusal table which is similar in width to that of the old denture (Fig. 8.6).

Labial contour and lip support

The labial contour of the upper denture determines the amount of support provided for the upper lip. If the lip support provided by the existing upper denture is acceptable, it is usually appropriate to shape the labial aspect of the upper record block to provide the same amount of support. The lip support provided by an upper record block is the product of three factors:

- The position of the incisal edge in the horizontal plane,
- The position of the incisal edge in the vertical plane,
- The inclination of the labial surface of the record rim.

The first two factors can be controlled accurately if the incisal relationship on the previous dentures is copied by following the method of shaping the upper rim as described previously.

An alternative and effective way of establishing the position of the incisal edge in the vertical plane is to measure the distance on the existing denture between the incisive papilla and the incisal edge with a specially designed gauge (Fig. 8.7). With the denture resting on the table of the gauge, and the locating needle positioned in the concavity produced by the incisive papilla, the relationship of the central incisors in both horizontal and vertical planes can be read on the scales attached to the gauge. The record rim is then shaped and the relationship of its midline to the incisive papilla is checked on the gauge.

Level and orientation of the occlusal plane

The level and orientation of the occlusal plane are critical for both the appearance and the function of dentures. The patient's experience with the existing dentures will again provide invaluable information on whether or not the occlusal plane is satisfactory. If the experience has been a happy one the level of the occlusal plane can be reproduced by shaping the record blocks as described above. If there have been problems with the existing dentures that can be attributed to the positioning of the occlusal plane then reference to the old dentures will allow measured changes to be introduced.

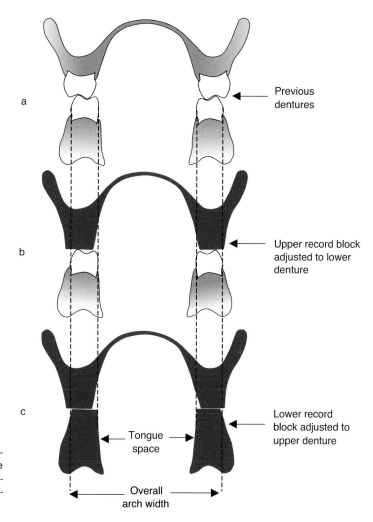

a

Previous dentures

b

Upper record block adjusted to lower denture

c

Lower record block adjusted to upper denture

Tongue space

Overall arch width

Figure 8.6 Procedure for reproducing the overall arch width and the tongue space on replacement dentures: (a), (b) and (c) illustrate the consecutive stages of the procedure.

Shaping the lower record block

It is essential that adequate tongue space is provided within the confines of the lower denture so that tongue function is unimpaired and the tongue can help rather than hinder the stability of the prosthesis. To maintain such a space when replacing a well-tolerated lower denture, the following aspects must be borne in mind while shaping the lower rim:

• The shape of the dental arch and its relationship to the underlying ridge;

• The width of the occlusal table;
• The height of the occlusal plane.

The method of shaping the upper record block has already been described. Continuing this process allows the transfer of the characteristics of the arch width and occlusal width of the old lower denture to the rim (Fig. 8.6).

If the replacement dentures are being made to a similar occlusal vertical dimension as the old denture, and the height of the upper rim has been correctly established, the desired height of

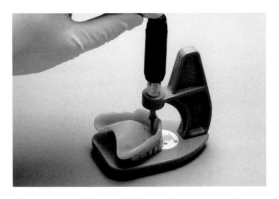

Figure 8.7 The incisal relationship measured in vertical and horizontal planes with an Alma gauge (see text for further details).

Selecting artificial teeth

Unless careful thought is given to this very important matter, the time given to the other aspects of denture construction is likely to be wasted because if incorrect choices are made the patient may reject the new dentures on the grounds of an unacceptable change in appearance. Decisions to be made at this stage concerning the artificial teeth are about the:

- Shade
- Mould
- Material
- Arrangement

the occlusal plane will be determined automatically once the lower rim is adjusted to the upper rim.

On many occasions, however, it is necessary to increase the occlusal vertical dimension to compensate for wear of the old occlusal surfaces and resorption of the alveolar bone, which allows the lower denture in particular to sink.

Should the increase be made on the upper or lower rim or shared between both? Each clinical case must be treated on its merits when making such a decision. It is necessary to have a clear idea of the magnitude of change required and to decide whether such an increase, if added to the upper rim, will improve or detract from the appearance of the patient or, if added to the lower rim, will so increase the height of the occlusal plane that the stability of the lower denture will be impaired. However, the patterns of bone resorption occurring in the upper and lower denture-bearing areas differ and it is usually the lower denture that has sunk most as a result. The upper denture benefits from continued support from the hard palate, which is relatively stable. Therefore, if the upper occlusal plane is to be kept unchanged and the lower occlusal plane is restored to its former level it is the lower denture that most commonly has to be increased in height.

When choosing the shade and mould of the upper anterior teeth, it is naturally very important to obtain the patient's thoughts on the appearance of the existing dentures. If, as a result of discussion, it is planned to maintain a similar appearance with the new dentures, it is necessary to choose the same or similar mould and shade for the upper anterior teeth. By taking an impression of the teeth of the old denture, it is possible to furnish the technician with a cast which provides guidance as to the arrangement of the teeth. However, it must be remembered that the cast only indicates the relationship between the artificial teeth and does not show the position of these teeth in relation to the underlying ridge. This latter relationship can only be obtained by correctly shaping the record rim.

There are occasions, of course, where it is necessary to alter the mould, shade or arrangement of the existing teeth. For example, the crown length may have been severely reduced by occlusal wear or the colour may have been altered by bleaching or staining. There is no problem if the patient has recognised the deterioration and requests an improvement. However, if the clinician is the first person to notice this state of affairs, it is important to explain and demonstrate the reason for a proposed change very carefully. If the ground is well prepared for an alteration in appearance and the patient's full agreement has been obtained, the change is likely to be accepted. It is particularly important to warn the patient that members of the family or close friends may comment on a change in facial appearance or even, tactlessly, enquire whether new dentures have been provided. Such comments are capable of turning the patient against the new dentures unless the ground has been prepared adequately in advance.

Positioning the posterior border of the upper denture

The clinician will normally wish to position the posterior border of the upper denture at the vibrating line. However, if an existing denture is under-extended in this region there may be uncertainty as to whether the patient can tolerate the desired correction of the under-extension. Under such circumstances, if a fully extended new denture is fitted which subsequently cannot be tolerated, the palate of the replacement denture will have to be shortened. As a result, the posterior palatal seal will be lost and the retention of the denture reduced. As an insurance against this eventuality it is a wise practice to produce two post-dam lines, one in the position of that on the old denture and one at the vibrating line. If, after wearing the new denture for a few days, the patient reports that the new position of the posterior border is intolerable, the extension of the palate can be cut back to the old post-dam line without the danger of breaking the continuity of the border seal.

Denture copying – clinical indications

So far in this chapter, discussion has been restricted to ways in which existing dentures can be used as a guide in the construction of replacement prostheses by conventional clinical procedures. However, none of these methods allow the features of an existing denture to be copied exactly. The ability to do this can be ex-

tremely useful, particularly in the treatment of older patients.

With increasing age, there is a progressive reduction in the ability to learn the new patterns of muscular behaviour upon which the successful control of complete dentures largely depends. An older person may therefore have difficulty in controlling a replacement denture if its shape differs from that of the old one. As more older patients are likely to require replacement dentures, a technique for copying the shape of dentures and so avoiding these problems of adaptation becomes increasingly valuable.

It must be stressed that it is rarely appropriate to copy all aspects of an old denture exactly. Strictly speaking therefore, 'copy technique' is something of a misnomer. Usually the method is used to copy selected aspects of denture design, which the clinician judges to be important to the success of treatment, while correcting other aspects which are considered to be unsatisfactory. For example, the overall shape of the dental arches and polished surfaces may be copied while a loss of fit and a worn occlusion are corrected.

The appropriate clinical work is undertaken on a copy of the old denture. This copy may be described as the copy template. The finished product becomes the copy denture.

Indications for copying dentures

It cannot be overemphasised that the correct application of a copying technique depends upon an accurate diagnosis, which itself is dependent upon a careful evaluation of the three surfaces of the existing denture. This examination allows a decision to be reached on the adequacy or otherwise of each surface and thus whether or not a copying technique is a feasible proposition, and, if it is, how best to employ that technique.

In general terms, an assessment of the three surfaces will allow the dentures to be placed into one of the categories shown in Table 8.1.

Table 8.1   Assessment of the adequacy of the three surfaces of the existing denture.

Category	Impression surface	Occlusal surface	Polished surface
a	Satisfactory	Satisfactory	Satisfactory
b	Unsatisfactory	Satisfactory	Satisfactory
c	Satisfactory	Unsatisfactory	Satisfactory
d	Unsatisfactory	Unsatisfactory	Satisfactory
e			Unsatisfactory
f	Questionable	Questionable	Questionable
g	Questionable	Questionable	Questionable

KEY	Satisfactory	Questionable	Unsatisfactory

Category (a) – all denture surfaces satisfactory

In this category, where all the denture surfaces are satisfactory, is the patient who is perfectly happy with existing dentures but wishes to have the added security of a 'spare set'. The copying technique may be used to produce the extra dentures.

Category (b) – deficiencies in the impression surface

Where an error is found only on the impression surface, the patient's complaint is normally best treated by relining or rebasing the denture (Chapter 15).

Category (c) – deficiencies in the occlusal surface

If a patient's complaint can be localised to a small defect on the occlusal surface, treatment may involve simple occlusal adjustment. If the defect is the result of general occlusal wear of posterior teeth, it may be advisable to avoid making new dentures, especially when treating patients whose advanced age and poor state of health suggest that there are advantages in reducing the number and complexity of treatment visits. Instead, the occlusal relationship can be recorded, the dentures articulated and the worn teeth replaced by new ones which are positioned in the corrected occlusal relationship and ultimately attached to the denture base with cold-curing resin.

Category (d) – deficiencies in the impression and occlusal surfaces

This category is perhaps the most common one where, over the years, there has been progressive wear of the occlusal surfaces and loss of fit as a consequence of bone resorption. A copying technique may be the ideal approach when providing new dentures that eliminate these faults. In this way, the well-accepted overall shape of the polished surface can be accurately retained. The clinical and technical stages required to deal with this situation will be described later in the chapter.

Category (e) – deficiencies in the polished surface

If it is concluded that a major error exists in the polished surface and that the denture is not positioned in the neutral zone, there is unlikely to be an indication for employing a copying technique. Having said this, a case can be argued for a modified copy technique in certain circumstances. For example, if a complaint of a loose lower denture is judged to be due to the lower anterior teeth being positioned too far labially, the desired change can be made on the wax replica teeth of the copy template and the effect of that change can be judged in the mouth. If the result is a more stable denture, the new well-defined prescription can be passed to the laboratory for the construction of trial dentures. An example whereby a copy technique allows changes in overall shape to be carefully controlled is shown in Figs. 8.8a–d.

Category (f) – the chronic denture patient with multiple deficiencies in the dentures

The typical scenario in this category is the patient who has experienced problems with many dentures and who is just about managing to wear a set which might be described as the least unsatisfactory of the collection. The clinician might conclude, not unreasonably, that obvious faults with the dentures are the cause of the problems and be tempted to try to correct them by adjusting the troublesome dentures. However, such a course of action can be misguided and a shortcut to disaster because, in such cases, it can never be guaranteed that the corrections will achieve the hoped-for result. They may even, as far as the patient is concerned, make things worse. The very difficult situation then arises of the patient who was just about managing with just one of the many sets of problematic dentures and now cannot manage any of them. Unfortunately, it is not usually possible to save the day by undoing the alterations that have failed in an attempt to return the denture to its original state.

Such a catastrophe can be avoided if the old dentures are first copied without any corrections being carried out. The copy dentures are then modified as appears to be appropriate and worn for a trial period. If the patient reports that the problems have been eliminated all is well and good. However, if the modifications do not work the patient still has the original denture to fall back on, so at the very least no harm has been done.

Category (g) – the older denture patient with deficiencies in the impression and occlusal surfaces

The patient with the following characteristics falls into this category:

- Older, and judged by the clinician to have a very limited ability to adapt to major changes in denture shape.
- Wearing dentures which have been successful for many years, but which have gradually deteriorated to the point where they now have a combination of faults creating problems for the patient.

A 'one-step' approach to the correction of the denture faults by providing new dentures may fail because of the very limited ability of the patient to adapt to the relatively substantial changes. This problem might be avoided by introducing the changes gradually. For example, the occlusal vertical dimension can be increased over a period by the repeated addition of small increments of cold cure acrylic resin to the occlusal surfaces. A new increment of resin is not added until the patient has adapted

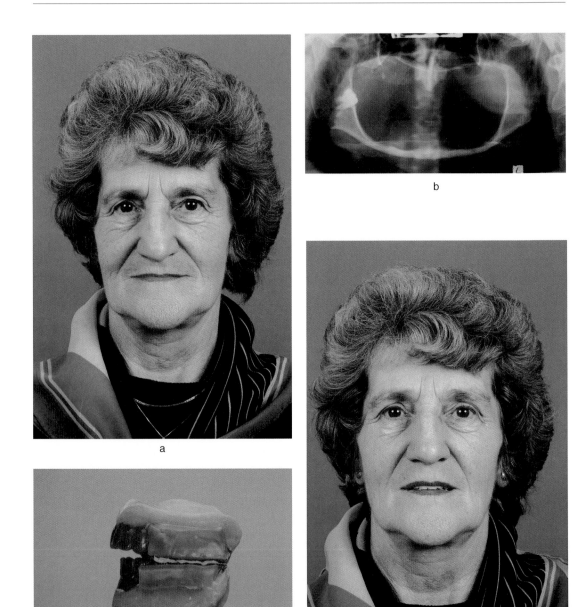

a

b

c

d

Figure 8.8   (*Continued*)

successfully to the previous one. Once the desired endpoint has been reached, the dentures with all their additions look rather like a patchwork quilt (Fig. 8.9). The copy technique can then be used to convert the corrected but untidy old dentures into the replacements.

To copy or not to copy?

In concluding this section, it should be stressed that a copying technique is but one approach to treatment – albeit a most valuable one. In general terms, the older the patient, the stronger the reasons for using the technique. In fact, this method of treatment may prove to be the only way of realising success for a patient whose powers of adaptation have deteriorated markedly. However, the copy technique must not be regarded by either clinician or dental technician as a shortcut to denture construction where relatively little care is needed. In fact, unless the decision to use the method is based on a sound diagnosis, and the clinical and technical procedures are undertaken with the greatest care, the course of treatment is highly likely to fail.

If the copy technique is used with care, a comprehensive prescription for the design of

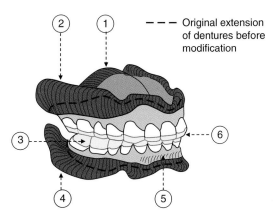

Figure 8.9 Diagram showing examples of diagnostic modifications which may be made to old dentures. (1) Addition to the posterior palatal border to extend the denture to the vibrating line. (2) Modifications to upper buccal flanges to: (a) correct underextension; (b) improve facial seal; (c) produce a form favourable for neuromuscular control of the denture. (3) Posterior occlusal additions to: (a) correct occlusal imbalance; (b) increase occlusal vertical dimension; (c) prevent postural protrusion of the mandible. (4) Extension of lower buccal flange to: (a) improve distribution of occlusal loads to the residual ridge; (b) increase resistance to posterior displacement by contact with the retromolar pad. (5) Hollowing the labial flange to reduce displacement by the mentalis muscle. (6) Additions to the incisal edges to: (a) improve appearance; (b) facilitate speech; (c) allow incision.

Figure 8.8 (a) This woman had worn the same set of dentures for many years. She requested replacements which would fit more satisfactorily and which would provide more support for her face. (b) A radiograph confirmed the extensive resorption of the lower ridge. Additionally, the upper ridge was flabby. The retained lower third molar was an incidental finding and did not require surgical extraction as it was causing no symptoms. The prosthetic risk was that if a significant increase in the occlusal vertical dimension was introduced and the dental arches expanded to support the facial muscles the resulting increase in the bulk of the new dentures would make them unstable. As part of the assessment, wax was added to the old dentures to mimic the changes that might be made. The patient was asked her opinion on the new appearance and whether she had noted any increase in looseness of the dentures. As she made no adverse comments it was concluded that the proposed changes were feasible. (c) Copy templates were made and wax was added to them as in Figure 2.1. This procedure ensured that changes to the denture shape were made in a controlled manner and that a detailed prescription was given to the dental technician. The trial denture stage was a routine matter. Wash impressions were taken in upper and lower copy templates before returning them to the laboratory for processing. (d) The finished copy dentures were stable and retentive and provided an improvement in appearance which was appreciated by the patient. The copy technique had provided a relatively easy solution to a potentially difficult clinical problem.

the replacement dentures is produced and the dental technician receives ample information for the decisions made at the treatment planning stage to be carried out reliably.

Scott et al. (2006) compared conventional and copy techniques for providing replacement of complete upper and lower dentures. They reported that the copy technique resulted in patients reporting greater improvement in functional satisfaction of lower dentures made with the copy technique as against the conventional approach. Clark et al. (2004) warned that the chances of losing control of the occlusion were potentially high if both upper and lower dentures were being copied.

A final point is worth making. As the lower denture is usually more dependent on muscular control than the upper, there are often stronger indications for copying it so that such features as the polished surface and the tongue space can be faithfully carried through to the replacement. In addition, it will be appreciated that the presence of the lower copy will help the clinician to shape the upper record rim to produce an appropriate arch shape for the upper denture which is being constructed in the conventional manner at the same time.

Denture copying – practical procedures

Various methods of constructing copy dentures have been described in the literature (Duthie et al. 1978; Davenport & Heath 1983; Murray & Wolland 1986); each one requires the existing denture to be invested in an elastic material which is adequately supported in some sort of container. Two different methods will be described. In both, the objective is to produce a copy template of existing dentures with wax teeth and acrylic resin bases using materials which are readily available in the dental surgery. Thus the first stage becomes a chair side procedure and not one which relies on laboratory facilities.

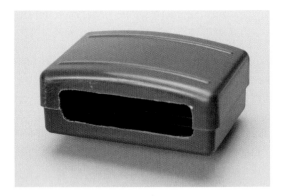

Figure 8.10 Soapbox suitable as a container for the copy technique.

Preparation of the copy template

Method 1

The patient's denture is invested in alginate, which is supported in a container such as a soapbox. A window is cut into its side to provide an exit for sprues as shown in Fig. 8.10. The technique is summarised in Fig. 8.11. A variation of this method utilises a specially designed aluminium flask (Fig. 8.12) (Murray & Wolland 1986).

After polymerisation, the copy is removed from the mould and the sprues are cut off. The resulting copy template has a rigid acrylic base together with wax teeth, which make the job of the dental technician very much easier when setting up teeth on the trial dentures. It has been shown that accurate copies can be constructed with this technique, the maximum dimensional change being –2.12% (Heath & Basker 1978).

Method 2

This technique uses stock impression trays and silicone putty (Duthie et al. 1978). First, the occlusal and polished surfaces of the denture are embedded in a mix of silicone putty held in an upper tray. The impression surface is then invested in a second mix of putty, which is supported on the reverse surface of another tray

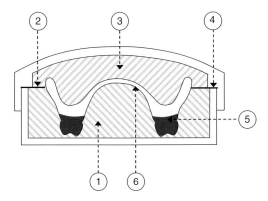

Figure 8.11 Diagrammatic summary of the copy denture technique. (1) First mix of alginate to obtain an impression of polished and occlusal surfaces. Adhesive is not applied to the walls of the container. (2) Alginate is trimmed at the level of the upper border of the box and just below the denture periphery. Petroleum jelly is smeared on the surface of the alginate to facilitate separation of the two halves of the mould. (3) Second mix of alginate to obtain a record of the impression surface. (4) Soap box closed on to stops. Denture removed when alginate set. Sprue channels cut with wax knife into heels of polished surface impression. (5) Wax poured to above level of gingival margin. Mould closed and held together with rubber band. (6) Base poured in a fluid mix of cold-curing acrylic resin.

(Fig. 8.13). Once the putty has set, the two impressions are separated and the denture is removed. Sprue holes are cut into the heels of the impression, and the copy template is produced as described above.

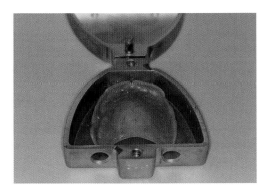

Figure 8.12 Specially designed aluminium flask for the copy technique (Murray & Wolland 1986).

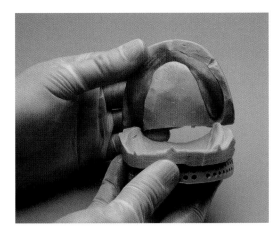

Figure 8.13 Silicone putty mould used for copy method 2 (Duthie et al. 1978) (see text for details).

Stages in copy denture production

The various clinical and technical stages are summarised in Table 8.2. It may be possible to undertake more than one clinical stage at the same appointment. It can be seen from Table 8.2 that the various stages are similar to those followed when constructing dentures in the conventional manner. Of course, if the occlusal surface is not to be altered and the copy templates can be interdigitated accurately, stage 4 (recording the occlusion) would not be required.

Communication with the dental technician

There is evidence to suggest that unless both the clinician and the dental technician have a clear understanding of the rationale behind the copy technique, and why the technique is being used for a particular patient, it is likely that the prescription will not be followed accurately by the dental laboratory (Kippax et al. 1998). The same study showed that not only can the quality of the copies be poor, but also that the replacement teeth are not positioned as requested.

Table 8.2   Summary of clinical and technical stages of the copy denture technique.

Stage	Clinical	Technical	Remarks
1	Diagnosis and treatment plan		List those aspects of the existing dentures that will be modified and those aspects that will be copied
2	Invest dentures to be copied		
3		Construct copy templates	Wax teeth on rigid bases
4	Record occlusion		If the impression surface deficiency is such that the copy templates are unstable in the mouth, border modifications and impressions in low viscosity silicone should be taken before recording the occlusion (Fig. 8.14)
5		Pour casts. Articulate copy templates. Make trial dentures.	It is important to remove only one or two wax teeth at a time so that the remainder act as effective guides to accurate positioning of the new denture teeth
6	Assess trial dentures. Take impression in low viscosity silicone if not done in stage 4.		If impressions were taken at Stage 4, sufficient silicone material will still be attached to the bases to ensure acceptable stability of the trial dentures (Fig. 8.15)
7		Finish dentures	It will be necessary to remove the acrylic palate of the upper trial denture and to lay down a wax palate of correct thickness before investing the denture. The remaining cold-curing resin and impression material are discarded and the flask is packed with heat-curing resin.
8	Fit dentures		
9	Recall		

It can hardly be stressed enough that the high quality of technical work needed to take a copy denture through to a successful completion is dependent upon a mutual appreciation of the benefits of the technique, an accurate prescription and a precise attention to detail of the technical work.

Quality control and enhancement

To audit the reaction of patients to replacement dentures the following questions might be asked of the patient at the appropriate stage of treatment:

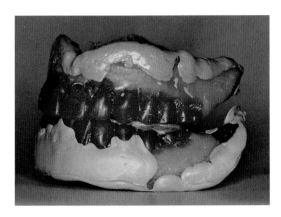

Figure 8.14 Wash impressions taken in the copy dentures at the stage of recording the occlusion.

- Do you prefer the new dentures to the old ones?
- How different do the new dentures feel? What particular difference do you notice?
- How similar to the old dentures do the new copy dentures feel?
- How long did it take you to get used to the new dentures?

The following questions might be asked of the dental technician:

- With regard to copy dentures, were you given sufficient information to allow you to

position the new artificial teeth in the correct position?
- With regard to copy dentures, were you given a clear indication of the objectives of treatment?

From a collection of patients' record cards the following points might be reviewed:

- Did the treatment plans clarify those aspects of the design of the existing dentures that required alteration and those aspects which should remain unchanged in the replacement dentures?
- Were the objectives of the treatment plans fulfilled?

References and additional reading

Clark, R.F.F., Radford, D.R. & Fenlon, M.R. (2004) The future of teaching complete denture construction to undergraduates in the UK: is a replacement denture technique the answer? *British Dental Journal*, 196, 571–5.

Davenport, J.C. & Heath, J.R. (1983) The copy denture technique – variables relevant to general dental practice. *British Dental Journal*, 155, 162–3.

Duthie, N. & Yemm, R. (1985) An alternative method for recording the occlusion of the edentulous patient during the construction of replacement dentures. *Journal of Oral Rehabilitation*, 12, 161–71.

Duthie, N., Lyon, F.F., Sturrock, K.C. & Yemm, R. (1978) A copying technique for replacement of complete dentures. *British Dental Journal*, 144, 248–52.

Heath, J.R. & Basker, R.M. (1978) The dimensional variability of duplicate dentures produced in an alginate investment. *British Dental Journal*, 144, 111–14.

Heath, J.R. & Davenport, J.C. (1982) A modification of the copy denture technique. *British Dental Journal*, 153, 300–2.

Heath, J.R. & Johnson, A. (1981) The versatility of the copy denture technique. *British Dental Journal*, 150, 189–93.

Kippax, A., Watson, C.J., Basker, R.M. &. Pentland, J.E. (1998) How well are complete dentures copied? *British Dental Journal*, 185, 129–33.

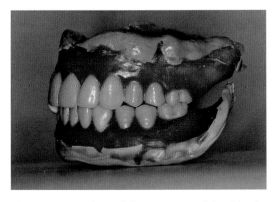

Figure 8.15 The trial dentures are stabilised by the wash impressions taken at the stage of recording the occlusion.

Murray, I.D & Wolland, A.W. (1986) New dentures for old. *Dental Practice*, 24, 1–6.

Osborne, J. (1960) The full lower denture. *British Dental Journal*, 109, 481–97.

Scher, E.A. & Ritchie, G.M. (1978) Prosthodontic treatment of the elderly by incremental modifications to old dentures. *Quintessence International*, 8, 47–53.

Scott, B.J.J., Forgie, A.H. & Davies, D.M. (2006) A study to compare the oral health impact profile and satisfaction before and after having replacement complete dentures constructed by either the copy or the conventional technique. *Gerodontology*, 23, 79-86.

Walker, A. & Cooper, I. (eds) (2000) *Adult Dental Health Survey*. Oral Health in the United Kingdom 1998. The Stationery Office, London.

Watt, D.M. & Lindsay, K.N. (1972) Occlusal pivot appliances. *British Dental Journal*, 132, 110–12.

Preparation of the Mouth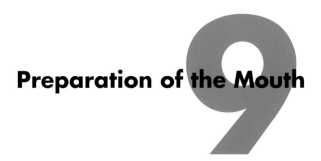

Preparation of the mouth is often necessary before dentures are made and may involve the elimination of pathology within the denture-bearing tissues or the creation of a more favourable anatomical environment.

The various conditions requiring treatment may be considered in two sections, those involving the oral mucosa and those involving bone.

(1) *Conditions involving the oral mucosa*
- Denture stomatitis
- Inflammatory papillary hyperplasia of the palate
- Angular stomatitis (angular cheilitis)
- Shallow sulci
- Denture-induced hyperplasia
- Prominent frena

(2) *Conditions involving the bone*
- Pathology within the bone
- Sharp and irregular bone
- Undercut ridges
- Prominent maxillary tuberosities
- Tori

Conditions involving the oral mucosa

Denture stomatitis

Clinical appearance

The clinical appearance of denture stomatitis varies from a patchy to a diffuse inflammation of the mucosa covered by a denture (Fig. 9.1). Newton (1962) classified denture stomatitis into three types on the basis of its clinical appearance:

- Type I: Pinpoint hyperaemia
- Type II: Diffuse inflammation
- Type III: Granular (palatal inflammatory papillary hyperplasia (p. 118)

The condition typically involves the mucosa of the maxillary denture-bearing area and does not extend beyond the borders of the denture. It may occur alone but is sometimes seen with two associated conditions, inflammatory palatal papillary hyperplasia and angular stomatitis.

Prosthetic Treatment of the Edentulous Patient, Fifth Edition, © R.M. Basker, J.C. Davenport and J.M. Thomason
Published 2011 by Blackwell Publishing Ltd.

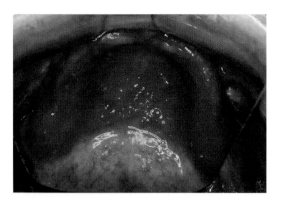

Figure 9.1   Denture stomatitis. The characteristically sharp delineation of the diffuse palatal inflammation by the borders of the denture is seen at the junction of the hard and soft palate, where the line separating the inflamed from normal tissue corresponds to the posterior border of the denture.

Nomenclature

In spite of the lesion's rather angry appearance the patient rarely complains of soreness, therefore the term 'denture sore mouth', which has been used in the past to describe this condition, is inappropriate. Other terms currently used in the literature to describe the condition are:

- Denture-related stomatitis.
- Denture-induced stomatitis – however, it has been argued that as the denture is rarely the primary aetiological agent this term is seldom appropriate.
- Stomatitis prothetica.
- Chronic atrophic candidiasis – for this and the following term to be appropriate it is necessary that a microbiological investigation should have confirmed the presence of candida.
- *Candida*-related stomatitis

Prevalence

Denture stomatitis is a common condition, having been reported in 10–60% of patients wearing complete dentures. However, in the general complete denture-wearing population the prevalence of the condition is likely to be closer to the lower limit of this range than to the upper (Radford et al. 1999).

Predisposing factors

Age
Denture stomatitis has been found to be more common in the elderly, particularly if hyposalivation is present (Figueiral et al. 2007; Campisi et al. 2008).

Gender
Denture stomatitis occurs more frequently in females than in males, the ratio being approximately 4:1 (Davenport 1970; Pires et al. 2002). Although the cause of this predisposition to denture stomatitis in females is not known, possible explanations include endocrine imbalance, iron deficiency anaemia, vaginal carriage of candida, a higher oral carrier rate of candida and a greater inclination than males to wear dentures at night.

Night wearing of dentures
It appears that behavioural factors, such as wearing the dentures at night and poor denture hygiene, are of major importance in the aetiology of denture stomatitis (Jeganathan et al. 1997; Sakki et al. 1997; Saulman et al. 2006). Wearing the dentures at night can aggravate the effect of both denture plaque and denture trauma by increasing the exposure of the palatal mucosa to both aetiological factors.

Poor denture hygiene
Poor denture hygiene allows the build-up of denture plaque containing candida and other microorganisms. A strong association between poor denture hygiene and denture stomatitis has been identified (Khasawneh & Al-Wahadni 2002; Kulak-Ozkan et al. 2002).

High-carbohydrate diet
Dentures with a reduced masticatory efficiency may encourage a patient to adopt a relatively

easily managed high-carbohydrate diet, which favours the growth of candida and increases the adhesion of the microorganism to the denture surface. An increase in the amount and frequency of intake of relatively inexpensive carbohydrates may also be encouraged by the patient's economic circumstances.

Systemic factors

Systemic conditions which can predispose to denture stomatitis include immunological deficiencies (Golecka et al. 2006), hormonal imbalance, e.g. diabetes, and nutritional deficiencies, e.g. vitamin B complex, vitamin C and iron.

Aetiology

Many different local and systemic factors have been incriminated in the aetiology of denture stomatitis, which is now widely accepted to be multifactorial in origin. The relative importance of microorganisms, in particular *Candida albicans*, and trauma from the dentures is still debated. However, the bulk of the relevant literature supports the view that the presence of candida organisms within plaque on the impression surface of the denture is the key local factor.

In 1885, G.V. Black, commenting on the condition we now know as denture stomatitis, stated that, 'Fungi grow readily under any plate irrespective of the material of what it is made. They produce acids which if the mouth and palate are not properly cleaned will cause sore mouth'. He sampled microorganisms from under the dentures of patients with this condition and expressed surprise at their abundance. He concluded that 'plates are not cleaned often enough and that cleanliness is the chief preventive measure'. Thus, well over 100 years ago Black summarised the modern view of both the aetiology and management of denture stomatitis.

In a study of 3450 patients wearing at least one removable denture the main risk factors associated with denture stomatitis were found to be wearing the dentures continuously, low levels of vitamin A and smoking (Shulman et al. 2005). The authors recommended improved denture cleaning and removing the dentures at night.

Candida albicans

The evidence suggests that the most important local causative factor of denture stomatitis is the presence of microorganisms within plaque on the impression surface of the denture (Davenport 1970; Budtz-Jørgensen 1974; Olsen 1974; Khasawneh et al. 2002; Ramage et al. 2004). The plaque is present in significant quantities because of inadequate denture hygiene and its effects are maximised if the patient wears the dentures at night. The fungus, *Candida albicans* (Fig. 9.2), is the organism most commonly associated with denture stomatitis and which has received the most attention in the literature, although other candida species may also be present (Marcos-Arias et al. 2009). This fungus is dimorphic, occurring as both yeast-like blastospores and filamentous pseudohyphae. In denture stomatitis, large numbers of both forms are usually found in plaque on the impression surface of the denture. Relatively few candida organisms are found on the

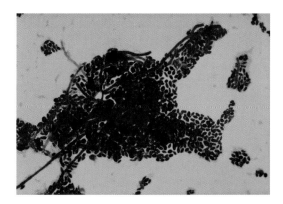

Figure 9.2 Mycelial and yeast forms of *Candida albicans* obtained from the impression surface of a denture.

mucosa and there is no evidence that candidal invasion of the mucosa occurs.

Bacteria

Although the evidence for a causal relationship between candida and denture stomatitis is strong, it has been suggested that a variety of bacteria may also play a part in the condition (Kulak et al. 1997).

Denture trauma

It has been proposed that trauma to the oral mucosa is a cause of denture stomatitis (Emami et al. 2008). Dentures can traumatise the mucosa either because of the presence of faults in the prostheses such as loss of fit or occlusal imbalance or because the patient exhibits parafunctional activity, such as bruxism, which overloads the tissues. It is sometimes argued that if trauma from the dentures was a major factor in the development of denture stomatitis then the condition would be more commonly seen under mandibular than maxillary dentures. This is because the area of mucosal support for the prosthesis is much less in the mandible than in the maxilla and therefore the load per unit area and potential degree of trauma is significantly greater in the mandible than in the maxilla. However, the widespread inflammation characteristic of denture stomatitis that is seen clinically is a feature of the maxillary, not the mandibular, denture-bearing mucosa.

Other factors

It should be remembered that palatal inflammation under dentures is a non-specific response to a variety of injurious agents. Therefore diffused inflammation of the denture-bearing mucosa may occasionally be seen, which is not the result of denture plaque or trauma. For example:

- *Raised residual monomer*. A faulty curing cycle when the dentures are processed can result in a residual monomer content high enough to produce mucosal inflammation (p. 116) (Austin & Basker 1980). This, unlike the classical denture stomatitis resulting from poor denture hygiene, is characteristically associated with discomfort from the inflamed mucosa.

- *Self-medication*. Palatal inflammation is sometimes caused by patients using topical agents in an inappropriate way. Certain mouthwashes, ointments, or other substances which are normally free of adverse effects in the mouth, can cause mucosal damage when applied beneath a denture. Examples of preparations that can behave in this way are chlorhexidine gel, salicylate ointments and even whisky – with which some more ingenious patients have been known to bathe their sore mucosa. The damage occurs because the exposure to the agents is increased by their being held against the mucosa for extended periods by the denture and because they are not diluted or washed away by the saliva. Also, a vicious cycle may be established in which the patient initially uses the preparation in a misguided attempt to relieve some discomfort; the preparation then causes further mucosal damage which increases the soreness and so the patient applies even more of the injurious agent.

Aetiological interactions

The possible interaction of the various predisposing and aetiological factors is complex and uncertain, but a possible scenario which is compatible with the bulk of the relevant literature is as follows (Fig. 9.3).

Toxins produced by the candida cells left on the denture surface by deficient hygiene measures, together with trauma from the denture initiate an inflammatory reaction. A resulting thinning of the epithelium results in increased permeability and escape of inflammatory exudates. The exudates, together with desquamated mucosal cells, form a favourable nutrient medium, which promotes the growth of

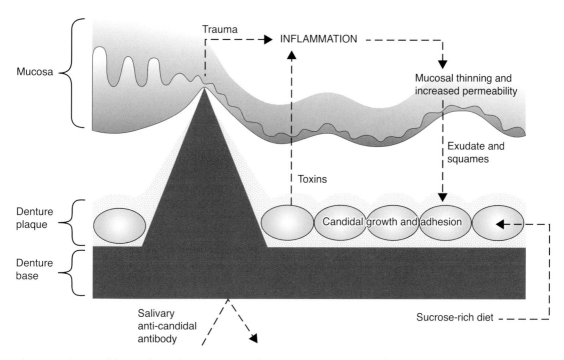

Figure 9.3   Possible aetiological interactions in denture stomatitis (see text for fuller explanation). (Reproduced with permission from Stephen Hancock. © 2000 *British Dental Journal*.)

Candida albicans. In addition, these exudates and the sucrose-rich diet which may result from the dietary selection sometimes associated with the wearing of dentures, may contribute to the condition by increasing the adhesiveness of the candidal cells, and thus encouraging the formation of denture plaque. As candidal proliferation occurs, the rate of production of potent toxins by the microorganisms increases. The passage of these toxins into the tissues is facilitated by the thinning and increased permeability of the mucosa. Aggravation of the inflammatory response occurs and so a vicious circle is set up. Anti-candidal antibody is secreted in parotid saliva but the denture base may restrict access of the antibody to the candida cells.

Diagnosis

The diagnosis of denture stomatitis is essentially a clinical one made on the basis of the ap-

pearance of the palatal mucosa. Identification of the aetiological factors responsible for a particular case may be achieved by noting the following.

Night-wearing of dentures

It should be noted routinely from the history whether or not the dentures are worn both day and night.

Denture hygiene

Details of the patient's denture cleaning regime should be obtained, including the method and frequency of cleaning together with the type of immersion cleanser used. The amount of plaque on the impression surface of the denture should be recorded. This assessment of the quantity and distribution of denture plaque is made easier by applying a disclosing solution to the denture (Fig. 14.10). In those cases where only a little plaque is seen, it should be realised that a patient will sometimes have made an effort to clean the dentures in readiness for the visit to the dentist, which is atypical of their normal denture hygiene regimen.

Denture trauma

The degree of denture trauma should be assessed. This can be estimated from the relative functional adequacy of the dentures in terms of occlusion and fit, and from evidence of the presence or absence of parafunctional activity.

Other local factors

- *Raised residual monomer*. If palatal inflammation and discomfort occur shortly after a new denture has been fitted, or an existing denture repaired or relined, then a raised residual monomer content might be suspected.
- *Self-medication*. Questioning the patient about any current oral medication such as mouthwashes or ointments might indicate if the condition is iatrogenic, resulting from mucosal irritation by these preparations.
- *Diet*. A dietary assessment can be carried out if it is suspected that a high carbohydrate diet is contributing to the condition.

Systemic factors

The medical history may provide clues that systemic factors are playing a part. If this is the case, or if the condition subsequently fails to respond to local treatment, appropriate investigations should be arranged.

It is important to obtain details of drug therapy in case a particular medication is causing conditions such as a dry mouth (see Chapter 16).

Treatment

Although denture stomatitis is symptomless and the patient is often unaware of its presence, it should be treated before new dentures are constructed because of the following:

- Swelling of the oral mucosa will have occurred as a result of the inflammation. Producing a new denture from an impression of the mucosa in this condition will compromise the fit of the prosthesis, especially if the new well-fitting denture brings about some resolution of the swelling.
- The mouth may be the source of candida organisms and other microorganisms responsible for infection in other parts of the body, such as nailbeds, the pharynx and the larynx (Nikawa et al. 1998). In debilitated patients, systemic spread of candida from the mouth can occur with fatal consequences.

    There is increasing evidence that the oral cavity, particularly in denture wearers, can be a reservoir for methicillin-resistant *Staphylococcus aureus* (MRSA) which clearly has serious implications for both patients and their carers (Lee et al. 2009). Commonly employed denture-cleaning solutions have been shown to be effective against MRSA in vitro (Maeda et al. 2007).

As behavioural factors are so important in the aetiology of denture stomatitis, appropriate modification of the patient's behaviour is essential for long-term success. Therefore the primary objectives of local treatment of denture stomatitis (Lombardi & Budtz-Jørgensen 1993) are to improve denture hygiene and discourage the patient from wearing the dentures at night.

In addition, in those cases where denture faults are identified and which could be traumatising the denture-bearing tissues, correction of the faults should be undertaken.

Improve denture hygiene

- *Motivating, instructing and monitoring the patient*. It is vital that the clinician convinces the patient of the need for meticulous cleaning of the dentures. The methods for carrying it out should be discussed using appropriate language, clearly demonstrated, subsequently monitored and reinforced if necessary. Once a high level of denture hygiene has been achieved it is essential that it is maintained otherwise recurrence of the denture stomatitis is likely (Cross et al. 2004).

- *Laboratory cleaning of the dentures.* Where deposits are heavy and possibly partly calcified, and where the surface polish of the denture has deteriorated, it is recommended that laboratory cleaning and polishing of the denture is carried out before home care by the patient is instituted.
- *Disinfection of the dentures.* The dentures should be regularly immersed by the patient in a suitable disinfectant. Two solutions have been shown to be effective in controlling denture plaque: alkaline hypochlorite and aqueous chlorhexidine gluconate (Hutchins & Parker 1973; Altman et al. 1979; Budtz-Jørgensen 1979; Abelson 1985; Webb et al. 1998c; Barnabe et al. 2004). The former solution has been shown to be effective in removing denture plaque while the latter inhibits its formation. Overnight immersion is necessary if either a hypochlorite solution containing 0.08% available chlorine or 0.1% aqueous chlorhexidine gluconate is used. When it is impossible to persuade a patient to leave the denture out at night, immersion in a hypochlorite solution containing 0.16% available chlorine for 20 minutes daily or in 2% aqueous chlorhexidine gluconate for approximately 5 minutes daily are alternatives. Before immersion, the denture should be brushed thoroughly to remove most of the plaque and then, if chlorhexidine is to be used, rinsed carefully to remove any soap which would otherwise inactivate the chlorhexidine. Patches of brown staining usually appear on a denture that has been immersed in chlorhexidine solution. As a rule, the staining is not severe and can be removed by subsequent immersion in a hypochlorite cleaner. The presence of a metal denture base complicates matters because hypochlorite can cause corrosion of the base. However, the recommended short immersion period can be used with safety.

Disinfection of dentures by short exposure to microwave irradiation has also been shown to be effective (Baysan et al. 1998; Webb et al. 1998c; Dixon et al. 1999; Webb et al. 2005). However the practicality of this approach remains uncertain: the procedure kills the organisms but does not remove the plaque, and there is the possibility that overexposure to the irradiation could have adverse effects on the denture materials.

Ultrasonic cleaning devices have been shown to be potentially useful for cleaning dentures (Hashiguchi et al. 2009; Arita et al. 2005).

Correction of denture faults

- *Occlusal faults.* An unbalanced occlusion should be corrected by occlusal adjustment or by the addition of cold-curing acrylic resin to the occlusal surfaces of the dentures (p. 95).
- *Impression surface faults.* Lack of fit in a denture can be corrected by applying a short-term soft lining material to the impression surface (p. 234). However, caution should be exercised in selecting this option as the presence of a temporary lining will make it much more difficult for the patient to maintain the all-important high level of denture hygiene. It has been reported that certain of these lining materials exhibit antifungal activity in vitro, but it is unlikely that this activity is significant in vivo.

Leaving the dentures out at night

All patients should be strongly advised to leave their dentures out as much as possible, ideally at night, although some will feel unable to conform to this timing for a variety of reasons. In some instances, successful treatment will not be possible unless the patient follows this advice. This regimen reduces the period the mucosa is in contact with denture plaque, reduces the intra-oral population of candida and other organisms (Williamson 1972), provides an opportunity for prolonged immersion of the dentures in a disinfectant and, for those cases where denture trauma is a contributory factor, reduces the period over which mucosal damage can occur.

Antifungal preparations

Antifungal agents such as nystatin, amphotericin B, fluconazole, itraconazole and miconazole have been advocated for the treatment of denture stomatitis and they have been shown to be effective in the short term. They are used topically as lozenges, mouthwashes or ointments applied to the denture and to the lesion. Where problems with patient compliance are anticipated, some of these agents can be applied to the denture by the clinician incorporating them into a tissue conditioner or a lacquer (Budtz-Jørgensen & Carlino 1994; Konsberg & Axell 1994; Parvinen et al. 1994; Truhlar et al. 1994; Dias et al. 1997; Chow et al. 1999; Geerts et al. 2008). However, these preparations do nothing to modify the oral conditions and patient behaviour responsible for the inflammation in the long term. Clinical studies have shown that a rapid relapse usually follows the cessation of such antifungal therapy if this is the sole treatment employed. There is no difference at 1 year following start of treatment between patients treated with antifungal antibiotics in combination with denture hygiene instruction and correction compared with those treated by denture measures alone (Bergendal 1982; Bissell et al. 1993; Webb et al. 1998c). The recurrence of denture stomatitis in patients who maintain a high level of denture cleanliness is low (Cross et al. 2004). The prescription of antifungal agents in the treatment of denture stomatitis is therefore not supported by the available evidence.

Systemic therapy

An appropriate combination of the simple therapeutic measures described above will usually effect a cure within 2–3 weeks if there are no underlying systemic factors. Therefore, if a cure is not achieved in this time, and if persistent local factors cannot be identified, systemic causes

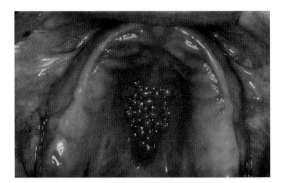

Figure 9.4 Inflammatory papillary hyperplasia of the palate.

should be suspected and the patient referred to a medical practitioner for further investigation.

Inflammatory papillary hyperplasia of the palate

This condition, alternatively known as hyperplastic or granular denture stomatitis, involves the palatal mucosa and appears as multiple elevations, usually bright red in colour. It is 'raspberry-like' in appearance and may involve the whole or part of the hard palate (Fig. 9.4). At one time, it was suggested that this condition might be premalignant; but malignant transformation has not been reported, nor is it associated with the cytological signs of dysplasia (Kaplan et al. 1998).

Aetiology

The condition is closely related to the simple atrophic form of denture stomatitis and shares the same aetiology (Kaplan et al. 1998). In addition, the presence of a relief chamber in an upper denture may predispose to this hyperplastic change (Ettinger 1975).

Treatment

Treatment may be considered to have two phases, as described in the following.

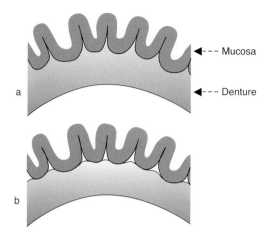

a — — — Mucosa

— — — Denture

b

Figure 9.5   The impression surface of the denture in palatal inflammatory papillary hyperplasia: (a) sharp spicules of acrylic penetrate the fissures between the hyperplastic papillae if the impression surface is not modified after processing; (b) the spicules of acrylic may be lightly stoned before fitting the denture to reduce the amount of trauma.

Elimination of the mucosal inflammation

Treatment of the inflammatory component of this condition is the same as that described for denture stomatitis. Antifungal agents have been reported to reduce the inflammatory component but the hyperplasia remains (Salonen et al. 1996).

Prosthetic or surgical management of the hyperplasia

When the inflammation has been successfully treated the hyperplastic nodules will still remain, although they will now be pale in colour and reduced in size. A decision then has to be made whether to construct a denture on this foundation or to remove the nodules surgically beforehand. The approach adopted in a particular case will depend on factors such as the size of the nodules, and the patient's age and medical history.

If an acrylic denture is constructed without prior surgical removal of the nodules, sharp spicules of acrylic resin will penetrate the fissures of the lesion (Fig. 9.5a). As all dentures move to a certain extent during function, these spicules have an abrasive effect on the mucosa and inflammation will recur. To prevent this happening, the spicules should be lightly polished to reduce their sharpness before fitting the denture (Fig. 9.5b).

Angular stomatitis

Angular stomatitis, sometimes described as angular cheilitis, is an erythematous, often erosive, non-vesicular skin lesion radiating from the angles of the mouth. It is usually bilateral, frequently painful and is rarely seen except in denture wearers (Fig. 9.6). It has been found to occur in 28% of long-term hospitalised elderly denture-wearers. It is more common in females. If left untreated, it can result in unsightly scarring. The majority of patients with angular stomatitis also have an associated denture stomatitis.

Aetiology

Common local and systemic factors which may contribute to the development of angular stomatitis are as follows.

Local
- Infection
- Inadequate lip support
- Maceration of the skin

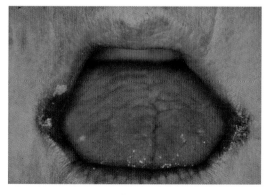

Figure 9.6   Angular stomatitis – clinical appearance before treatment.

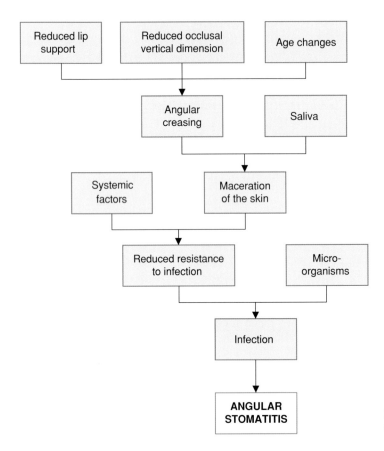

Figure 9.7 The multifactorial aetiology of angular stomatitis.

Systemic
- Iron deficiency
- Vitamin B and C deficiency
- Insulin-dependent diabetes mellitus

The aetiological factors listed above are closely interrelated as indicated in Fig. 9.7. Maceration results from the continuous bathing by saliva of the skin at the corners of the mouth, which lowers the resistance of the skin to infection. Maceration is encouraged by the presence of skin creases which draw saliva from the mouth by capillary action and which may be due to inadequate lip support being provided by the upper denture or to the presence of an excessive freeway space. However, an increased freeway space should never be assumed to be present simply on the evidence of angular stomatitis.

Microorganisms may be carried in the saliva to the lips from intra-oral sites, of which the main ones are the denture and the dorsum of the tongue. The significance of microbial plaque on the dentures is demonstrated by the observation that if patients with angular stomatitis do not wear their dentures, a complete cure usually results in 2 weeks even though all dental support to the lips has been lost. *Candida albicans* is frequently isolated from the lesion of angular stomatitis where denture stomatitis is also present. However, if angular stomatitis occurs alone, *Staphylococcus aureus* is recovered from the lesion twice as often as candida (McFarlane & Helnarska 1976) In such cases, the nose may be the source of secondary infection with carriage on the fingers being the method of transmission.

Treatment

The treatment of angular stomatitis in the first instance involves the elimination of local infection and the reduction of the intra-oral population of micro-organisms.

Denture hygiene

Denture hygiene instruction and immersion of the dentures in a hypochlorite denture cleaner, as described for denture stomatitis, should be instituted. In many cases, such simple measures will effect a cure in about 2 weeks.

Antimicrobial agents

Improved denture hygiene may be supplemented where necessary by prescribing one of the broad-spectrum antimicrobial agents, such as miconazole oral gel or a tetracycline/nystatin ointment, which are active against both fungi and bacteria. However, it is not advisable to prescribe one of the many compound skin preparations which contain steroids, as topical steroids have been shown to be the commonest cause of perioral dermatitis and may therefore aggravate the condition.

If specific antimicrobial therapy is to be employed, a swab from the angles of the lips should be cultured to allow identification of the responsible organisms. If the cultures are positive for candidal organisms, amphotericin B lozenges (10 mg) or nystatin pastilles (100 000 units) may be sucked four times a day. These preparations are of value in the treatment of angular stomatitis because candidal organisms not only grow in large numbers on the denture but also proliferate on the dorsum of the tongue. Both reservoirs could be contributing to the high salivary count predisposing to the angular stomatitis.

If swabs from the lesion indicate that a bacterial infection is present, benefit may be gained from the topical application of a tetracycline ointment or miconazole gel (an antifungal with some antibacterial properties). Treatment should be continued for 2–4 weeks.

Denture modifications

When it appears that the skin folds are due to a reduced occlusal vertical dimension or inadequate lip support, the existing dentures can be modified to test the diagnosis. This can be done by temporarily correcting the suspect denture surface by the addition of wax to see whether a subsequent permanent correction would eliminate or reduce the folds. If the temporary wax modification does result in an improvement, new dentures should be made accordingly. As an interim measure, it is sometimes possible to correct the existing dentures in the short term by the addition of cold-curing acrylic resin at the chair side (p. 95). If the occlusal vertical dimension of the old dentures is reduced it can be corrected by adding tooth-coloured resin to the occlusal surfaces of the posterior teeth.

However, if the temporary modifications have little, or no effect on the folds, it must be accepted that they are the result of an irreversible tissue change, such as loss of tissue tone associated with ageing. The persistence of the folds makes treatment more difficult and recurrence of the condition more likely.

Failure to respond to local measures suggests that systemic factors are playing a part and that further investigations are required.

A suggested interrelation between the local causative factors leading to denture stomatitis, angular stomatitis and inflammatory papillary hyperplasia is shown in Fig. 9.8.

Shallow sulci

The problems characteristically created by a shallow sulcus are twofold:

* Denture instability
* Unfavourable load distribution – a problem occurring primarily in the lower jaw

Treatment

Prosthetic treatment

The main approach to treatment is prosthetic – to go over the dentures again with a fine

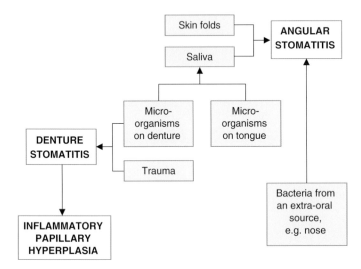

Figure 9.8 A suggested relationship between the local causative factors leading to denture stomatitis, angular stomatitis and inflammatory palatal hyperplasia.

toothcomb and to undertake any corrections that offer the possibility of improving stability or obtaining more tissue coverage. Where overloading has resulted in persistent discomfort a long-term soft lining may be provided (p. 238).

Surgical treatment

If prosthetic measures fail, then surgery to improve the quality of the denture-bearing tissues might be of benefit. The most obvious interventions currently undertaken are implants to support the prostheses. Other forms of pre-prosthetic surgery have largely fallen out of favour because the advanced alveolar resorption which commonly creates the need also limits what can be achieved by surgical intervention.

Soft tissue surgery is now largely confined to removal of denture hyperplasia and, less frequently, frenectomy to reduce prominent frena.

Denture-induced hyperplasia

Denture-induced hyperplasia takes the form of single or multiple flaps of fibrous tissue related to the border of a denture (Fig. 9.9). It is found in up to 10% of denture wearers (Axell 1976; Budtz-Jørgensen 1981).

Aetiology

The primary cause of this condition is overextension of the denture border causing chronic irritation of the sulcus tissues. The lesion characteristically develops slowly as a result of the gradual resorption of alveolar bone causing the denture to sink so that its borders dig into the mucosa. The chronic nature of the process means that discomfort is often not a prominent feature and therefore the patient continues wearing the offending denture for far too long. Hyperplastic lesions of considerable size

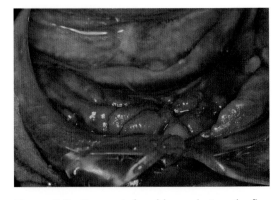

Figure 9.9 Denture-induced hyperplasia – the flap of fibrous tissue is situated in the lower labial sulcus.

can develop before the patient becomes aware of the need for treatment.

This situation contrasts with tissue damage produced by overextension present when a denture is first fitted. Here mucosal injury occurs rapidly, usually within a day or two, and presents commonly in the form of frank ulceration with associated pain. Because of the discomfort, the patient seeks treatment to alleviate the problem before hyperplasia has had time to develop.

Treatment

Treatment should be undertaken in the following sequence:

(i) *Eliminate denture trauma*. The hyperplastic tissue diminishes in size if the denture is not worn for a period of time or if the flange is cut away from the affected area. Other denture adjustments to reduce the level of trauma may be indicated, such as applying a short-term soft lining material to improve the fit and stability of the denture, or correcting occlusal imbalance.

(ii) *Review at 2 weeks*. In some cases, the degree of resolution resulting from the elimination of denture trauma is sufficient to allow satisfactory dentures to be made without the necessity for surgical intervention.

(iii) *Surgical excision if required*. If the size of the lesion remaining after correction of the denture is still too large to allow adequate extension of the denture, surgical removal is indicated. It must be remembered that the swelling of an oral malignancy in the sulcus could masquerade as a denture-induced hyperplasia and therefore all excised hyperplastic tissue should routinely be sent for histological examination.

Prominent frena

These are bands of fibrous tissue whose attachments are close to the crest of the alveolar ridge.

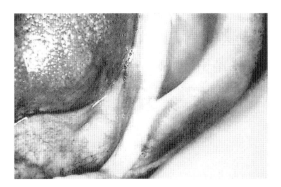

Figure 9.10 A prominent frenum attached to the crest of the ridge in the lower left premolar region.

Prominent frena may be found in both jaws labially and buccally in the premolar regions (Fig. 9.10). In order to accommodate this fibrous tissue, it is necessary to make a deep notch in the denture flange. The stress concentrations which are set up at the apex of the notch predispose to fracture of the denture base. In addition, there may be difficulty in achieving an efficient border seal.

Surgical excision of a prominent frenum may be necessary in extreme cases.

Conditions involving the bone

Pathology within the bone

Pathology within the bone should be suspected if one or more of the following are present:

- A sinus
- A swelling
- Irregularity of the shape of the ridge

Radiographs should not usually be taken of edentulous patients in the absence of signs or symptoms. However, the existence of clinical evidence, such as that listed above, justifies the taking of full-mouth radiographs to confirm or allay the suspicion that there is pathology within the bone. For this purpose, panoramic radiography has the advantage of a relatively low-radiation dosage to the patient compared with a full set of intra-oral films.

Treatment

Radiographic surveys have revealed the presence of such items as unerupted teeth, retained roots and dental cysts in 30–40% of edentulous patients. However, this finding should be qualified with the fact that the significant diagnostic yield in these surveys was low, as only a small percentage of these patients actually required surgical treatment. For example, if an unerupted tooth is deeply embedded in healthy bone with no associated pathology evident, future complications are unlikely. Surgical removal is not only unnecessary but positively contraindicated, as it would involve a considerable loss of alveolar bone. On the other hand, a tooth or tooth fragment lying close to the surface should usually be removed, because the pressure from a denture is likely to induce resorption of the overlying bone so that the tooth or fragment is exposed to the oral cavity (Fig. 9.11).

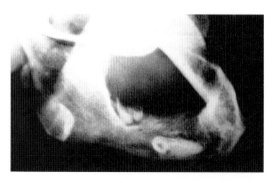

Figure 9.11 A radiograph showing a tooth deeply embedded in bone and a root on the surface. Before making complete dentures, removal of the root is essential: the tooth, however, should be left undisturbed.

Sharp and irregular bone

Bony spicules

Where sharp spicules of bone are present on the crest of a ridge which is covered by thin atrophic mucosa, pain may be produced by pressure from a denture. One reason for the presence of the sharp spicules is that insufficient care was taken when the teeth were extracted, such as the failure to compress the sockets adequately. Another possible reason is irregular bone resorption resulting from previous periodontal disease. The most common area for these spicules to occur is in the lower anterior region.

Treatment

The insertion of a short-term soft lining material into an existing denture may be sufficient to relieve the symptoms; if so, the material can be replaced by a long-term soft lining material. Occasionally, however, prosthetic treatment is unsuccessful and it becomes necessary to smooth the bone surgically. A conservative approach to bone removal is recommended, as in many cases excessive resorption has already occurred and little ridge remains.

Mylohyoid ridges and genial tubercles

Bony prominences associated with muscle attachments are another cause of discomfort beneath dentures. The prominences that occasionally cause trouble are:

* The mylohyoid ridges
* The genial tubercles

When the natural teeth are present these bony projections are well down in the depths of the sulci, but after the teeth are extracted and the associated alveolar bone is resorbed the projections come to lie within the denture-bearing area and become progressively more prominent with increasing age. Discomfort is caused by the denture exerting pressure on the thin layer of mucosa covering these sharp bony projections.

Treatment

(i) *Prosthetic treatment*. Prosthetic measures to resolve the problem should be attempted first. These include the following:

- A thorough re-appraisal of the dentures and correction of any design faults.
- Reducing masticatory load on the denture-bearing tissues by reducing the area of the occlusal table, for example, by reducing the width of the posterior teeth so that they penetrate the bolus of food more easily.
- Localised relief or adjustment of the impression surface of the denture in the region of the bony projections.
- Smoothing the impression surface of the denture so that movement of the denture is less traumatic to the mucosa.
- Placing a soft lining.

(ii) *Surgical treatment*. If prosthetic treatment of the condition is unsuccessful surgical removal of the bony projections may be required.

Undercut ridges

If ridges are grossly undercut (Fig. 9.12), complete seating of a denture may be impossible without extensive cutting back of the flange and the risk of reduced retention. To avoid this problem, surgical reduction of the undercut may be necessary. In some instances, the reduction can be carried out unilaterally so as to allow the denture to be rotated into position (see Fig. 4.11).

Prominent maxillary tuberosities

These may be composed of either fibrous tissue or bone and may in extreme cases be so large as to completely eliminate the inter-alveolar space. In such cases, it is impossible for fully

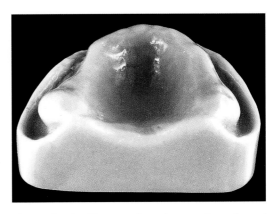

Figure 9.12 There is a large bony undercut buccal to the right tuberosity. A denture can be inserted only if the flange is extensively reduced or the undercut eliminated surgically.

extended denture bases to be accommodated and so retention and support of the dentures is likely to be compromised.

Treatment

Prosthetic treatment

(i) *Re-assessment of the occlusal vertical dimension*. This re-assessment should be carried out routinely, because, if the patient is able to accept a small increase in occlusal vertical dimension, sufficient inter-alveolar space might be created to allow full extension of the denture bases.

(ii) *Accept posterior under-extension of both upper and lower dentures*. This might well be successful for the upper denture because the ridges are normally well developed so the denture is well retained and stable as a result. However, the approach is much more likely to compromise the lower denture and therefore should not be adopted in this case.

(iii) *Use a thin denture base*. It may be possible to extend the dentures fully if a very thin metal base is used in the area of the reduced inter-alveolar space.

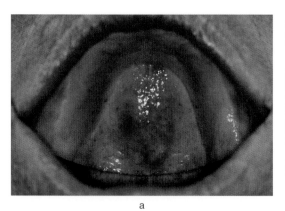
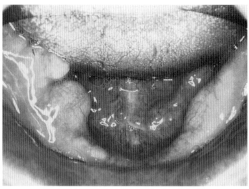

a   b

Figure 9.13   Prominent tori. (a) A palatine torus; (b) mandibular tori situated lingually in left and right premolar areas.

Tori

Tori are developmental bony prominences occurring in the maxilla and mandible that can adversely affect denture function and comfort.

Palatine torus

A palatine torus occurs in the midline of the hard palate and when covered by a thin, relatively incompressible layer of mucosa may lead to problems of discomfort, instability and midline fracture of the upper denture (Fig. 9.13a).

Treatment

If it is considered that a palatine torus is likely to give rise to the difficulties mentioned above a palatal relief is commonly placed in the denture. This approach is discussed further on p. 162. Only in exceptional cases would surgical removal of the torus be contemplated.

Mandibular tori

Mandibular tori usually occur bilaterally on the lingual aspect of the mandible, frequently in the premolar region; they are situated close to the mucosal reflection in the lingual sulcus (Fig. 9.13b). Their presence may make it difficult to provide comfortable dentures as the bor-

der of the denture readily traumatises the mucosa overlying the bony protuberances. In such instances, surgical removal of the tori may be necessary.

References and additional reading

Abelson, D.C. (1985) Denture plaque and denture cleansers. *Gerodontics*, 1, 202–6.

Altman, D.M., Yost, K.G. & Pitts, G. (1979) A spectrofluorometric protein assay of plaque on dentures and of denture cleaning efficiency. *Journal of Prosthetic Dentistry*, 42, 502–6.

Arendorf, T.M. & Walker, D.M. (1987) Denture stomatitis: a review. *Journal of Oral Rehabilitation*, 14, 217–27.

Arita, M., Nagayoshi, M., Fukuizumi, T., Okinaga, T., Masumi, S., Morikawa, M., Kakinoki, Y. & Nishihara T. (2005) Microbicicidal efficacy of ozonated water against *Candida albicans* adhering to acrylic denture pales. *Oral Microbiology and Immunology*, 20, 206–10.

Austin, A.T. & Basker, R.M. (1980) The level of residual monomer in acrylic denture base material. *British Dental Journal*, 149, 281–6.

Axell, T. (1976) A prevalence study of oral mucosal lesions in an adult Swedish population. *Odontologisk Revy*, 27 (Suppl. 36), 1–103.

Barnabe W., de Mendonca N., Pimenta F., Pegoraro L. & Scolaro J. (2004) Efficacy of sodium hypochlorite and coconut soap used as disinfecting agents in the reduction of denture stomatitis, *Streptococcus mutans* and *Candida albicans*. *Journal of Oral Rehabilitation*, 31, 453–9.

Baysan, A., Whiley, R. & Wright, P.S. (1998) Use of microwave energy to disinfect a long-term soft lining material contaminated with *Candida albicans* or *Staphylococcus aureus*. *Journal of Prosthetic Dentistry*, 79, 454–8.

Bergendal, T. (1982) Status and treatment of denture stomatitis patients – a 1 year follow-up study. *Scandinavian Journal of Dental Research*, 90, 227–38.

Bergendal, T., Hiemdahl, A. & Isacsson, G. (1980) Surgery in the treatment of denture-related inflammatory papillary hyperplasia of the palate. *International Journal of Oral Surgery*, 9, 312–19.

Bissell, V., Felix, D.H. & Wray, D. (1993) Comparative trial of fluconazole and amphotericin in the treatment of denture stomatitis. *Oral Surgery, Oral Medicine, Oral Pathology*, 76, 35–9.

Black, G.V. (1885) Sore mouth under plates. *Dental Items of Interest*, 7, 492.

Brook, I.M. & Lamb, D.J. (1987) Treatment of denture-induced hyperplasia. *Dental Update*, 14, 288–95.

Budtz-Jørgensen, E. & Carlino, P. (1994) A miconazole lacquer in the treatment of *Candida*-associated denture stomatitis. *Mycoses*, 37, 131–5.

Budtz-Jørgensen, E. (1974) The significance of *Candida albicans* in denture stomatitis. *Scandinavian Journal of Dental Research*, 82, 151–90.

Budtz-Jørgensen, E. (1979) Materials and methods for cleaning dentures. *Journal of Prosthetic Dentistry*, 42, 619–23.

Budtz-Jørgensen, E. (1981) Oral mucosal lesions associated with the wearing of removable dentures. *Journal of Oral Pathology*, 10, 65–80.

Campisi, G., Panzarella, V., Matranga, D., Calvino, F., Pizzo, G., Lo Muzio, L., & Porter, S. (2003) Risk factors of oral candidosis: a twofold approach of study by fuzzy logic and traditional statistic. *Archives of Oral Biology*, 53, 388–97.

Chow, C.K., Matear, D.W. & Lawrence, H.P. (1999) Efficacy of antifungal agents in tissue conditioners in treating candidiasis. *Gerodontology*, 16, 110–18.

Cross, L., Williams, D., Sweeney, C., Jackson, M., Lewis, M. & Bagg, J. (2004) Evaluation of the recurrence of denture stomatitis and Candida colonization in a small group of patients who received itraconazole. *Oral Surgery Oral Medicine Oral Pathology Oral Radiology and Endodontics*, 97, 351–8.

Davenport, J.C. (1970) The oral distribution of *Candida* in denture stomatitis. *British Dental Journal*, 129, 151–6.

Davenport, J.C. (1972) The denture surface. *British Dental Journal*, 133, 101–5.

Dias, A.P., Samaranayake, L.P. & Lee, M.T. (1997) Miconazole lacquer in the treatment of denture stomatitis: clinical and microbiological findings in Chinese patients. *Clinical Oral Investigations*, 1, 47–52.

Dixon, D.L., Breeding, L.C. & Faler, T.A. (1999) Microwave disinfection of denture base materials colonized with *Candida albicans*. *Journal of Prosthetic Dentistry*, 81, 207–14.

Emami, P., de Grandmont, P., Rompré, P., Barbeau, J., Pan, S. & Feine, J. (2008) Favouring trauma as an etiological factor in denture stomatitis. *Journal of Dental Research*, 87, 440–4.

Ettinger, R.L. (1975) The etiology of inflammatory papillary hyperplasia. *Journal of Prosthetic Dentistry*, 34, 254–259.

Figueiral, M.H., Azul, A., Pinto, E., Fonseca, P.A., Branco, F.M. & Scully, C. (2007) Denture-related stomatitis: identification of aetiological and predisposing factors – a large cohort. *Journal of Oral Rehabilitation*, 34, 448–55.

Geerts, G., Stuhlinger, M. & Basson, N. (2008) Effect of an antifungal denture liner on the saliva yeast count in patients with denture stomatitis – a pilot study. *Journal of Oral Rehabilitation*. 35: 664–9.

Golecka, M., Oldakowska-Jedynak, U., Mierzwinska-Nastalska, E. & Adamczyk-Sosinska, E. (2006) Candida-associated denture stomatitis in patients after immunosupression therapy. *Transplantation Proceedings*. 38: 155–6.

Hashiguchi, M., Nishi, Y., Kania, T., Ban, S. & Nagaoka, E. (2009) Bactericidal efficacy of glycine-type amphoteric surfactant as a denture cleaner and its influence on properties of denture base resins. *Dental Materials Journal*. 28: 307–14.

Hopkins, R. (1987) *A Colour Atlas of Pre-prosthetic Surgery*. Wolfe, London.

Hopkins, R., Stafford, G.D. & Gregory, M.C. (1980) Preprosthetic surgery of the edentulous mandible. *British Dental Journal*, 148, 183–8.

Hutchins, D.W. & Parker, W.A. (1973) A clinical evaluation of the ability of denture cleaning solutions to remove dental plaque from prosthetic devices. *New York State Dental Journal*, 39, 363–7.

Infanta-Cossio, P., Martinez-de-Fuentes, R., Torres-Carranza, E. & Gutierrez-Peerez, J.L. (2007) *British Journal of Oral and Maxillofacial Surgery*, 45, 658–60.

Jeganathan, S., Payne, J.A. & Thean, H.P. (1997) Denture stomatitis in an elderly edentulous Asian population. *Journal of Oral Rehabilitation*, 24, 468–72.

Kaplan, I., Vered, M., Moskona, D., Buchner, A. & Dayan, D. (1998) An immunohistochemical study of p53 and PCNA in inflammatory papillary hyperplasia of the palate: a dilemma of interpretation. *Oral Diseases*, 4, 194–9.

Keur, J.J., Campbell, J.P.S., McCarthy, J.F. & Ralph, W.J. (1987) Radiological findings in 1135 edentulous patients. *Journal of Oral Rehabilitation*, 14, 183–91.

Khasawneh, S. & Al-Wahadni, A. (2002) Control of denture plaque and mucosal inflammation in denture wearers. *Journal of the Irish Dental Association*, 48: 132–8.

Konsberg, R. & Axell, T. (1994) Treatment of *Candida*-infected denture stomatitis with a miconazole lacquer. *Oral Surgery, Oral Medicine, Oral Pathology*, 78, 306–11.

Kulak, Y., Arikan, A. & Kazazoglu, E. (1997) Existence of *Candida albicans* and micro-organisms in denture stomatitis patients. *Journal of Oral Rehabilitation*, 24, 788–90.

Kulak-Ozkan, Y., Kazazoglu, E. & Arikan, A. (2002) Oral hygiene habits, denture cleanliness, presence of yeasts and stomatitis in elderly people. *Journal of Oral Rehabilitation*. 29: 300–4.

Lamey, P.J. & Lewis, M.A.O. (1989) Oral medicine in practice: angular cheilitis. *British Dental Journal*, 187, 15–18.

Lee, D., Howlett, J., Pratten, J., Mordan, N., McDonald, A., Wilson, M. & Ready, D. (2009) Susceptibility of MRSA biofilms to denture-cleansing agents. *FEMS Microbiology Letters*. 291: 241–6.

Lombardi, T. & Budtz-Jørgensen, E. (1993) Treatment of denture-induced stomatitis: a review. *European Journal of Prosthodontics & Restorative Dentistry*, 2, 17–22.

MacFarlane, T.W. & Helnarska, S.J. (1976) The microbiology of angular cheilitis. *British Dental Journal*, 140, 403–6.

Maeda, Y., Kenny, F., Coulter, W., Loughrey, A., Nagano, Y., Goldsmith, C., Millar, B., Dooley, J., Lowery, C., Rooney, P., Matsuda, M. & Moore, J. (2007) Bactericidal activity of denture-cleaning formulations against planktonic health-care associated and community-associated methicillin-resistant *Staphylococcus aureus*. *American Journal of Infection Control*, 35: 619–22.

Marcos-Arias, C., Vicente, J., Sahand, I., Eguia, A., De-Juan, A., Madariaga, L., Aguirre, J., Eraso, E. & Quindos, G. (2009) Isolation of *Candida dubliniensis* in denture stomatitis. *Archives of Oral Biology*, 54: 127–31.

Moore, T.C., Smith, D.E. & Kenny, G.E. (1984) Sanitization of dentures by several denture hygiene methods. *Journal of Prosthetic Dentistry*, 52, 158–63.

Nikawa, H., Hamada, T. & Yamamoto, T. (1998) Denture plaque – past and recent concerns. *Journal of Dentistry*, 26, 299–304.

O'Driscoll, P.M. (1965) Papillary hyperplasia of the palate. *British Dental Journal*, 118, 77–80.

Olsen, I. (1974) Denture stomatitis – occurrence and distribution of fungi. *Acta Odontologica Scandinavica*, 32, 329–33.

Parvinen, T. Kokko, J. & Yli-Urpo, A. (1994) Miconazole lacquer compared with gel in treatment of denture stomatitis. *Scandinavian Journal of Dental Research*, 102, 361–6.

Peltola, P., Vehkalahti, M. & Wuolijoki-Saaristo, K. (2004) Oral health and treatment needs of the long-term hospitalized elderly. *Gerodontology*, 21: 93–9.

Pires, F.R., Santos, E.B.D., Bonan, P.R.F., De Almeida, O.P. & Lopez, M.A. (2002) Denture stomatitis and salivary Candida in Brazilian edentulous patients. *Journal of Oral Rehabilitation*, 29: 1115–9.

Radford, D.R., Challacombe, S.J. & Walter, J.D. (1999) Denture plaque and adherence of *Candida albicans* to denture-base materials in vivo and in vitro. *Critical Reviews in Oral Biology & Medicine*, 10, 99–116.

Ralph, J.P. & Stenhouse, D. (1972) Denture-induced hyperplasia of the oral soft tissues. *British Dental Journal*, 132, 68–70.

Ramage, G., Tomsett, K., Wickes, B., Lopez-Ribot, J. & Redding, S. (2004) Denture stomatitis – a role for Candida biofilms. *Oral Sugery, Oral medicine, Oral Pathology Oral Radiology & Endodontics*. 98: 53–9.

Sachdeo, A., Haffajee, A.D. & Socranski, S.S. (2008) Biofilms in the edentulous oral cavity. *Journal of Prosthodontics*, 17, 348–56

Sakki, T.K., Knuuttila, M.L., Laara, E. & Anttila, S.S. (1997) The association of yeasts and denture stomatitis with behavioral and biologic factors. *Oral Surgery, Oral Medicine, Oral Pathology, Oral Radiology, & Endodontics*, 84, 624–9.

Salonen, M.A., Raustia, A.M. & Oikarinen, K.S. (1996) Effect of treatment of palatal inflammatory papillary hyperplasia with local and systemic antifungal agents accompanied by renewal of complete dentures. *Acta Odontologica Scandinavica*, 54, 87–91.

Samaranayake, L.P. & MacFarlane, T.W. (1981) A retrospective study of patients with recurrent chronic atrophic candidosis. *Oral Surgery, Oral Medicine, Oral Pathology*, 52, 150–3.

Samaranayake, L.P. (1986) Nutritional factors and oral candidosis. *Journal of Oral Pathology*, 15, 61–5.

Shulman, J.D., Rivera-Hidalgo, F. & Beach, M.M. (2005) Risk factors associated with denture stomatitis in the United States. *Journal of Oral Pathology and Medicine*, 34: 340–6.

Theilade, E. & Budtz-Jørgensen, E. (1988) Predominant cultivable microflora on removable dentures in patients with denture-induced stomatitis. *Oral Microbiology and Immunology*, 3, 8–13.

Truhlar, M.R., Shay, K. & Sohnle, P. (1994) Use of a new assay technique for quantification of antifungal activity of nystatin incorporated in denture liners. *Journal of Prosthetic Dentistry*, 71, 517–24.

Webb, B.C., Thomas, C.J. & Whittle, T. (2005) A two-year study of *Candida*-associated stomatitis treatment in aged care patients. *Gerodontology*, 22, 168–76.

Webb, B.C., Thomas, C.J., Willcox, M.D., Harty, D.W. & Knox, K.W. (1998a) *Candida*-associated denture stomatitis. Aetiology and management: a review. Part 1. Factors influencing distribution of *Candida* species in the oral cavity. *Australian Dental Journal*, 43, 45–50.

Webb, B.C., Thomas, C.J., Willcox, M.D., Harty, D.W. & Knox, K.W. (1998b) *Candida*-associated denture stomatitis. Aetiology and management: a review. Part 2. Oral diseases caused by *Candida* species. *Australian Dental Journal*, 43, 160–6.

Webb, B.C., Thomas, C.J., Willcox, M.D., Harty, D.W. & Knox, K.W. (1998c) *Candida*-associated denture stomatitis. Aetiology and management: a review. Part 3. Treatment of oral candidosis. *Australian Dental Journal*, 43, 244–9.

Williamson, J.J. (1972) Diurnal variation of *Candida albicans* counts in saliva. *Australian Dental Journal*, 17, 54–60.

Wilson, J. (1998) The aetiology and management of denture stomatitis. *British Dental Journal*, 185, 380–4.

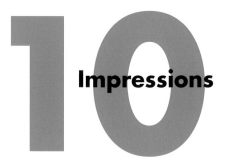

Impressions

This chapter describes the clinical techniques necessary for obtaining accurate preliminary and master impressions. The information presented here is directly related to the theoretical discussion on stability in Chapter 4.

A denture is constructed on a cast of the denture-bearing tissues. Before this cast can be made, an impression, or negative likeness, of these tissues is obtained. The impression material, which is held against the tissues and supported by an impression tray, exhibits plastic flow in the initial stages and then subsequently hardens or sets. Either plaster of Paris or model stone is then poured into the impression to form the cast, or positive likeness, of the denture-bearing tissues.

If maximum accuracy of the casts is to be achieved, a two-stage impression procedure is required. First, preliminary impressions are taken using stock 'off the peg' impression trays and second, the more accurate master impressions are taken using trays which have been 'tailor-made' for a particular patient on casts obtained from the preliminary impressions.

The denture-bearing areas

The surface anatomy of the denture-bearing areas is illustrated in Figs. 10.1 and 10.2.

The upper denture is normally extended posteriorly to the vibrating line, which is the junction between the moving tissues of the soft palate and the static tissues anteriorly (Fig. 10.3). Two small depressions in the mucosal surface, the foveae palatinae, common collecting ducts from minor salivary glands, are often seen in this region and are therefore a useful landmark for this junction.

The fibrous band running along the residual ridge is the vestige of the palatal gingivae and, like the incisive papilla, remains relatively constant in position during the remodelling of the ridge which follows extraction of the natural teeth. These two structures can therefore be used as landmarks allowing teeth on complete dentures to be placed in positions similar to those of their natural predecessors (Fig. 10.4). This biometric approach also requires specific design features to be incorporated into the impression trays – for details of these the reader

Prosthetic Treatment of the Edentulous Patient, Fifth Edition, © R.M. Basker, J.C. Davenport and J.M. Thomason
Published 2011 by Blackwell Publishing Ltd.

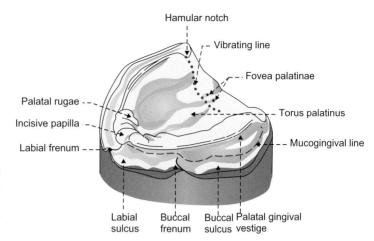

Figure 10.1 Surface anatomy of the upper denture-bearing area. The vibrating line indicates the normal posterior extension of the upper denture.

is referred to the relevant bibliography (Watt & MacGregor 1976).

In the lower jaw, the denture should extend over the pear-shaped pads. These pads are very important as buttresses helping to resist distal movement of the denture.

As explained in Chapter 4, it is important that the borders of the denture conform to the functional form of the sulci so that a good facial seal can be produced and maximum phys-

ical retention obtained. Broad coverage of the tissues by the denture also ensures that the occlusal loads are distributed as widely as possible.

Anatomy of the sulcus tissues

When recording the functional shape of the sulci, it is necessary to have an understanding of the anatomical structures that influence this shape. These are shown diagrammatically in Figs. 10.5–10.10.

The form of the sulcus changes markedly during function and the shape of the denture must make allowance for these changes, otherwise discomfort or displacement of the denture is likely to result. The required shape of the denture borders is obtained by careful border moulding of the impression. The following areas require particular attention.

Mentalis muscle

Contraction of the mentalis muscle raises the soft tissues of the chin, thus reducing the depth and width of the labial sulcus (Fig. 10.7). If there has been marked resorption of the underlying bone, this muscle can exert considerable pressure on the labial flange, resulting in its posterior and upward displacement.

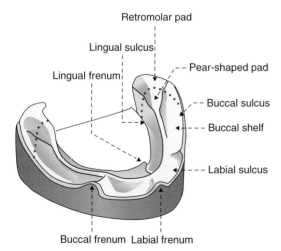

Figure 10.2 Surface anatomy of the lower denture-bearing area. The heavy dotted line indicates the normal posterior extension of the lower denture.

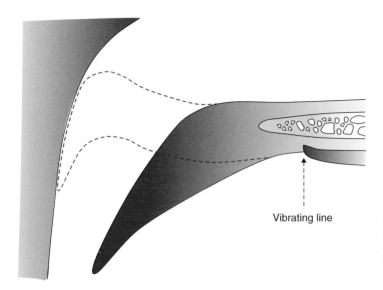

Figure 10.3 Longitudinal section through the palate showing correct relationship of the posterior border of the upper denture to the junction between the moving and static tissues (vibrating line).

Vibrating line

Modiolus

The area of strong muscle activity in the lower labial sulcus is bounded distally on each side by the modiolus, a decussation of muscle fibres at the corner of the mouth (Fig. 10.8). Narrowing of the lower denture base related to the modiolus is usually necessary to avoid displacement (Fig. 10.5). The muscles contributing to the modiolus are able to move or fix the corner of the mouth in any required position during function. For example, approxima-

tion of the modiolus to the buccal surface of the denture closes the buccal sulci anteriorly during mastication, so helping to contain the bolus of food as it is being crushed between the posterior teeth.

Masseter muscle

On clenching the teeth the anterior border of the masseter muscle bulges into the disto-buccal sulcus area (Fig. 10.5).

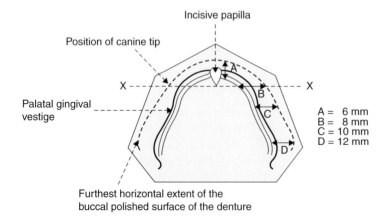

Incisive papilla

Position of canine tip

X

Palatal gingival vestige

A = 6 mm
B = 8 mm
C = 10 mm
D = 12 mm

Furthest horizontal extent of the buccal polished surface of the denture

Figure 10.4 Diagram of the upper arch showing average distances from the palatal gingival vestige of the furthest horizontal extent of the polished surface of the denture in the incisal (A), canine (B), premolar (C) and molar (D) regions (the biometric approach). The line (X–X) passing through the posterior border of the incisive papilla can be used as a guide to positioning the tips of the canines.

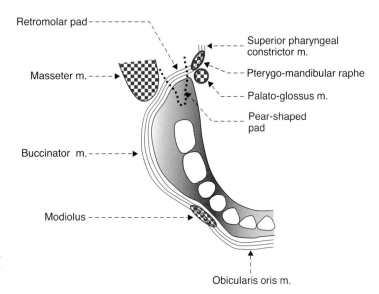

Figure 10.5 The buccal and distal anatomical relations of the lower denture.

Floor of mouth

When the tongue is elevated, the sublingual folds are raised and may greatly reduce the depth and width of the lingual sulcus. This phenomenon is most marked when advanced resorption of the ridge has occurred.

Zygomatic process of the maxilla

The anatomical structures determining the form of the sulcus in the upper jaw are shown in Fig. 10.9. Particular care must be taken to avoid vertical over-extension in the first molar region, as mucosal injury may result from a

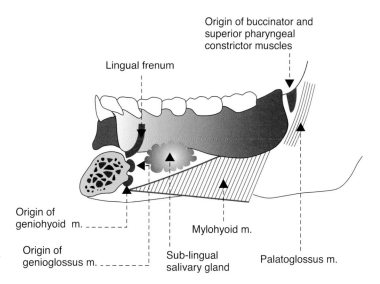

Figure 10.6 The lingual anatomical relations of the lower denture.

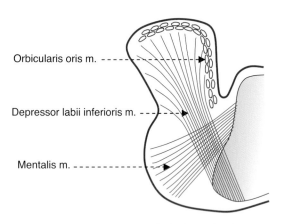

Figure 10.7 Section through the lower lip showing the muscles which influence the shape of the labial sulcus.

sandwiching of the soft tissues between the denture border and the zygomatic process of the maxilla.

Coronoid process

Buccal to the tuberosities, the sulcus often reaches its deepest point; however, its width is reduced when the mouth is opened because of the close proximity of the coronoid process of the mandible (Fig. 10.9). If the buccal flanges of the eventual denture are too wide posteriorly, they will either restrict mandibular opening or be displaced by the coronoid process. Thus, the borders of the impression in this re-

gion should be moulded to the correct width by the patient moving the mandible from side to side when the mouth is open.

Buccinator muscle

A certain amount of lateral displacement of the buccinator muscle by the denture in other areas can occur without causing instability of the denture. In fact, such displacement can be desirable as it can increase retention by improving the facial seal (Fig. 10.10). It can also make it easier to create a favourable slope of the polished surface for effective muscular control of the denture.

The preliminary impression

Stock trays

Stock trays are available in a range of sizes and shapes. These trays are constructed in metal or plastic and may be perforated or unperforated. Certain types of plastic trays are intended to be disposable.

Ideally, a stock tray should cover the entire denture-bearing area and allow a uniform space of a few millimetres in between it and the underlying mucosa (Fig. 10.11).

However, as the range of sizes and shapes of stock trays is limited and the shape of the denture-bearing areas so varied, the fit of the

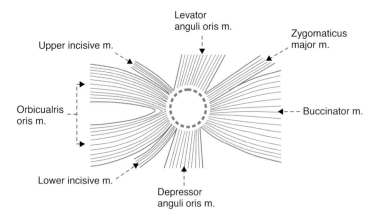

Figure 10.8 The muscles contributing to the modiolus (dotted circle).

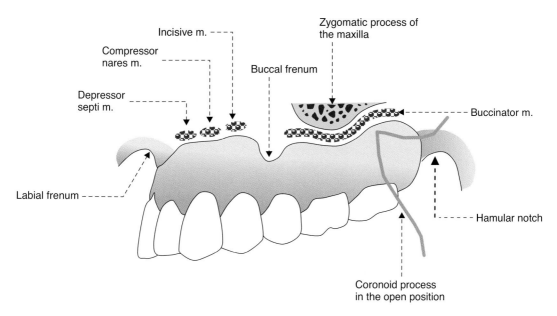

Figure 10.9   The buccal anatomical relations of the upper denture.

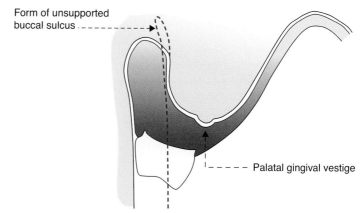

Figure 10.10   Lateral displacement of the buccinator muscle by the denture to improve facial seal.

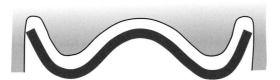

Figure 10.11   The ideal relationship of a stock tray to the sulci and denture-bearing mucosa.

tray is usually less than perfect. The tray may be too wide or too narrow; it may not cover the denture-bearing tissues posteriorly; the tray flange may be under-extended, finishing short of the mucosal reflection in the sulcus, or may be over-extended so that it digs into and distorts the sulcus tissues.

It is a common misconception amongst novice clinicians that accuracy of the preliminary impressions is not particularly important as it is assumed, incorrectly, that any faults can be easily corrected when obtaining the master impressions. However, this is far from the truth. It is very important that the preliminary impression is as accurate as the limitations of the stock tray allow, because the more faults there are in this impression, the more time-consuming and difficult will be the modifications of the special trays at the next visit. As a result the quality of the master impression is likely to be compromised.

When it has been decided to use a relatively low viscosity impression material such as alginate for the preliminary impression it is often necessary to modify the extension of the stock tray. Under-extension of the tray can be corrected by the addition of impression compound or pink wax to the deficient flange, while over-extension can be corrected, if the tray is plastic, by trimming back the flange with a bur.

Impression materials and techniques

As even a correctly selected and modified stock tray is very unlikely to have a perfect relationship to the denture-bearing tissues, it is desirable for the impression material chosen for a preliminary impression to have a relatively high viscosity, as this allows it to compensate better for the shortcomings in fit and extension of the stock tray.

Alginate

Alginates vary considerably in their viscosity and the high viscosity type is most suitable for preliminary impressions. Alternatively, the powder–water ratio of the more fluid alginates can be increased to achieve the required consistency.

Retention of alginate to the impression tray

Alginate does not adhere to the tray surface and so retention must be provided by means of a perforated tray or an adhesive. Perforations allow alginate to flow through and 'rivet' the body of the impression to the tray. If adhesive is used, it should be applied thinly to the entire inner surface of the tray and also carried over the peripheries to include a few millimetres of the outer surface. Time should be allowed after application of the adhesive for it to become tacky, a process which can be speeded up considerably by dispersing the adhesive over the surface of the tray with a stream of air from a triple syringe.

Border moulding the lower impression

The lower impression is usually taken first as it is easier for the patient to tolerate than the upper. When the impression is seated in the mouth the patient is asked to raise the tongue to contact the upper lip and to sweep the tongue to touch each cheek in turn before returning to maintain contact with the upper lip until the alginate has set. This tongue movement will raise the floor of the mouth and tense the lingual frenum, causing the alginate in the over-extended parts of the lingual periphery to be moulded to conform more closely to the functional depth of the sulcus. If the tongue is allowed to relax and fall back into the floor of the mouth while the impression material is still fluid, the material may flow down into the floor of the mouth and the impression will become overextended once more. Buccal and labial border moulding is achieved by firm stretching of the relaxed lips and cheeks with the fingers. It is essential that the clinician supports the tray carefully during these border moulding manoeuvres.

Border moulding the upper impression

If the sulci buccal to the maxillary tuberosities are deep, air may be trapped as the loaded impression tray is inserted. To overcome this problem, these areas can be pre-packed with alginate before seating the tray. The tray is first loaded and placed to one side; then with the cheek reflected and the patient's mouth half closed, alginate is placed into the buccal sulcus with a spatula or finger. The loaded tray is then quickly inserted into the mouth, positioned over the ridge and seated with sufficient pressure to cause the alginate to flow and record the shape of the tissues. Excess alginate will flow into the sulci, producing an over-extended impression. This over-extension must be corrected by carrying out border moulding.

Removing the impression from the mouth

When the border moulding is complete, the tray must be kept perfectly still until the alginate has set, otherwise strains will be induced in the impression. Then when the impression has been removed from the mouth, gradual release of these strains will take place, causing distortion. In order to remove the set impression from the mouth, the border seal must be broken. This is achieved by first asking the patient to half close the mouth; the cheek is then reflected away from the buccal surface of the impression on one side to allow access of air to the periphery, and a sharp jerk is applied to the tray handle. If the impression is removed slowly, distortion of the alginate is more likely to occur.

The completed impression

Saliva should be removed from the impression surface by rinsing briefly under a cold tap. Excess water is shaken off and the impression is inspected carefully. A satisfactory completed impression will include the entire denture-bearing area. The surface of the impression should be smooth and show evidence

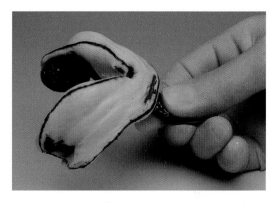

Figure 10.12   A lower impression in alginate showing a border which has been molded by the adjacent tissues. Correct extension in the lingual pouches has been achieved by suitable extension of the tray. The line drawn on the impression provides a useful guide when the cast is trimmed.

of having been moulded by the tissues (Fig. 10.12). The border areas should be rounded and include impressions of the frenal attachments.

The dimensional instability of alginate

An alginate impression is particularly susceptible to dimensional change developing as a result of an increase or a decrease in its water content. These two processes are:

1. Imbibition – the absorption of water
2. Syneresis – the loss of water

If water is left on the surface of the impression imbibition will take place causing the alginate to swell. If the impression is left in a dry atmosphere syneresis will occur with consequent shrinkage of the alginate. Therefore it is essential that a satisfactory impression is rinsed, disinfected, covered as soon as possible with a damp napkin and placed in a plastic bag. Casts should be poured as soon as possible. While the impression is waiting to be poured, it must not be allowed to rest on any surplus alginate which has flowed over the posterior border of the tray, as this will cause distortion.

Impression compound

This is a thermoplastic material which softens when heated in a water-bath to temperatures between 55°C and 70°C. The high viscosity of the material and the fact that it becomes rigid when chilled make it unnecessary to correct any under-extensions of a stock tray before taking the impression.

Preparing the material

As the impression compound softens in the water-bath, a portion of sufficient size to take the planned impression is kneaded with the fingers by folding the material inwards from the periphery of the mass to the centre. This produces a smooth, crease-free, surface on one side of the compound; it also improves flow and helps to give the material a uniform consistency.

Obtaining the lower impression

The lower impression is usually obtained before the upper. The portion of compound is formed into a cylinder and then extended to the length of the tray by pulling on either end. This creates a dumb-bell-shaped specimen which distributes the material along the tray in a fashion corresponding to the width of the denture-bearing area to be recorded – narrow anteriorly and broad posteriorly. The compound is placed in the dried tray so that the smooth side will be towards the tissues and is then moulded with the fingers to the approximate shape of the ridge. The surface of the compound can be lightly flamed to improve its flow and then tempered in warm water to avoid burning the patient. Coating with petroleum jelly is sometimes recommended to improve surface flow. The tray is then seated firmly in the mouth and supported while border moulding is carried out as described for the alginate preliminary impression. However, in this instance, as the impression compound is more viscous than alginate, the moulding must be executed with greater firmness, otherwise over-extension of

the impression will occur. When the impression has cooled and hardened, it is removed from the mouth and inspected. If minor faults are present, corrections can be carried out by trimming away excess material with a hot wax knife, or by adding new compound to repair deficiencies and then resoftening the surface of the impression before reseating it in the mouth. If there are major faults, for instance in positioning the tray, the impression is retaken. Once a satisfactory impression has been obtained, it must be hardened by thoroughly chilling it in cold water.

Obtaining the upper impression

The impression for the upper jaw is obtained by placing a golf-ball-sized portion of softened compound into the centre of a dried tray and pre-forming it with the fingers to the shape of the ridge and palate. The procedure then is as described for the lower impression. Completed impressions in compound are shown in Fig. 10.13.

The alginate wash impression technique

A satisfactory impression in compound is often quite adequate for producing a cast on which to construct a special tray. However, there are occasions when the clinician might require a more accurate picture of the mucosa so that the potential denture-bearing area can be visualised more easily. This can be achieved by refining the initial compound impression with a wash impression in alginate as follows:

- Obtain the best possible impression in compound and dry it thoroughly.
- Trim back the borders of the impression by 1–2 mm with a heated wax knife.
- Apply a thin layer of alginate adhesive to the impression surface.
- Load the compound impression with a small amount of low viscosity alginate, seat it fully on the tissues and complete border trimming as before.

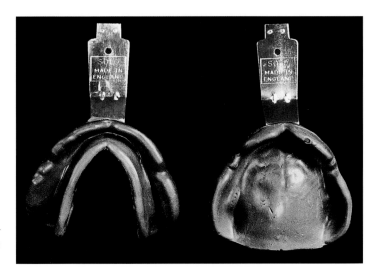

Figure 10.13 Upper and lower impressions taken in impression compound.

The completed impressions

The completed satisfactory impressions are disinfected before being sent to the laboratory.

Communication with the dental technician

In order to achieve the best possible treatment outcome, it is essential that the clinician and dental technician work together as a team. An adequate understanding of each other's work and contribution, together with effective two-way communication, are of paramount importance in achieving success. The clinician therefore needs to ensure that at the end of each clinical stage, when sending items to the laboratory, all the information required by the dental technician is provided together with a clear indication of the clinician's requirements for the next clinical stage. This communication traditionally takes the form of a comprehensive written prescription, but on occasion the dental technician will need additional information or clarification. Under such circumstances, the value of discussing the case face to face, or on the telephone cannot be underestimated. Increasingly, electronic links are likely to play a significant part in contributing to effective communication between the dental surgery and the laboratory.

The laboratory prescription

After the preliminary impressions have been obtained, the following information should normally be entered on the laboratory prescription by the clinician:

- Confirmation that all items sent from the clinic to the laboratory have been disinfected.
- Materials to be used for the special trays.
- Details of the design of the special trays including:
  - Spaced or close fitting.
  - Size and location of any stops to be preformed in spaced special trays.
  - Perforated or not.
  - Type of handle and any finger rests.
  - Any special requirements, e.g. a special tray for a flabby ridge.
- The written prescription can be supplemented by the clinician marking the required extension of the special trays on the preliminary impressions with an indelible

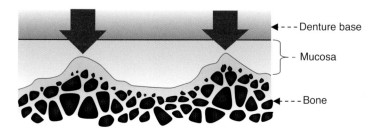

Figure 10.14 Occlusal loads transmitted by the denture to the mucosa will tend to be greatest (arrows) where the mucosa is thinnest.

pencil if the impression is in alginate, or with the tip of a wax knife if the impression is in impression compound.

Quality control and enhancement

An audit of the quality of this clinical stage can be most fruitful if the quality of the end product – the special tray – is assessed. The audit might include the following:

- Is there avoidable over-extension or under-extension of the special tray, particularly in the 'high risk' areas such as the upper posterior border and tuberosity regions and, in the lower, the pear-shaped pads and lingual pouches?
- Has the dental technician been provided with sufficient information in the prescription?
- Has the dental technician produced what was asked for?

The master impression

Mucostatic and mucodisplacive impression techniques

The clinician's goal when taking master impressions is to record as accurately as possible the shape of the mucosa overlying the alveolar ridges and hard palate together with the functional depth and width of the sulci. However, there is some disagreement as to the best method of achieving this goal.

Mucostatic impression

The mucosa overlying the alveolar ridges and hard palate is not of uniform thickness. Consequently, if the clinician uses a mucostatic technique which applies minimal pressure to the tissues, and therefore records their resting shape, there is a possibility that the subsequent distribution of occlusal loads by the finished dentures will be uneven (Fig. 10.14). However, as the impression surface of the denture conforms closely to the mucosa surface of the underlying mucosa, both when the denture is under load and when it is not, physical retention will be optimal.

Mucodisplacive impression

The alternative approach, a mucodisplacive technique, applies pressure to the mucosa during the impression-taking procedure so that the shape of the tissues under load is recorded. This approach may have the advantage that occlusal loads are more evenly dispersed over the tissues, but has the disadvantage that the physical retention of the denture when the teeth are apart is likely to be less than that obtained with a mucostatic impression technique (Fig. 10.15).

Selecting the appropriate impression technique

Should the mucosa be recorded in its resting state or in its displaced state? In most cases, it will be found that the best results may be most simply obtained by a mucostatic technique. Pressure on the tissues is reduced as far

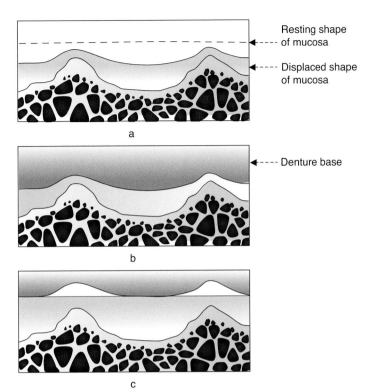

Figure 10.15 The mucodisplacive impression technique: (a) the difference in the shape of the mucosal surface produced by a mucostatic technique (dotted line) and a mucodisplacive technique (continuous line); (b) the impression surface, obtained by a mucodisplacive technique, fits the mucosa closely when the denture is under occlusal load; (c) when the occlusal load is removed the mucosa returns to its resting shape and the denture ceases to fit accurately.

as possible by using an impression material of low viscosity. Impression plaster, zinc oxide-eugenol impression paste and low viscosity alginate or silicone rubber are examples of suitable materials.

In some patients, a moderate variation in mucosal compressibility may be present and a mucostatic impression, particularly in the case of the lower jaw, results in a denture that distributes the occlusal loads unevenly with consequent mucosal injury and associated discomfort. In this situation, it may be advisable to record the shape of the mucosa in a displaced state by using an impression material of high viscosity. The load applied during the impression-taking procedure should be the same as that occurring during function. A method which fulfils these requirements is known as a functional impression technique and is described on p. 237.

Special trays

To ensure accuracy of the master impression special trays must be made of a material that is dimensionally stable and rigid enough not to deform under the stresses of impression taking. Light-cured or cold-curing acrylic resins satisfy these requirements and are the tray materials of choice.

Spaced trays

In order to avoid permanent distortion of an elastic impression material as it is withdrawn from undercut areas, an adequate uniform thickness of the material is required. The special tray should be constructed on the preliminary cast after a spacer of appropriate thickness for the planned impression material has been adapted to it (Fig. 10.16). Alginate

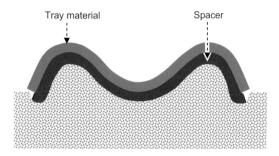

Figure 10.16 A spaced special tray is constructed by adapting the tray material over a spacer which has been applied to the cast.

is the most commonly used elastic impression material for edentulous patients and this requires a spacer of about 3 mm. The elastomers have a better elastic recovery than alginate and so require less spacing of the special tray.

Close-fitting trays

Close-fitting trays are used with impression materials that are used in thin section such as zinc oxide-eugenol impression paste and light-bodied elastomers.

It is an advantage if a lower acrylic close-fitting tray has vertical pillars in the premolar regions to act as finger rests (Fig. 10.17).

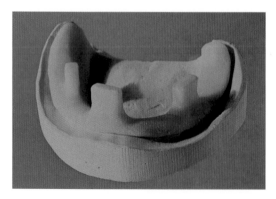

Figure 10.17 A lower close-fitting acrylic tray showing the position of the finger rests in the premolar regions.

These rests keep the fingers, which stabilise the tray and support the impression, well clear of critical border areas of the impression while it sets. If this is not done, inaccuracies will result from the fingers restricting the border moulding movements of the soft tissues. They can also displace excess impression material into the sulci. The anterior stub handle is for holding and manipulating the tray. Its shape avoids interference with the lower lip which otherwise can make placement of the tray difficult and can hinder border trimming of the impression in that area.

The use of stops

If an unmodified spaced special tray is tried in the mouth to check its border extension, it will be seated in contact with the underlying mucosa (Fig. 10.18a). In this position, the borders of the tray bear a different relationship to the sulcus to the one that will exist when the impression is taken. In this latter instance, the tray will be separated from the mucosa by a few millimetres of impression material (Fig. 10.18b). Thus, a border that appears to be correctly extended on first inspection may be under-extended when the impression is taken.

Placing stops in the tray before checking and correcting the borders will overcome this problem, ensuring a uniform thickness of about 2–3 mm of impression material, and stabilising the tray during impression taking.

In the lower tray these stops are placed in the incisal region and over the pear-shaped pads. In

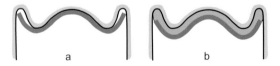

Figure 10.18 (a) Tray in contact with the mucosa – the border appears to be correctly extended. (b) Tray separated from the mucosa by the impression material – tray border under-extended.

the upper tray the stops are placed in the incisal region and along the line of the post-dam.

There are several ways that stops can be produced:

- *During construction of an acrylic tray in the laboratory.* Windows are cut in the wax spacer at appropriate locations on the cast used to manufacture the impression tray (Fig. 10.19). The stops are produced by the acrylic dough flowing into these windows and contacting the model. This is the preferred method of producing stops as it is accurate and saves chair side time.
- *At the chair side in the mouth.* Tracing compound is applied to the tray and tempered in warm water to avoid burning the mucosa. The tray is then seated in the mouth to mould the tracing compound to the ridge

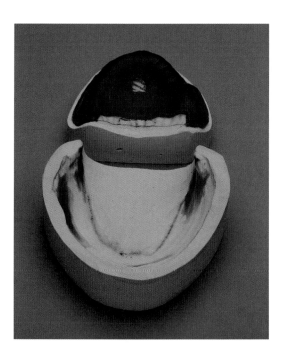

Figure 10.19 The upper cast and wax spacer, showing where the stops will be created (see text for details).

tissues creating the required space between the tray and mucosa.
- *At the chair side on the cast.* Tracing compound is applied to the tray as in the previous paragraph and the tray is then seated on the wet cast. This approach has the advantage that it is easier to visually check that the tray is centred correctly on the ridge while the stops are being formed than it is when seating the tray in the mouth.

Once the stops have been prepared the border extension of the tray is checked intra-orally.

Checking the special tray

As a special tray is made on a cast poured from a relatively inaccurate preliminary impression, it will commonly be found on checking the tray in the mouth that the periphery does not conform to the shape of the sulcus tissues in all areas. Both over-extension and under-extension may be present.

Visual assessment

The tray can be checked visually in most areas of the mouth with the exception of the lingual sulcus where the tongue obscures the view in the posterior regions. Over-extension in these regions is present if the tray is displaced upwards when the patient raises the tongue to contact the upper lip. However, as under-extension is the more common fault, it is wise to assume its presence if over-extension cannot be demonstrated.

The diagnostic impression

A rapid and effective way of checking tray extension is to take a diagnostic impression with alginate. For this it is not necessary to apply adhesive to the tray, which simplifies subsequent removal of the impression material from the tray once it has served its purpose. Careful border moulding of the diagnostic impression is carried out and subsequent inspection of the completed impression gives a very clear record of the accuracy of the tray extension in all areas. The tray can then be corrected as necessary.

Correcting the special tray

Correction of over-extension

Over-extension must be corrected by trimming away the offending acrylic resin with a bur or stone until the height of the flange has been reduced by the appropriate amount. If over-extension of the special tray is not corrected, the sulcus tissues will be stretched and the master impression will be over-extended. If this fault is not recognised before the denture is finished, the over-extended flange will injure the tissues; in addition, elastic recoil of the displaced sulcus tissues will cause instability of the denture.

Correction of under-extension

Under-extension is corrected by extending the tray in the region of the deficiency with a border-trimming material. These additions to the tray must then be carefully border moulded. It should be remembered that the common areas of under-extension of the upper denture are the posterior border and around the tuberosities, while the lower denture is often under-extended in the regions of the pear-shaped pads and lingual pouches (Basker et al. 1993). So whatever technique is used, the greatest care must be taken to ensure that the impression includes these vital areas.

If an under-extended tray is not corrected, there are two possible sequelae:

1. The impression material is not carried to the full depth of the sulcus, so that the finished denture is under-extended.
2. The impression material reaches the full functional depth of the sulcus but is not supported by the under-extended tray. When the cast is poured, the weight of the artifi-

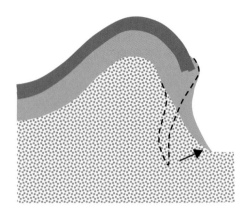

Figure 10.20   Distortion of unsupported elastic impression material by the artificial stone.

cial stone will distort the unsupported part of the elastic impression material, resulting in a denture which is an inaccurate fit (Fig. 10.20).

In order to obtain the best possible recording of the lingual sulcus, it is essential to train the patient to make the following tongue movements before making additions lingually to the lower tray: the tip of the tongue is placed in one cheek and then swept round anteriorly to the other cheek; this is repeated two or three times and then the tongue is raised to contact the upper lip. The tongue should not be protruded further than the lip as such a movement is rarely used in normal function and only results in an excessive and unnecessary reduction in depth of the lingual flange of the eventual denture. Another useful technique is to ask the patient to push the tongue against the hard palate. This movement activates the muscles in the floor of the mouth and assists in obtaining accurate border extension.

If biometric guides (mentioned briefly on p. 130), are being followed in the design of a denture, a border-trimming material should be used to extend the tray flanges laterally to support the cheek and lips in the positions shown in Fig. 10.4.

Creating a post-dam

If the post-dam (p. 101) is to be created by compressing the mucosa while obtaining the final impression, rather than by cutting a groove into the palate of the master cast, the following procedure is adopted. Firstly, tracing compound is placed along the posterior border on the inner aspect of the adjusted tray so that when the tray is seated with sufficient pressure, the mucosa will be compressed by the tracing material. Secondly, after trimming the tracing compound back to the posterior border of the tray, a relatively low viscosity impression material is selected for the definitive impression. The tray is then inserted with enough pressure to displace the impression material from over the tracing compound. If this has been done correctly the tracing compound will be visible through a thin veneer of the set impression material. This compression caused during impression taking will result in a permanent denture base which has a raised lip along the posterior border on its impression surface. This projection, the post-dam, compresses the palatal mucosa once the denture is placed in the mouth and thus creates the border seal.

Border trimming materials

Materials available for the correction of under-extended impression trays include tracing compound and high viscosity elastomers.

Tracing compound, which is thermoplastic, has the advantage that it can be progressively corrected, by resoftening or by adding further material, until the tray extension is satisfactory. The setting of the high viscosity elastomers, on the other hand, is by an irreversible chemical reaction and requires a 'one shot' approach; thus, if the border trimming is deficient at the first attempt the entire procedure will have to be repeated.

The technique for using tracing compound is summarised in Fig. 10.21. The tracing compound should be applied in increments to the tray border, with each increment being border

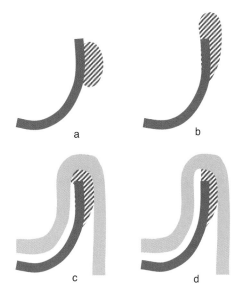

Figure 10.21 A method of applying tracing compound for correction of under-extension: (a) the tracing compound is softened and placed on the outer surface of the tray – sufficient bulk of material should be used to allow a broad area of attachment and to retain heat so that there is an adequate working time for border moulding; (b) the compound is tempered in warm water and moulded with the fingers to produce a flange; (c) border moulding is carried out and then the tray is chilled in cold water; (d) finally, the space between the tracing compound and the alveolar ridge is re-established by removing material with a wax knife.

moulded before the next addition is made. If adequate moulding has not been achieved at the first attempt, the over-extended compound is resoftened using a fine flame, tempered in warm water to avoid burning the mucosa, and border moulded once more. When the adjustment is complete, the tracing compound is chilled in cold water. The finished result is shown in Fig. 10.19.

Impression materials and techniques

Alginate

This material is elastic when set and therefore is indicated where bony undercuts are present.

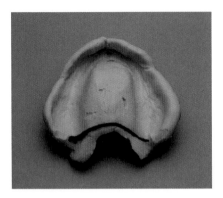

Figure 10.22   A satisfactory upper alginate impression.

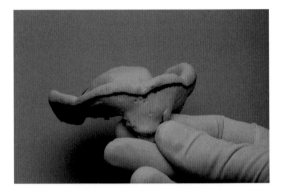

Figure 10.23   An alginate impression showing the position of the indelible pencil line placed as a guide to subsequent trimming of the cast.

Whereas high viscosity alginates are indicated for the preliminary impression, they are not recommended for master impressions as they readily cause mucosal displacement, particularly in the border areas. Thus, a low viscosity type should be used.

The procedures for manipulating the alginate and obtaining the impression are the same as those described for the alginate preliminary impression (p. 134).

Figure 10.22 shows a satisfactory impression in which the borders are rounded and well defined.

It is important that having carefully recorded the shape of the borders this valuable information is reproduced on the cast. A useful guide can be given to the dental technician by drawing a line on the alginate with indelible pencil 3–4 mm beyond the border of the impression (Fig. 10.23). This line is transferred to the cast material and acts as a landmark, discouraging over-trimming of the cast which would otherwise result in loss of information concerning the functional width of the sulcus (Fig. 10.24).

Zinc oxide-eugenol impression paste

This excellent impression material is rigid when set and is dimensionally stable, so it is preferred to alginate in all cases where there are no bony undercuts. Other advantages of this material

accrue from the fact that it is used in a close-fitting, rather than a spaced tray, i.e.:

- The overall bulk of the impression is kept to a minimum and so is better tolerated by the patient.
- Where the sulcus is narrow, it is easier to avoid displacement of the buccal mucosa (Fig. 10.25).
- It is easier to obtain an impression of a resorbed lower ridge without the mucosa of the floor of the mouth becoming trapped within the border of the tray.

Checking and correcting the tray extension

As zinc oxide-eugenol impression paste is used in a thin film, stops are not added to the special tray. Instead, the borders should be

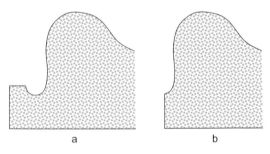

a   b

Figure 10.24   Cross section through (a) a correctly trimmed and (b) an overtrimmed cast.

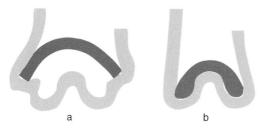

Figure 10.25 (a) A spaced tray may displace the buccal mucosa laterally from its normal position. (b) A more accurate recording of the sulcus width is possible with a close-fitting tray.

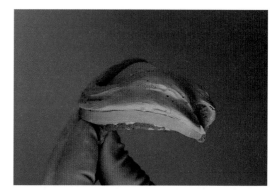

Figure 10.27 The addition of a wax beading to guide the cast trimming.

checked with the tray held in contact with the mucosa. Again a diagnostic impression in low viscosity alginate is an excellent way of carrying out a comprehensive check on the tray extension. Over-extension of acrylic trays may be corrected with an acrylic bur, while under-extension may be corrected with any of the border-trimming materials mentioned previously. The procedure differs from that described for spaced trays in that when the border-trimming material has set, a space does not need to be re-created in that area.

A completed impression is shown in Fig. 10.26. A clear guide to the correct trimming of the cast is created by the wax beading which adheres easily to the impression paste (Fig. 10.27).

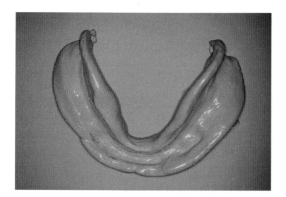

Figure 10.26 A satisfactory lower zinc oxide-eugenol impression paste impression.

Impression plaster

Impression plaster is a good impression material primarily for the upper edentulous jaw where there are no bony undercuts. A spaced special tray should be used so that the impression has adequate strength when set, and any fragments which break off when the impression is removed from the mouth are large enough to be relocated accurately and to be attached to the main part of the impression.

Impression plaster has the following properties which are clinically relevant:

- *Rigid when set.* However, if small bony undercuts are present the use of impression plaster is not ruled out. The material which enters the undercut area will break off when the impression is removed from the mouth and can then be re-attached to the impression as mentioned above.
- *Dimensionally stable.*
- *Low viscosity.* Impression plaster is therefore a good material to use when a mucostatic impression is required.
- *Susceptible to excess saliva.* It is difficult to obtain a satisfactory lower impression in patients who salivate profusely because the saliva mixes with the plaster and a rough, friable surface is produced.

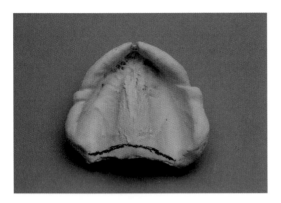

Figure 10.28 An upper plaster master impression on which a pencil line has been drawn at the posterior border to indicate the position of the post-dam.

A satisfactory plaster impression is shown in Fig. 10.28 and the position of the post dam has been indicated on the impression with an indelible pencil. The completed impression is disinfected before being sent to the laboratory.

Elastomers

The elastomers include the following impression materials:

- Condensation-cured silicone rubbers
- Addition-cured silicone rubbers
- Polysulphide rubbers
- Polyethers

The silicone materials are relatively expensive, but in spite of the modest cost penalty compared with alginate and zinc oxide-eugenol impression paste they are becoming increasingly popular for complete denture impressions. The silicone elastomers have the following desirable clinical properties:

- *Excellent elastic recovery.*
- *Excellent dimensional stability.*
- *A wide range of viscosities.* The silicone materials vary from heavy-bodied putties to light-bodied perfecting pastes, creating a versatile group of materials suitable for a wide variety

of clinical applications. These range from the use of putties for border trimming to perfecting pastes for wash impressions.
- *They are clean and easy to handle.*
- *A wide range of working and setting times.* This versatility makes them appropriate for most techniques. For example, some materials with an extended setting time are suitable for functional impressions of both the denture-bearing mucosa and the neutral zone. Other materials with short setting times allow conventional impressions to be taken rapidly and thus reduce patient discomfort.
- *Non-adherence to dry mucosa.* The low viscosity silicone materials are preferred alternatives to zinc oxide-eugenol impression paste for patients with dry mouths, as the latter material can adhere to and irritate the dry mucosa.

Communication with the dental technician

The laboratory prescription

After the master impressions have been obtained the following information should normally be entered on the laboratory prescription by the dental clinician:

- Confirmation that all items sent from the clinic to the laboratory have been disinfected.
- Materials to be used for the bases of the record blocks. Normally, these are acrylic resin or shellac. The relative merits of these materials and the indications for their use are discussed at the beginning of the next chapter.
- The written prescription can be supplemented by the dental clinician delineating the borders of the impression with a pencil line or wax beading to indicate to the dental technician the required limit of cast trimming. It is worth emphasising in this context

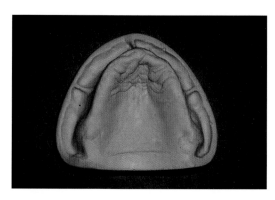

Figure 10.29 Upper cast with the full depth and width of sulci carefully maintained.

that the best prescription for the eventual denture border is an accurately trimmed cast which has been produced from a carefully taken impression (Fig. 10.29).

Quality control and enhancement

An audit of a series of cases at the appropriate time might include the following:

- Did the recording of the functional width and depth of the sulcus ensure that the borders of the eventual denture covered the maximum area?
- Did the borders of the bases of the record blocks/eventual dentures require no more than minimal adjustment?
- Did the dental technician maintain the full sulcus depth and width on the master casts?

Were the bases of the record blocks extended to the full depth of the sulcus on the master cast?
- Was the dental technician provided with all the information necessary to provide the next item of work?

References and additional reading

Basker, R.M., Ogden, A.R. & Ralph, J.P. (1993) Complete denture prescription – an audit of performance. *British Dental Journal*, 174, 278–84.

Lawson, W.A. (1978) Current concepts and practice in complete dentures. Impressions: principles and practice. *Journal of Dentistry*, 6, 43–58.

Nairn, R.I. (1964) The posterior lingual area of the complete lower denture. *Dental Practitioner and Dental Record*, 15, 123–30.

Shannon, J.L. (1972) The mentalis muscle in relation to edentulous mandibles. *Journal of Prosthetic Dentistry*, 27, 477–84.

Strang, R., Whitters, C.J., Brown, D., et al. (1998) Dental materials: 1996 literature review. Part 2. *Journal of Dentistry*, 26, 273–91.

Watt, D.M. (1978) Tooth positions on complete dentures. *Journal of Dentistry*, 6, 147–60.

Watt, D.M. & MacGregor, A.R. (1976) *Designing Complete Dentures*. W.B. Saunders, Philadelphia.

Wilson, H.J. (1966a) Elastomeric impression materials. Part 1: The setting material. *British Dental Journal*, 121, 277–83.

Wilson, H.J. (1966b) Elastomeric impression materials. Part 2: The set material. *British Dental Journal*, 121, 322–8.

Wilson, H.J. (1966c) Some properties of alginate impression materials relevant to clinical practice. *British Dental Journal*, 121, 463–7.

Recording Jaw Relations – Clinical Procedures

This chapter describes the basic technique for recording the jaw relationship. This clinical stage is, in fact, concerned with far more than establishing the relationship between maxilla and mandible. It is the process by which the information essential for the production of new dentures is transferred from the patient to the dental laboratory so that the dental technician is provided with what amounts to a blueprint for the prostheses.

This chapter focuses primarily on recording the jaw relationship for patients without existing dentures. However, in Chapter 8 the point was made that most patients require replacement dentures, and that the existing ones provide a great deal of information which will be invaluable at this clinical stage. Therefore we recommend that the reader also refer to Chapter 8 to obtain a more comprehensive picture of the clinical procedure.

Measuring the rest vertical dimension

The rest vertical dimension is recorded to provide a point of reference from which the occlusal vertical dimension of the dentures can be calculated by subtracting the required freeway space (usually approximately 3 mm). Determining the rest vertical dimension is one of the more difficult tasks in dentistry, as indicated by the large number of denture problems that can be attributed to errors in this dimension.

To reduce the chance of error and to coax the mandible into the rest position, the patient must be completely relaxed. This can be encouraged by paying particular attention to the following points:

- Many patients are apprehensive when they enter a dental surgery. The clinician

Prosthetic Treatment of the Edentulous Patient, Fifth Edition, © R.M. Basker, J.C. Davenport and J.M. Thomason
Published 2011 by Blackwell Publishing Ltd.

therefore needs to make every effort to reassure the patient and allay any feelings of anxiety.

- The patient should be seated in a comfortable, upright position in the dental chair.
- External stimuli should be reduced to a minimum, as disturbing noises, or a bright light shining in the patient's eyes, are likely to increase activity of the mandibular musculature and thus reduce the rest vertical dimension.
- Relaxation may be further promoted if the patient's eyes are closed, although it is important that the clinician explains what is to be done at the time, otherwise this exercise may achieve quite the opposite effect and induce a state of apprehension.
- Some patients are helped if they are asked to swallow, lick their lips, or make the sound 'm' before trying to relax the mandible.

Before measuring the rest vertical dimension, the clinician must be satisfied that the patient is truly relaxed. Visual assessment of facial features and proportions assists the clinician in judging the progressive development of this state of mind. It is pointless making a measurement if the patient appears tense, or if the lower third of the face is clearly reduced or increased in height.

The rest vertical dimension is measured as the distance between two selected points, one related to the upper jaw and one to the lower jaw. Two methods are commonly used to make this measurement, the Willis gauge and the 'two-dot' technique (Fig. 11.1). It is most important to appreciate the inherent inaccuracies of both measuring methods. As a general rule, it is advisable to repeat measurements of the rest vertical dimension on several occasions during the appointment. This gives the clinician an idea of the reproducibility and reliability of the recordings. Above all, it should be borne in mind that all clinical methods of measuring the rest vertical dimension are based to a greater

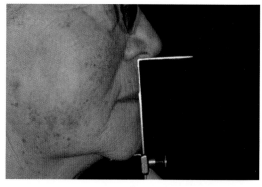

a

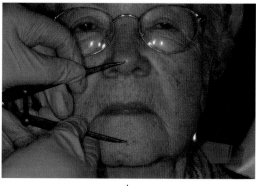

b

Figure 11.1   Two methods of measuring the rest vertical dimension and the occlusal vertical dimension. (a) The Willis gauge. (b) The two-dot technique; the distance between the dots is measured with a pair of dividers.

or lesser extent on what is in reality intelligent guesswork.

The Willis gauge

In the case of the Willis gauge, three points require attention to minimise the potential errors of this technique.

The position of the fixed arm under the nose

If the patient has a well-defined naso-labial angle, the fixed arm can be positioned with

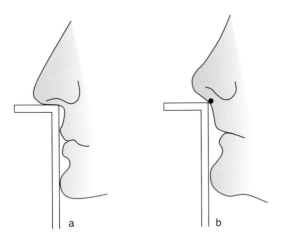

Figure 11.2 (a) The shape of the naso-labial angle allows the fixed arm of the Willis gauge to be located accurately. (b) A location mark may be used where the naso-labial angle is obtuse.

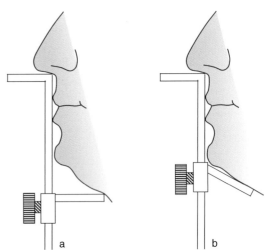

Figure 11.3 (a) The shape of the chin prevents positive location of the sliding arm of the Willis gauge. (b) Sliding arm modified to allow more accurate positioning.

reasonable accuracy. However, if the naso-labial angle is obtuse, positioning of the gauge becomes less precise. Under these circumstances it helps if a small mark is made on the skin at the angle so that the fixed arm can be positioned in relation to it (Fig. 11.2).

The position of the sliding arm under the chin

The sliding arm should be moved so that it only just touches the under-surface of the chin, because if pressure is applied to the sub-mental tissues by the gauge, errors will result from the mandible being pushed upwards. Also, the tissues will be compressed by an amount that will be impossible to reproduce consistently on subsequent measurements. Further inaccuracies may arise if the shape of the chin is such that it prevents positive location of the sliding arm. However, this difficulty can be avoided by modifying the gauge to reduce the length of the arm and to alter its angle (Fig. 11.3).

The vertical orientation of the gauge

The vertical orientation of the gauge should be such that it makes contact with the face both

above and below the lips. The handle contacts the upper lip under the nose and also contacts the chin in the mental region, so that its long axis is in line with the long axis of the face. This keeps any variation in vertical orientation of the gauge to a minimum during successive measurements (Fig. 11.4). However, consistent orientation of the gauge is difficult to achieve with facial profiles associated with full lips or a severe skeletal class II jaw relationship, because the handle of the gauge cannot be placed in contact with the chin.

The two-dot technique

When the two-dot technique is used, the dot related to the upper jaw is best placed on the tip of the nose and not on the upper lip because the latter is too mobile to provide a reliable location. The rest vertical dimension is then measured using dividers. This technique has been shown to be particularly subject to error. The cause is usually movement of the dot on the chin due to an inability by the patient to thoroughly relax the muscles of facial expression.

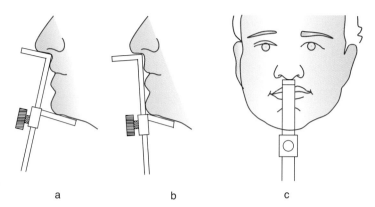

Figure 11.4 (a) Incorrect; (b) and (c) correct positioning and orientation of the Willis gauge.

a   b   c

A particular complication is that an increase in occlusal vertical dimension will not necessarily be associated with a corresponding increase in the distance between the dots because, as the mandible moves down away from the maxilla, there is a tendency for the patient to try to maintain a lip seal. The effort by the circum-oral musculature needed to keep the lips together pulls the dot on the chin upwards.

However, in spite of these limitations, the technique remains a useful one to have in reserve for certain types of facial profile and for bearded patients for whom consistent positioning of the Willis gauge may be difficult or impossible.

The post-dam

Before discussing the construction of record blocks, it is helpful to consider a related subject, the post-dam.

The physical forces of retention are created and maintained in the sulci by a valve-like seal between the flange of the denture and the mucosa. Obviously, this kind of seal cannot be produced along the posterior border of the upper denture as it crosses the palate and so it has to be completed by other means.

To obtain this posterior seal, either a groove is cut into the palate of the master cast, or the mucosa in this area is compressed during impression taking so that when the permanent denture base is processed a raised lip is created on its impression surface. This projection, the post-dam, compresses the palatal mucosa once the denture is placed in the mouth and thus creates a border seal. At the same time, the polished surface of the denture can be bevelled in this region so that the edge of the denture is not so noticeable to the patient's tongue (Fig. 11.5).

When cutting the post-dam it should normally be completed at the appointment for recording the jaw relationship so that the post-dam will be incorporated into the trial denture. However, when problems with retention of the

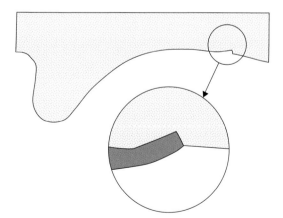

Figure 11.5 The post-dam region of an upper denture. Inset: the bevelled polished surface allows the denture to merge with the mucosa.

upper record blocks are anticipated, it is advantageous to have a post-dam on the upper record block. In such cases the post-dam will need to be prepared on the master cast before the record block is constructed.

It is the clinician, rather than the dental technician, who should be responsible for creating the post-dam because only the clinician can make the essential clinical assessments regarding its position and depth.

The position of the post-dam

The orthodox position of the post-dam is at the junction of the moving tissues of the soft palate and the static tissues of the hard palate anteriorly (Fig. 11.3). It should extend laterally to the mucosa overlying the hamular notches. If the border of the denture is taken further posteriorly, the patient may well complain of nausea. Furthermore, the continual movement of the soft palate in relation to the posterior border of the denture will repeatedly break the seal and is likely to result in inflammation and even ulceration of the mucosa. If the post-dam is placed anteriorly to the junction, it terminates on relatively incompressible tissue. It is then impossible to achieve a reasonable depth to the post-dam and, as a result, the seal is less efficient.

The depth of the post-dam

The depth to which a post-dam can be cut depends upon the compressibility of the mucosa and this varies across the palate. For example, the mucosa in the midline of the palate is bound tightly to the underlying periosteum, while laterally the presence of a submucosa gives rise to much greater compressibility. Such variation is detected clinically by palpation and the depth of the post-dam is modified accordingly.

The record blocks

It is essential that the wax record rims should be placed on well-fitting rigid bases. A non-rigid wax base is likely to change shape during the recording procedure and thus prevent accurate location both in the mouth and subsequently on the casts.

Suitable materials for the bases are:

- Light-curing acrylic resin
- Heat-curing acrylic resin
- Shellac

Aspects of the advantages and disadvantages of the materials compared in Table 11.1 are discussed below:

Table 11.1   A comparison of materials used in the construction of bases for record rims.

	Rigidity	Ease of manufacture	Retention	Ease of modification
Light-curing acrylic resin				
Heat-curing acrylic resin				
Shellac				
KEY	Good	Satisfactory		

Rigidity and strength

Although both types of acrylic resin are more rigid than shellac, the latter material is rigid enough to use as a base for upper blocks. However, where the lower ridge is narrow in cross-sectional shellac is unreliable as it may easily deform or fracture in use.

Ease of manufacture

Light-curing acrylic is the quickest and easiest of the materials for the dental technician to use.

Accuracy of fit

Heat-curing acrylic resin bases provide the best fit and allow maximum retention to be established. Thus, when the rims have been carved to their final shape, it should be possible to engage the patient in conversation without the blocks becoming dislodged. Observing a patient talking is of immense value in judging the occlusal vertical dimension, as discussed in 'Adjusting the lower record rim' later in this chapter.

A heat-curing acrylic base can be particularly valuable when the prognosis for retention in the upper jaw is very poor. It helps to first try the denture base in the mouth alone. Any perfecting of the extension of the base can then be completed and a baseline estimate of retention obtained. The wax rim can then be added. If the retention is significantly reduced the most obvious cause is that the superstructure of the rim is not in muscle balance and must therefore be modified.

Ease of modification

Before positioning a post-dam the clinician needs to be confident about the patient's tolerance to that degree of posterior extension. Where there is uncertainty about tolerance the use of a shellac base allows the base extension to be modified easily at the chairside.

Where the inter-ridge distance is small the thinness and adjustability of a shellac base can make life easier for both the clinician, when recording the jaw relationship, and the dental technician, when setting up the teeth for the trial denture.

It will be appreciated that the matters just discussed need to be considered immediately after the master impressions have been taken, as they will influence the prescription for the material to be used by the dental technician to construct the record blocks.

Adjusting the upper record rim

Before starting any adjustment, upper and lower record blocks should be placed in the mouth in turn and checked for stability, retention, extension and comfort. It is important to appreciate that a loose or uncomfortable record block will almost certainly disturb normal mandibular movement and invoke such a feeling of insecurity in the patient that the essential relaxation is not achieved and is perhaps the strongest reason for suggesting the use of 'permanent' acrylic bases. If there are problems with any of these aspects it is essential that corrections are carried out before proceeding any further.

There are two basic objectives when adjusting the upper record rim:

- To establish the correct orientation and level of the occlusal plane.
- To produce the correct shape for the labial, buccal and palatal surfaces.

Although the procedures are described below in sequence, in practice the final form of the record blocks is most often achieved as a result of a coordinated process in which earlier adjustments are reviewed and modified in the light of the results of later adjustments.

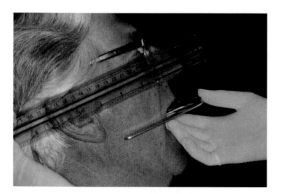

Figure 11.6 A Fox's occlusal plane indicator; the intra-oral portion is held against the occlusal surface of the upper record block; the extra-oral extension allows the clinician to judge the orientation of the occlusal plane with the interpupillary line and with the ala-tragal line. The latter line is indicated by the ruler held against the patient's face.

Establishing the orientation of the occlusal plane

The orientation of the occlusal plane of the upper rim is conveniently judged by using a Fox's occlusal plane indicator (Fig. 11.6) or a disposable wooden tongue spatula. The intra-oral part of the instrument rests on the occlusal surface of the record rim while the extra-oral extension allows the clinician to judge the relationship of the plane to the facial guidelines.

Adjustment in the coronal plane

The rim is adjusted so that the occlusal plane is parallel to the interpupillary line, or alternatively, at right angles to the long axis of the patient's face. Failure to follow these guidelines, which ensure that the occlusal plane appears horizontal in relation to the general symmetry of the face, will result in an unsightly, lopsided appearance of the finished dentures.

Adjustment in the sagittal plane

A useful guideline for sagittal orientation of the occlusal plane is the ala-tragal line, an imaginary line joining the lower border of the ala of the nose with the midpoint of the tragus of the ear, to which the occlusal plane is made parallel (Fig. 11.6). Failure to conform to this guideline is likely to detract from the aesthetic result. It can also have adverse consequences for stability; for example, if the occlusal plane on the lower denture is tilted up posteriorly it may become so high that the denture is displaced by the tongue rather than being controlled by it.

Establishing the level of the occlusal plane

The incisal level of the upper rim is related to the upper lip, but it is impossible to describe hard and fast rules for determining this relationship. For example, whereas a patient with a long upper lip may show very little of the upper teeth during normal function, the patient with a short upper lip is likely to display more of the teeth. For those patients who don't have existing dentures, a baseline from which to start is to modify the incisal edge so that it is just visible when the lip is at rest. As the rim is then either reduced or added to, errors in appearance are easy enough to identify. It is important, as part of this assessment, to look at the relationship of the rim to the lip during function by getting the patient to smile and say a few words whilst wearing the record block. The eventual answer comes as the result of trial and error and by exercising a little visual common sense.

Correct shaping of the labial, buccal and palatal surfaces of the wax rim

Shaping the labial surface

Adequate lip support depends upon the position and inclination of the labial face of the wax rim. The biometric guides mentioned in Chapter 10 can help in achieving the correct shape. For example, the incisal edges of the upper central incisors can be placed up to 1 cm in front

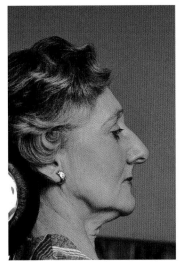 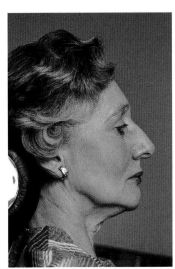

Figure 11.7 (a) An upper record block providing inadequate support to the upper lip – the naso-labial angle is obtuse. (b) Addition of wax to the labial face of the upper record block providing more support for the upper lip – the naso-labial angle is 90°.

a

b

of the centre of the incisive papilla to compensate for the resorption of the alveolar ridge. Another useful guide is the naso-labial angle. A study of dentate adults (Brunton & McCord 1993) suggests that if the angle is within the range 102°–116° the upper lip is adequately supported by the record block (Fig. 11.7). It is essential that the position of the labial surface of the rim is compatible with the stability of the record block. The further forward the rim the greater will be the displacing force of the lip muscles acting on the labial surface. Also, it should be remembered that the displacing force occurring on incising food when the finished denture is worn will also be increased. If the prognosis for retention of the upper denture is unfavourable as a result of extensive post-extraction resorption of bone, it may be necessary to effect a compromise between function and appearance by positioning the rim further palatally if this gives greater stability.

Shaping the buccal surface

The record rim posteriorly should be shaped so that it fills the buccal sulcus and slightly dis-places the buccal mucosa laterally as shown for the denture in Fig. 11.10. This will contribute to retention by achieving an efficient facial seal. The rim itself will usually be buccal to the crest of the ridge by an amount proportional to the amount of resorption that has occurred. Reference to the biometric guides (Chapter 10) will help to identify an appropriate position. However, care should be taken not to place the rim too far buccally, as it will then be outside the neutral zone and increased force from the buccinator muscle will cause displacement. The buccal and palatal surfaces of the rim should be shaped to converge occlusally so that pressure from the cheeks and tongue has a resultant force towards the ridge, thus aiding neuromuscular control.

Shaping the palatal surface

It is essential to create adequate space for the tongue by ensuring that the rim is not placed too far lingually and by reducing the width of the rim where necessary by removing wax from the palatal aspect until it corresponds to the width of the artificial teeth which will replace it.

If the record block is too bulky, the constriction of the tongue and the resulting abnormal sensory feedback is likely to influence mandibular posture and so lead to inaccuracies in recording the jaw relationship. In addition, speech quality, which can be most valuable in confirming the accuracy of jaw relationship recordings, can only make a contribution to this assessment if the dimensions of the rims are similar to those of the eventual dentures.

Adjusting the lower record rim

The adjustment of the lower rim may be considered to have three aspects, as discussed in the following.

Adjusting the height of the rim to the required occlusal vertical dimension

The orientation of the occlusal plane has already been established on the upper rim, while the overall height of the lower rim will be governed by the existing height of the upper and the need to fit both into the required occlusal vertical dimension. However, the clinician should be prepared to modify the upper occlusal plane further if problems arise when shaping the lower one. For example, if it becomes increasingly apparent that the lower rim is going to be so high that stability will be poor, or so low that there will be no room for the teeth, then appropriate modifications must be carried out on the upper block.

Shaping the labial, buccal and lingual surfaces to conform to the neutral zone

These surfaces of the rim are shaped to accommodate the surrounding musculature, because the lower rim will be unstable until it is positioned in the neutral zone. First, it is necessary to adjust the buccal and labial surfaces of the

rim so that they lie close to, but do not displace, the cheek and lip mucosa. Second, it is vital to allow adequate tongue space by carving the rim on the lingual side so that it is of a width similar to the denture teeth that will eventually replace it. Failure to adequately carve the lower rim to the neutral zone is a common error resulting in instability, inaccurate recording of the jaw relationship and an incomplete prescription for the dental technician.

When judging the relationship of the rim to the neutral zone, it is important that the tongue takes up a normal resting position forwards in the mouth with the tip contacting the lingual surface of the rim anteriorly. This may be difficult to achieve clinically because as soon as the tongue is mentioned to the patient there is a tendency for it to take on a 'life of its own'. Occasionally, the tongue is drawn towards the back of the mouth to adopt a posture which has been aptly described as a 'defensive tongue'. This is probably the result of a subconscious wish to guard the pharynx against the foreign body in the mouth. It is impossible to achieve muscular balance with such tongue behaviour and therefore it is necessary to coax the patient to position the tongue in a more anterior position before the stability of the record block can be assessed adequately.

Re-assessment of the occlusal vertical dimension

Having largely completed the adjustment of the record blocks, it is vital to undertake a re-assessment of their occlusal vertical dimension before finalising the recording of the jaw relationship. This is achieved by the following:

- *Measuring the rest vertical dimension.* Reference was made on pp. 72–73 to the increase in the rest vertical dimension that takes place when a lower denture is inserted into the mouth. The observation is of particular significance at the stage now reached. Once the lower rim has been adjusted to the oral musculature and its shape and size are judged to be comparable to the new denture which will eventually replace it, the recording of the rest vertical dimension must be re-checked with the lower block in situ. If, as is likely, the rest vertical dimension is found to have increased, the new reading should be used to re-calculate the occlusal vertical dimension. The record blocks are then adjusted accordingly.

- *Assessment of facial proportion.* With the record blocks in occlusion the clinician should make a judgement as to whether the facial proportions look correct, or whether the lower third of the face appears too long (excessive occlusal vertical dimension), or too short (reduced occlusal vertical dimension). Noting other facial features such as creases at the corner of the mouth, loss of red margin of the lips, incompetence of the lips and degree of mandibular protrusion will also provide clues to help in this assessment. With increasing clinical experience it is not unusual for a clinician to rely more and more on an assessment of facial appearance rather than direct measurement to decide whether or not a satisfactory occlusal vertical dimension has been produced.
- *Assessing speech with the record blocks in situ.* If the record rims have been constructed on well-fitting, stable bases and have been shaped correctly it should be possible to engage the patient in conversation. Frequent contact of the rims during speech indicates that the occlusal vertical dimension is excessive. On the other hand, if the patient can talk without making such contacts, the closest speaking distance has not been obliterated and the clinician has obtained additional valuable evidence that the occlusal vertical dimension is not too great.
- *Reference to previous dentures.* Where previous dentures exist the patient's experience with them will often provide clues as to whether their occlusal vertical dimension is satisfactory or not (Chapter 8). Depending upon the

findings, the occlusal vertical dimension of the record blocks can be adjusted to copy or modify the freeway space of these dentures.

If the patient has no existing dentures to which one can refer to for additional information, it is acceptable to initially establish the occlusal vertical dimension approximately 3 mm less than the rest vertical dimension. The freeway space so produced is satisfactory for the vast majority of patients. However, this should then be re-evaluated having observed speech and facial appearance.

Recording the retruded jaw relationship

The next stage is to establish even occlusal contact between the record rims at the chosen vertical dimension with the mandible in the retruded position.

Preparation of the patient

Every effort is made to get the patient to relax so that jaw muscle activity is reduced as much as possible. By adopting a relaxed manner, by gently guiding the mandible and by giving instructions such as, 'close together on your back teeth', the clinician is most likely to encourage the mandible to fall back into its retruded position. An additional procedure which may be of help in obtaining the retruded position is to ask the patient to curl the tongue to the back of the mouth and to touch the posterior border of the upper record block while closing. The patient may be assisted in this by placing a small blob of wax in the centre of the posterior border to act as a 'target' for the tongue so that the patient will be aware of when it is in the correct position. Whatever technique is used, it is wise to get the patient to close from an open position of around 1 cm only as the condyle will be more easily located in the glenoid fossa and closure will be a rotational rather than a translational movement

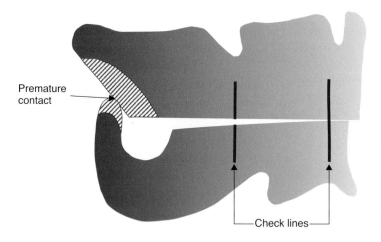

Premature contact

Check lines

Figure 11.8 Record blocks located extra-orally by using check lines showing premature contact between the bases posteriorly. The shaded areas indicate where wax can be removed from the bases to eliminate the premature contact.

Preliminary recording

Initially, in order to make large adjustments to a lower rim, the occlusal surface of the rim should be thoroughly softened and the patient asked to close together. Closure is stopped when the occlusal vertical dimension appears to be correct. However, as a means of making the final recording of the retruded position, this method is fraught with danger. Unless the patient is able to close into a surface of uniform softness, there is every chance that contact on a harder portion of wax will create an error in the recording by causing uneven compression of the underlying mucosa and effectively causing the record blocks to tip. In addition, contact on the harder wax is likely to result in an abnormal path of closure. It is necessary therefore to separate the two rims after chilling and cut away the excess wax that has been squeezed out. The record blocks are then reinserted and even occlusion is checked by asking the patient to close very gently into initial contact.

After any necessary corrections have been carried out, three check lines are drawn with a wax knife from one rim to the other, one in the midline and one either side in the premolar regions. These lines enable the blocks to be located outside the mouth to establish whether there is any premature contact on the posterior

aspects of the rims or bases (Fig. 11.8). In addition, the check lines allow the clinician to judge whether the patient continues to close in a consistent manner.

The patient may be further encouraged at this stage to make contact in the retruded position by reducing the height of the lower rim anteriorly by about 1 mm so that the rims occlude only in the premolar and molar regions (Fig. 11.9)

Definitive recording

Before the rims are finally located together, it is wise to consider five basic questions:

1. Are the rims stable?
2. Is there adequate freeway space?
3. Has a consistent retruded jaw relationship been established?
4. Is there even occlusal contact?
5. With the rims in the mouth and the lips brought together, is there a pleasing appearance?

Bearing in mind that the record rims are the blueprint for the eventual dentures, if any fault is left uncorrected at this stage, it will re-appear on the trial dentures.

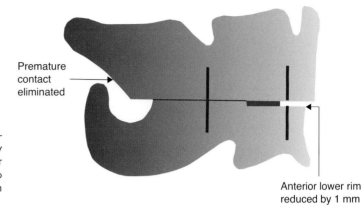

Premature
contact
eliminated

Anterior lower rim
reduced by 1 mm

Figure 11.9 The premature contact between the bases posteriorly has been eliminated and the lower rim has been reduced in height to encourage the patient to occlude in the retruded position.

For the definitive recording it is advisable to use a recording medium which initially is of low viscosity, thus offering little resistance to closure of the jaws, but which subsequently hardens sufficiently not to be distorted when the casts are mounted on the articulator. Suitable materials include a zinc oxide-eugenol occlusal registration paste, silicone registration paste, impression plaster and a wax containing fine metal particles.

The clinical procedure is as follows:

- Two locating notches are cut into the occlusal surface of the upper rim, one either side of the arch in the premolar areas.
- If a zinc oxide-eugenol paste is being used the occlusal surface of the upper rim is coated with a thin film of petroleum jelly which acts as a separating medium. If using a silicone registration paste this step is not required, but additional notches should be placed in the lower rim to allow accurate localisation.
- The registration medium is applied to the premolar and molar regions of the lower rim and the patient is guided into the retruded position. The patient must keep the mandible absolutely still until the registration medium has set – a requirement that can be a problem for older patients.

An alternative technique

An alternative, very rapid method for recording the jaw relationship is to start by reducing the lower rim to two occlusal pillars about 1 cm in length in the second premolar region. These pillars can be adjusted quickly by softening or adding wax to achieve balanced occlusal contact in the retruded jaw relation at the appropriate occlusal vertical dimension. The missing sections of the lower rim are then reconstructed by placing impression plaster into the spaces with a spatula and getting the patient to close into the plaster until the wax pillars occlude with the upper rim (Fig. 11.10). This particular technique has the advantage that the clinician has only two small areas of wax to adjust in order to establish even occlusal contact. As the contact is restricted to the premolar/molar region it encourages the patient to close in the retruded jaw relationship and also helps to stabilise the lower record block.

Having recorded the jaw relationship, the following questions need to be answered:

- Is a palatal relief chamber required, and if so what is its location and extent?
- What artificial teeth are appropriate?

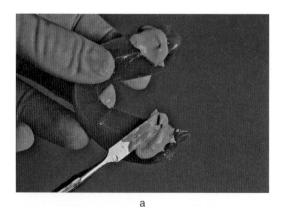

a

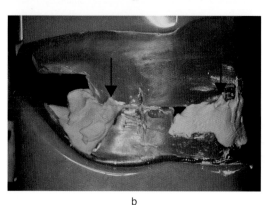

b

Figure 11.10 (a) Lower record block with occlusal contact area restricted to the premolar areas. Impression plaster is being applied to fill the spaces posteriorly. (b) Completed registration. Note that the impression plaster has filled locating notches (arrows) cut into the upper rim.

Palatal relief

If a relief chamber is required but has not been prescribed at the master impression stage then it should be done here. Very occasionally, when the upper denture-bearing tissues are palpated, the mucosa covering the ridge will be found to be more compressible than the mucosa in the middle of the palate. If an impression records these tissues in an undistorted state and a denture is constructed on the resulting cast then, when the denture is fitted, the compressible ridges will offer less support than the centre of

the palate. As a result, occlusal contact will result in pivoting and flexing of the denture about the midline. Initially, this pivoting may cause loss of border seal or inflammation of the mucosa. Over a longer period of time, the continual flexing of the denture is likely to produce fatigue of the acrylic resin resulting in a midline fracture (p. 246).

There are two ways of avoiding these problems. A more viscous impression material may be used for the master impression so that the shape of the tissues over the ridge is recorded in a compressed state. Alternatively, if a less viscous impression material is used, a sheet of tin foil, trimmed to correspond to the area of incompressible mucosa, may be cemented to the resulting cast in the midline so that when the denture is processed, a relief chamber is created. That part of the denture base overlying the incompressible midline will stand away from the mucosal surface and will only contact the tissues when the ridge mucosa is compressed.

As the authors favour an impression technique which records the shape of the mucosa with minimal distortion, for reasons discussed on p. 146, they prefer to use relief as a means of overcoming the problem of varying compressibility. However, this approach has its drawback because air may be trapped in the relief chamber, so potentially reducing the physical forces of retention. For this reason, it is important that relief is provided only when positively indicated. For example, although a palatine torus might be present, there is no need to provide a palatal relief over it unless the covering mucosa is found to be less compressible than that over the ridges.

The decision as to whether to provide a relief is the responsibility of the clinician, not the dental technician. If the clinical situation warrants a palatal relief, the size and shape of the area requiring it should be identified by palpation. The corresponding area on the cast is then outlined as a guide to the dental technician when laying down the tin foil of appropriate thickness. If a heat-cured acrylic base is to be used for the upper record block, a decision on palatal relief must be made after the working impression has been taken. If a palatal relief is required the relevant area can be marked on the impression with an indelible pencil. This mark is transferred to the master cast and acts as a guide to the laying down of the tin foil before the permanent base is constructed.

It should be said that the occasions when relief is not needed far exceed the occasions when it is required.

Choice of teeth

The information required to produce a pleasing and natural appearance for complete dentures includes the following:

- Incisal level
- Amount of lip support provided by the anterior teeth and labial flange
- Occlusal vertical dimension
- Colour, shape, size and material of the artificial teeth
- Arrangement of the artificial teeth

Incisal level, lip support and occlusal vertical dimension are indicated by the shape of the adjusted record rims as discussed previously. A decision on the colour, shape, size and material of the teeth must now be made. With this information, the technician is able to produce a basic set-up for the trial dentures. The final stage in refining the appearance, creating the detailed arrangement of the anterior teeth within the dental arch, is completed on the trial dentures at the chairside as discussed in Chapter 13.

The comments which follow, with the exception of those concerned with the choice of material of the denture teeth, are concerned primarily with the selection of anterior rather than posterior teeth.

Colour of teeth

An appropriate colour of artificial tooth is selected from a shade guide. When making the choice, it is advisable to moisten the teeth with water and hold them just inside the patient's open mouth. Care should be taken to avoid letting the patient view the teeth against a light background such as pale clothing. Under such conditions the shade will appear darker than it will when the denture is eventually in the mouth. As a result, the patient is likely to choose a shade that is too light; indeed for this reason alone, there is a lot to say in favour of the patient seeing the teeth against a dark background when viewing them out of the mouth.

It is, of course, important that a decision on colour should be influenced by the patient's comments and by the patient's opinion of previous dentures. However, as it is often difficult for the patient to forecast the final result from the appearance of one tooth positioned in the mouth, the clinician should offer guidance on the colour that is likely to be most suitable.

It is not possible to provide hard and fast rules on choice of colour in view of the variation in the natural dentition. However, the following comments are offered as useful guidelines:

- Natural teeth tend to become darker with increasing age. Therefore, it is appropriate to choose a shade of denture tooth which is in keeping with the patient's age.
- A more natural appearance is likely to be obtained if people with dark complexions are provided with darker teeth, while those with paler complexions are given lighter teeth.

Shape and size of teeth

Because of the enormous variation found in the natural dentition, it is possible to offer only very general guidelines for choosing the shape and size of artificial teeth.

Shape

Age, sex and personality

Over the years several papers have offered guidance on the choice and arrangement of artificial teeth to reflect the sex, age and personality of the patient (Chapter 13). As a generalisation, it has been stated that masculinity is associated with 'vigour, boldness and hardness' while femininity, in contrast, is described in terms of 'roundness, softness and smoothness'. Whereas larger and more angular tooth shapes indicate strength and masculinity, a delicate and more feminine impression is created by moulds that have curved outlines and are somewhat smaller. There is only limited hard evidence to suggest that these stereotypes are genetically derived and probably owe more to years of social conditioning. Anterior denture teeth can and probably should be made to reflect advancing years by introducing incisal grinding to simulate tooth wear.

Facial morphology

One cannot state categorically that patients with large faces and strong features have large teeth, or vice versa, because jaw size and tooth size have different genetic origins (which is a primary reason for the need for orthodontists). Nevertheless, when choosing artificial replacements in the absence of any other information, a large tooth mould is usually appropriate for those patients with a heavier skeletal makeup, and vice versa.

A further suggestion that has been made is that the shape of the upper anterior teeth should complement the shape of the patient's face. Three basic facial shapes have been described – square, ovoid and tapering – and corresponding tooth moulds have been produced which are an inverted version of these shapes.

A recent review of the literature (Sellen et al. 1999) concluded that there was no scientific basis for any of these proposals. Nevertheless these guidelines are worth bearing in mind on purely aesthetic grounds when selecting denture teeth, as their application can increase the chance of creating dentures which harmonise with the patient's facial appearance.

Size

Crown width

It is possible to use photographs of the patient (taken when still dentate) to calculate the width of the central incisor by measuring the width of that tooth and the interpupillary distance on the photograph and the interpupillary distance on the patient and then substituting the values in the following equation:

$$\text{Calculated width of incisor} = \frac{\text{photographic width of incisor} \times \text{actual PD}}{\text{photographic PD}}$$

where PD is the interpupillary distance. It has been shown that this technique is of proven value only if the pre-extraction photograph is a full-face portrait and of sufficient size, approximately 13 cm × 18 cm (Bindra et al. 2001).

Two further suggestions are offered as guidance when choosing the width of the anterior teeth:

1. The combined width of the two central incisors is frequently similar to the width of the philtrum of the upper lip (Fig. 11.11).
2. The projection of a line drawn from the inner canthus of the eye to the ala of the nose passes through the upper canine tooth (Fig. 11.11). These lines can be scribed onto the correctly contoured record block and then a flexible ruler curved around the labial surface of the rim to measure the distance between the lines. Tooth moulds which will fit into this distance can be identified from a chart.

Crown length

The crown length of the upper artificial teeth is indicated by the distance between inferior and superior reference points:

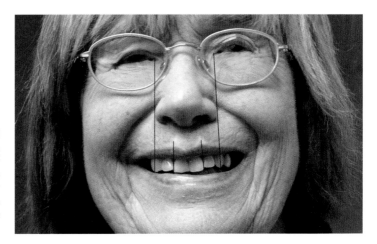

Figure 11.11 The combined width of the two central incisors tends to be similar to the width of the philtrum of the upper lip. The projection of a line from the inner canthus of the eye to the ala of the nose passes through the tip of the upper canine tooth.

1. The inferior reference point is the incisal level of the recording rim that has been carved to produce an appropriate relationship to the upper lip.
2. The superior reference point is the level to which the upper lip is raised on smiling. The further the necks of the teeth are placed below this 'smile line' the more gum will be shown when smiling. If an excessive amount of gum is displayed this can appear unsightly.

Mould guides

The choice of mould for the upper anterior teeth can be made from actual samples of moulds available, or from a printed mould guide. If the clinician has a selection of upper tooth moulds set in conventional tooth arrangements, they can be positioned inside the upper lip. It is preferable to use only half the anterior segment so that the set-up can be rotated in the mouth to follow the shape of the dental arch (Fig. 11.12). The full complement of anterior teeth may be so unlike the shape of the dental arch that the appearance resembles the teeth found in a Christmas cracker and thus offers little guidance to the clinician and even less to the patient.

Tooth arrangement

Patient history

Having recorded the information on colour and shape of the artificial teeth, it is advisable to ask patients if they remember any particular characteristic in the arrangement of the natural teeth which they would like to be included in the artificial set-up. For example, if a request is made to reproduce a fondly remembered median diastema or imbricated incisors this can be passed to the dental technician for inclusion in the trial

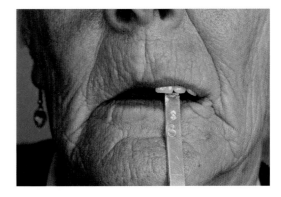

Figure 11.12 Choosing the mould for the anterior teeth. More guidance on the width of the teeth can be gained from trying in three anterior teeth only rather than a set-up of all six whose arch shape may be quite inappropriate for the patient.

dentures. However, it is commonly found that this line of questioning is of limited help. So often, patients remember only gross irregularities, which in any case they want modified in the artificial dentition.

Pre-extraction records

Most of the process of tooth selection and arrangement is a matter of inspired, creative guesswork helped by applying principles of proven clinical value. The uncertainty of this approach underlines the value of pre-extraction records, such as good-quality photographs, notes and dental casts. Immediate dentures are also an excellent way of transferring the desirable features of the natural dentition to the artificial one. Whenever possible, records such as these should be included in the decision-making process.

Tooth material – a comparison of acrylic and porcelain teeth

As consideration should be given as to whether acrylic or porcelain teeth should be used, it is appropriate to consider their respective qualities at this stage. However, it should be pointed out that very few porcelain teeth are used nowadays.

Appearance

A very satisfactory appearance can be obtained from both good-quality acrylic and porcelain teeth. In the manufacture of both types of teeth, it is possible to produce a satisfactory gradation of colour throughout the length of the crown and to introduce striations and stains to mimic the imperfections of natural teeth. However, the acrylic tooth may deteriorate more rapidly in some patients' mouths because of its lower resistance to wear.

Attachment to the denture base

The attachment of acrylic teeth to the denture base is by chemical union, while porcelain teeth are retained by means of pins or holes. Under normal circumstances, both methods work perfectly satisfactorily. However, in cases where the inter-ridge distance is small, it may be necessary to reduce the length of the tooth so much that, in the case of porcelain, the retentive element is removed. Under these circumstances acrylic teeth must be used. As a denture cools following processing, the denture base polymer contracts 20 times more than porcelain. This means that around the necks of porcelain teeth, where contraction is restricted, areas of strain are set up, which reduce the resistance of the polymer to fracture.

Transmission of masticatory forces

Porcelain teeth transmit a greater proportion of the masticatory forces to the underlying mucosa. This is because of the widely differing values in the modulus of elasticity of the two materials, that for porcelain being about nine times greater than the value for acrylic resin. Thus, the use of porcelain teeth can be a disadvantage in those patients whose denture-bearing tissues are less able to tolerate the higher forces.

Response to function

Noise
As porcelain teeth are approximately ten times harder than acrylic teeth they can make more noise on contact. In spite of this, as only a small percentage of patients complain of noise from porcelain teeth, it is a point of little importance. Possible reasons for this are that during mastication, a layer of food separates the two occluding surfaces for much of the time, and before the teeth eventually make contact there is always a deceleration of the mandible which limits the force on impact. In addition, during speech the teeth do not come into contact with each other at all provided an adequate freeway space has been provided.

Resistance to chipping
As acrylic resin has a lower modulus of elasticity than porcelain, it will absorb much more

energy before fracturing; thus, a sudden impact is more likely to chip porcelain teeth.

Occlusal wear

The resistance of the two materials to occlusal wear is perhaps the most significant difference between the two types of teeth from a clinical standpoint. As porcelain teeth are so much harder, their occlusal surfaces wear out only very slowly. Thus, the established jaw relationship in both horizontal and vertical planes is maintained for longer. Some people believe that the more rapid wear of acrylic teeth allows the patient to 'grind in' a personal occlusal pattern. This may be a justifiable view in the early stages of wear. However, further deterioration of the occlusal surfaces leads to irregular occlusal contact and loss of the original jaw relationship. Another argument put forward in favour of acrylic teeth is that the masticatory forces wear the teeth away rather than cause resorption of the underlying bone. However, anything more than minimal occlusal wear can result in an unbalanced occlusion which is itself a potent cause of resorption.

Obtaining balanced occlusal contact during function

The remainder of this chapter deals with the important topic of the relevance of balanced occlusion and the role played by the articulator. But first, it may be of help to the reader to have an understanding of a few definitions.

Definition of terms

Balanced occlusion

Balanced occlusion is present when there are simultaneous contacts between opposing artificial teeth on both sides of the dental arches. This term describes a static situation and applies when upper and lower dentures meet in any position.

Balanced articulation

Balanced articulation is a dynamic situation in which there are bilateral, simultaneous contacts of opposing teeth in central and eccentric positions as the mandible moves into and away from the intercuspal position.

Working and non-working sides

The working side is that to which the mandible moves, for example, in order to break up a bolus of food. The opposite side of the arch is termed the non-working, or balancing side.

Condylar path

The condylar path (Fig. 11.13) is the route taken by the mandibular condyle as it moves forwards and downwards from the glenoid fossa to the articular eminence.

Condylar angle

The condylar angle (Fig. 11.13) is the angle between the condylar path and the Frankfort plane.

Condylar axis

The condylar axis (Fig. 11.13) is a line between the mandibular condyles close to a hinge axis around which the mandible can rotate without translatory movement.

Advantages of occlusal balance

If occlusal balance exists, the masticatory forces are transmitted as widely as possible over the denture-bearing tissues. Furthermore, the even, bilateral contact positively assists in retaining the dentures. As the patient closes together, bilateral contact actively seats the dentures on the underlying tissues. Occlusal contact on only one side will usually result in either or both dentures tipping with resultant loss of retention. In addition, if the occlusion is unbalanced,

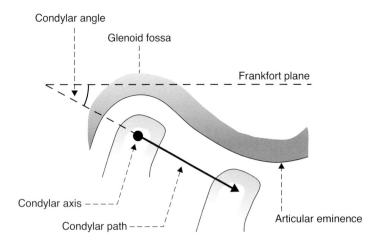

Figure 11.13 Diagrammatic representation of the relationship of the Frankfurt plane, the condylar path and the condylar angle.

the masticatory forces are transmitted initially to a reduced area of tissue. The likely consequences of this are inflammation of the mucosa, discomfort and, ultimately, an increased rate of resorption of the underlying bone.

It is important to make the point that balanced occlusion and articulation are relevant only when the teeth make contact. This situation occurs during the so-called 'empty mouth contacts' while swallowing saliva, clenching or grinding the teeth. During mastication, in the early stages of the chewing process, the bolus is generally too large or too firm for the upper and lower teeth to penetrate fully and to come into contact. Thus, occlusal balance does not operate at this stage, a situation reflected in the old adage, 'Enter bolus, exit balance.' It is only in the later stages of comminution of the bolus that the food is broken down and softened enough for the teeth to contact and for occlusal balance to come into play.

Articulators

If complete dentures are to be constructed with a balanced articulation, the articulator on which they are constructed has to be capable of reproducing certain basic characteristics of the patient, namely:

- The condylar angle
- The relationship of the maxilla to the condylar axis

Examples of three types of articulators commonly used are shown in Fig. 11.14.

The simple hinge articulator

If complete dentures are constructed on a simple hinge articulator, all that can be produced with certainty is balanced occlusion in the position in which the jaw relationship was recorded.

The average-movement articulator

The value for the condylar angle and the relationship of the maxilla to the hinge axis on this type of articulator are fixed to conform to average measurements obtained from many patients. The upper arm can be moved in the horizontal plane; thus, on the articulator the technician is able to simulate lateral and protrusive movements of the mandible and check that the arrangement of the artificial teeth provides a balanced articulation.

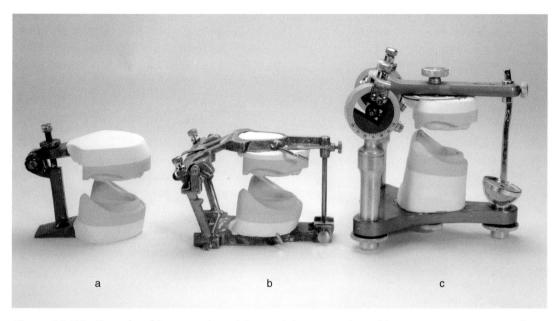

Figure 11.14   Examples of three articulators (a) a simple hinge articulator; (b) an average-movement articulator; and (c) a semi-adjustable articulator.

The semi-adjustable articulator

The semi-adjustable articulator allows the mounting of the casts in the anatomically correct relationship to the condylar axis using a face bow record. Also, by obtaining an interocclusal record of the jaw relationship with the mandible in protrusion the condylar path can be adjusted so that it more closely corresponds to that of the patient. Lateral and protrusive movements of the mandible can therefore be simulated on the articulator, allowing dentures to be constructed with occlusal balance in eccentric positions.

Limitations of articulators

Hinge articulator

In spite of the limitations of the simple hinge articulators, many dentures are made on this instrument and function quite satisfactorily. The likely reason for success is the ability of most patients to adapt to the limitations of the occlusal surface. The patient recognises that certain functional movements cause instability or discomfort and cease to make them. It will, of course, be apparent that such dentures may fail in those patients whose ability to adapt is more restricted.

Semi-adjustable articulator

Although the semi-adjustable articulator is a more complex instrument, there are features of its design which prevent it from reproducing mandibular movement with complete accuracy. For example, when a patient's mandible moves in protrusion, the head of the condyles move downwards, forwards and medially along an articular surface whose shape is a sigmoid curve. In contrast, the condylar spheres of the articulator move forwards, downwards and medially along a straight path. It should also be pointed out that the successful use of this type of articulator is dependent upon the accuracy of the face-bow record and the inter-occlusal record. In this respect it is worth emphasising the point that the accuracy is restricted to a degree by the varying compressibility of the mucosa on which the record rim sits

Average movement articulator

The average-movement articulator may be considered as lying somewhere between the two other instruments. As far as clinical tasks are concerned, it is less complicated to use than the semi-adjustable articulator whilst, at the same time, allowing the dental technician to position artificial teeth in such a way as to produce an articulation that has a level of balance which will satisfy most patients.

Selecting an articulator

Faced with the alternative approaches mentioned above, which articulator is most appropriate for the edentulous patient? Is the sophistication of the semi-adjustable articulator justified for all patients, or can satisfactory results be obtained with the less complicated instruments?

To help answer these questions, it is logical to consider what actually happens to complete dentures during normal function.

The first point to realise is that although a perfectly balanced articulation may be produced on the articulator when the dentures are fixed rigidly to the underlying casts, the situation is likely to be very different in the mouth. Once in the mouth, dentures are placed on a compressible foundation and they inevitably move when occlusal contact is made. Even if the mucosa is firm, there is the possibility of up to 1 mm of movement in the horizontal plane. With increasing compressibility, greater movement will occur.

The stability of complete dentures has received considerable attention in the literature. Research has shown that, during normal function, complete dentures are remarkably unstable. During incision, the posterior border of an upper denture usually drops. When the bolus of food is transferred to the posterior teeth for chewing, the upper denture commonly slides

towards the working side and the balancing side tends to drop. The lower denture is often seen to lift bodily. Muscular control of the dentures comes to the rescue and enables reasonably normal function to be established. This set of circumstances is probably one of the reasons behind the observation that long-term success of dentures does not appear to be related to sophisticated articulator systems (Carlsson 2006). The frequency of occlusal contact increases as the bolus of food is broken down. It appears that most of this contact occurs in the proximity of the retruded position. The results of these experimental observations may now be applied to the clinical situation and the following conclusions drawn and recommendations made.

- Due to the compressibility of the denture foundation and the inevitable movement of the dentures, the apparent precision of the more sophisticated semi-adjustable articulator seems to be superfluous. The use of an average-movement articulator makes for a simpler technique, while at the same time providing the facility to produce a level of balanced articulation that is acceptable for most patients.
- As it appears that functional tooth contact occurs in the region of the retruded position, it is usually sufficient to develop an occlusion which minimises the possibility of imbalance in an area 2–3 mm lateral and anterior to this position.
- In lateral occlusion, there should be contact on the working side and a balancing contact, or contacts, on the opposite side (Fig. 11.15a). It is important to avoid a premature contact or complete lack of contact on the balancing side (Figs. 11.15b and 11.15c).
- In protrusive occlusion, it would seem wise to aim for bilateral balancing contacts on one or more posterior teeth (Fig. 11.15d). It may be more difficult to produce a balancing contact in instances where the anterior tooth arrangement appropriate for the patient necessitates an anterior deep vertical overlap

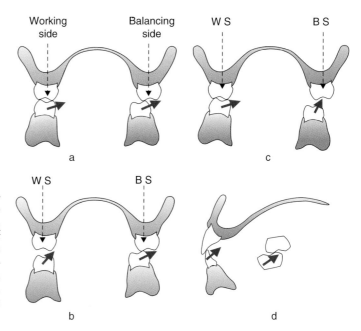

Figure 11.15 (a) Balanced occlusion with contact on the working side (left) and on the balancing side (right). The arrows indicate the direction of movement of the mandible as it returns to the intercuspal position. (b) A premature contact on the balancing side. (c) A premature contact on the working side. (d) Balancing contact on posterior teeth in protrusion.

(Chapter 12). However, within the zone in which balance is advantageous, the problem is frequently solved by a slight reduction in height of the lower incisors.

Selecting posterior teeth

With regard to the choice of posterior teeth, studies into patients' satisfaction and ability to chew tougher foods with cusped or cuspless types have indicated preference for the former (Heydecke et al., 2007; Sutton & McCord, 2007). It has been argued that cuspless teeth are better able to accommodate positional changes of the dentures relative to the supporting tissues brought about by resorption of alveolar bone and that cuspless teeth might be particularly suitable for older patients because an increased variation in occlusal contact positions is characteristic of this group. However, others argue that the positive interdigitation offered by cusped teeth helps to reduce the variation and that this can provide functional benefits for the older patient. If it is considered desirable to create a fully balanced articulation, than cusped teeth will facilitate the task.

Communication with the dental technician

The technician requires a detailed blueprint from which the trial dentures can be constructed. The following information should be included:

- Confirmation that all items sent from the clinic to the laboratory have been disinfected.
- The adjusted record blocks to indicate the following:
  - Jaw relationship
  - Relationship of the teeth to the underlying ridges
  - Arch relationship in both the anterior and posterior regions
  - Overall shape of the dentures

- Location, shape and depth of the post-dam.
- The location, size and shape of palatal relief if required.
- Type of articulator required.
- Face bow and protrusive interocclusal records if required.
- Shade, mould and material of anterior and posterior teeth.
- Any special instructions, e.g. regarding appearance and the setting of anterior teeth.

Quality control and enhancement

The accuracy with which this clinical stage has been accomplished, and how well the information has been transferred from the patient in the dental chair to the dental technician in the laboratory, can be judged at the subsequent stage of trial dentures.

Suggestions for topics that might be investigated in a series of cases include the following:

- In what percentage of cases was the amount of freeway space found to be appropriate and correct?
- In what percentage of cases was even occlusal contact established and a consistent antero-posterior jaw relationship recorded?
- In what percentage of cases did the posterior teeth appear to be positioned correctly in the neutral zone?
- In what percentage of cases had the prescription for the appearance of the anterior teeth been followed satisfactorily?
- In what percentage of cases was the dental technician satisfied with the information provided in the record rims and in the written prescription?

References and additional reading

Bindra, B., Basker, R.M. & Besford, J.S. (2001) A study of the use of photographs for denture tooth selection. *International Journal of Prosthodontics*, 14, 173–7.

Brewer, A.A., Reibel, P.R. & Nassif, N.J. (1967) Comparison of zero degree teeth and anatomic teeth on complete dentures. *Journal of Prosthetic Dentistry*, 17, 28–35.

Brill, N. (1957) Reflexes, registrations, and prosthetic therapy. *Journal of Prosthetic Dentistry*, 7, 341–60.

Brunton, P.A. & McCord, J.F. (1993) An analysis of nasiolabial angles and their relevance to tooth position in the edentulous patient. *European Journal of Prosthodontics and Restorative Dentistry*, 2, 53–6.

Carlsson, G.E. (2006) Facts and fallacies: An evidence base for complete dentures. *Dental Update*, 33, 134–42.

Feldmann, E.E. (1971) Tooth contacts in denture occlusion – centric occlusion only. *Dental Clinics of North America*, 15, 875–87.

Harcourt, J.K. (1974) Accuracy in registration and transfer of prosthetic records. *Australian Dental Journal*, 19, 182–90.

Helkimo, M., Ingervall, B. & Carlsson, G.E. (1973) Comparison of different methods in active and passive recording of the retruded position of the mandible. *Scandinavian Journal of Dental Research*, 81, 265–71.

Heydecke, G., Akkad, A.S., Wolkewitz, M., Vogeler, M., Türp, J.C. & Strub, J.R. (2007) Patient ratings of chewing ability from a randomised crossover trial: lingualised vs. first premolar/canine-guided occlusion for complete dentures. *Gerodontology*, 24, 77–86.

Kobowicz, W.E. & Geering, A.H. (1972) Transfer of maxillomandibular relations to the articulator. In: *International Prosthodontic Workshop on Complete Denture Occlusion* (eds B.R. Lang & C.C. Kelsey). Ann Arbor, Michigan.

McMillan, D.R. & Imber, S. (1968) The accuracy of facial measurements using the Willis bite gauge. *Dental Practitioner and Dental Record*, 18, 213–17.

McMillan, D.R., Barbenel, J.C. & Quinn, D.M. (1969) Measurement of occlusal face height by dividers. *Dental Practitioner and Dental Record*, 20, 177–9.

Nairn, R.L. (1973) Lateral and protrusive occlusions. *Journal of Dentistry*, 1, 181–7.

Preiskel, H.W. (1967) Anteroposterior jaw relations in complete denture construction. *Dental Practitioner and Dental Record*, 18, 39–44.

Sellen, P.N, Jagger, D.C. & Harrison, A. (1999) Methods used to select artificial anterior teeth for the edentulous patient: a historical overview. *International Journal of Prosthodontics*, 12, 51–8.

Sutton, A.F. & McCord, J.F. (2007) A randomized clinical trial comparing anatomic, lingualized, and zero-degree posterior occlusal forms for complete dentures. *Journal of Prosthetic Dentistry,* 97, 292–8.

Tryde, G., McMillan, D.R., Christensen, J. & Brill, N. (1976) The fallacy of facial measurements of occlusal face height in edentulous subjects. *Journal of Oral Rehabilitation,* 3, 353–8.

Yurkstas, A.A. & Kapur, K.K. (1964) Factors influencing centric relation records in edentulous mouths. *Journal of Prosthetic Dentistry,* 14, 1054–65.

Dentures and Muscles 12

Earlier in the book (Chapter 2), mention was made of the importance of the muscular control of dentures. Success in achieving this, as in so many aspects of prosthetic dentistry, is dependent upon the efforts of three people:

(1) *The clinician* – in recognising the importance of muscular control as well as designing and prescribing the shapes of dentures to be compatible with oral function.
(2) *The dental technician* – in also appreciating the importance of muscular control, following the clinician's prescription accurately and translating it into correctly designed dentures.
(3) *The patient* – in literally getting to grips with the final product and, with the clinician's support, persevering with the often-challenging task of learning the techniques for controlling the prostheses.

This chapter focuses on two aspects of denture design which are important in influencing how dentures function within the muscular environment into which they are placed:

- The positioning of incisor teeth
- Recording the position of the neutral zone

The relevance of a patient's natural incisal relationship

In dental publications it is common for photographs of dentitions or casts to depict a Class I incisal relationship and consequently there is a temptation to think, mistakenly, of this as the norm. A key objective of this chapter is to make the point that if such a relationship is provided for all complete dentures, treatment will fail in a sizeable proportion of patients. To prevent this from happening, there is a need to assess the patient carefully so as to establish a diagnosis of the skeletal relationship and the former incisal classification as both will influence the subsequent clinical and technical procedures.

A consideration of natural and artificial incisal relationships reveals a close similarity between orthodontic and prosthetic knowledge. At first thought, the two specialities might appear to be poles apart, as they are concerned largely with patients from opposite ends of

Prosthetic Treatment of the Edentulous Patient, Fifth Edition, © R.M. Basker, J.C. Davenport and J.M. Thomason
Published 2011 by Blackwell Publishing Ltd.

the age range. However, a study of the factors which govern the development of the natural occlusion – particularly the influence of the surrounding muscles – reveals fundamental similarities. Furthermore, it becomes increasingly apparent that prosthetic dentistry can be practised successfully only if this orthodontic knowledge is applied to the clinical prosthetic situation.

Development of the natural occlusion

As teeth erupt into the oral environment, their position is influenced by the activity and posture of the surrounding muscles, the size, shape and relationship of the jaws, and the occlusal forces produced by tooth contact. The shape and size of the jaws are inherited and, after growth has ceased, cannot be changed other than by surgical intervention. The functional behaviour of the muscles is partly inherited but may also be modified by treatment. It is important to consider the muscles and jaws as one unit because the muscles function from their skeletal origins and insertions.

The position of natural teeth is influenced more by the long-term forces associated with muscle posture than by the short-term forces occurring during function. As the teeth erupt

into a mould of muscular tissue created by the lips, cheeks and tongue, they eventually take up positions of relative stability related to the relaxed posture of these muscles. This situation contrasts with that occurring with complete dentures, which are all too readily displaced both by the short-term functional forces and also perhaps by the long-term postural forces. The design of complete dentures, particularly that of the lower prosthesis, therefore has to take muscular displacement into account if stability is to be achieved.

The prosthetic problem

When both clinician and dental technician are first taught to set up artificial teeth for complete dentures, it is traditional to position them in a Class I incisal relationship with a horizontal overlap of 2 mm and a vertical overlap of 2 mm. But for how many edentulous patients does this 'normal' incisal relationship resemble the previous natural dentition? In a survey of English school children aged 11–12 years, the percentages for the various dental arch relationships assessed on a modified Angle's classification were as shown in Fig. 12.1 (Foster & Walpole Day 1974). Thus, 52% of the children possessed a Class II incisal relationship. Of course, it is possible to correct some of the incisal

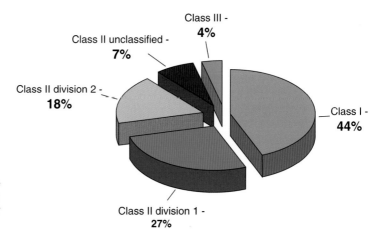

Figure 12.1 Percentages of the dental arch relationships occurring in English school children. (After Foster & Walpole Day 1974.)

Class III - **4%**

Class II unclassified - **7%**

Class II division 2 - **18%**

Class I - **44%**

Class II division 1 - **27%**

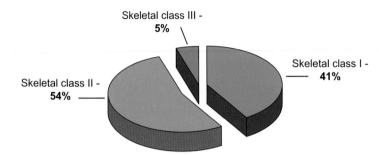

Figure 12.2 Percentages of the skeletal patterns occurring in English school children. (After Foster & Walpole Day 1974.)

relationships, but it must be remembered that the success of such treatment depends upon the underlying jaw relationship. The greater the discrepancy in jaw size and relationship, the harder it is to produce an ideal incisal relationship. More significant, therefore, are the results of the survey showing the variation in skeletal pattern, as shown in Fig. 12.2 (Foster & Walpole Day 1974).

It must be pointed out that these figures are representative of a group of young adolescents and that further growth of the mandible may reduce the number of those possessing a skeletal Class II pattern in a small percentage of cases; however, in the majority of patients the underlying Class II skeletal pattern is maintained into adulthood. The point being made is that parity will not be established between this group and the skeletal Class I group.

The results of the surveys suggest that, in the UK, the most common occlusion is a Class II tooth relationship superimposed upon a skeletal Class II jaw relationship. As a result, it would be expected that if all edentulous patients were provided with dentures which had a Class I incisal relationship, many such artificial dentitions would be in a different class from the previous natural ones. Some modification of the artificial arrangement is, of course, permissible and even requested by the patient – just as orthodontic treatment can be undertaken to modify a malocclusion where the prognosis is favourable. Of the remainder, the patient will either adapt to the dentures with difficulty or

find them quite intolerable. However, as discussed fully in Chapter 2, the success of prosthetic treatment depends so much upon the adaptability of a patient that if additional demands are made by creating an incisal relationship completely divorced from the natural state the chances of prosthetic treatment succeeding are reduced. The reasons for possible failure will be discussed in the next section, after which ways of preventing failure will be described.

Reasons for failure of treatment

To discover why prosthetic treatment may fail as a result of providing dentures with an incorrect incisal relationship, it is logical to consider each type of incisal relationship in turn and ask the following questions:

- How can a Class I artificial incisal relationship be produced?
- What is likely to happen as a result?

Class I

Figure 12.3 illustrates the tracing from a lateral skull radiograph of a dentate adult subject possessing a Class I incisal relationship. Of course, if complete dentures are constructed with the same incisal relationship, the artificial occlusion will be similar to the previous natural one, and few problems will be expected.

overlap may be reduced by moving either the lower incisors labially or the upper incisors palatally. If there is a deep overbite the vertical overlap can be altered by reducing the crown length or increasing the occlusal vertical dimension of the dentures. This latter option would mean that the freeway space is substantially reduced or eliminated altogether and so is not feasible. Complications which are likely to arise when following the other possibilities become apparent when considering the example in the same figure.

In Fig. 12.4b, the upper artificial teeth are placed in the same position as the natural ones while the lower teeth are placed further forwards. The result of this modification is to position the lower labial segment anterior to the neutral zone. The force exerted by the lower lip is no longer balanced by that of the tongue and so the lower denture becomes unstable. This error is not an uncommon one and is illustrated by the clinical case shown in Fig. 12.5.

In Fig. 12.4c, the lower incisors are placed in the position of the natural teeth and the upper anterior segment is moved backwards. This treatment may be quite acceptable if the skeletal relationship is favourable, just as orthodontic treatment in the natural dentition may successfully reduce a large horizontal overlap. However, there is the possibility of a marked change in appearance – including reduced support for the upper lip – which might be for the worse, as shown in Fig. 12.6, where the

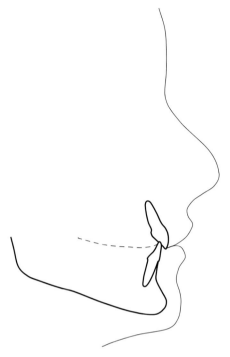

Figure 12.3 Tracing from a lateral skull radiograph of a dentate patient showing a Class I incisal relationship.

Class II division I

In order to convert a Class II division 1 incisal relationship (Fig. 12.4a) into a Class I relationship, it is necessary to modify the horizontal incisor overlap and, if there is an increased overbite, the vertical overlap as well. The horizontal

Figure 12.4 (a) Class II division 1 natural incisal relationship. (b) Upper artificial teeth placed in the same position as the natural ones; lower teeth proclined forwards. (c) Lower artificial teeth placed in the same position as the natural ones although the crown length is reduced; upper teeth moved back.

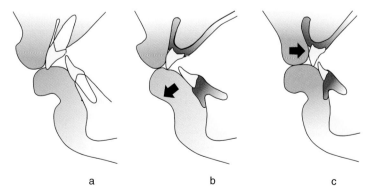

a   b   c

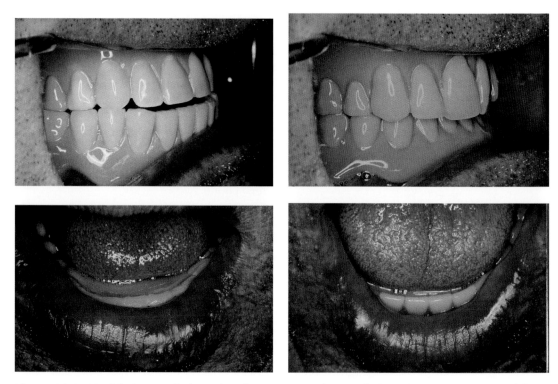

Figure 12.5   Top left: the incisal relationship of a patient complaining of a loose lower denture. Bottom left: the lower anterior teeth are positioned forwards of the neutral zone. Pressure from the lip results in mobility of the denture. Bottom right: replacement denture with the lower incisors placed in muscle balance. Top right: as a result of this change in incisal position, a Class II division 1 relationship is produced.

anterior teeth and upper lip almost appear to be strangers. A treatment possibility that can be explored to overcome these problems is to retrocline the upper incisors rather than move them palatally. This produces a Class II division 2 relationship, which reduces the horizontal overlap while retaining a realistic relationship of the necks of the teeth to the underlying ridge.

If the natural horizontal incisal overlap was large, allowing the lower lip to fall behind the upper incisors, a partial reduction of the overlap in the subsequent dentures may result in a very unsatisfactory 'half-way house' where the lower lip is unable to take up a comfortable position either behind or in front of the incisors.

This results in the persistent irritation of the lip by the incisal edge.

There is a group of patients possessing a severe skeletal Class II relationship, which is the result of a prominent maxilla rather than an underdeveloped mandible, where treatment can be carried out to correct a horizontal overlap which may be in the region of 10–20 mm. Although a combination of prosthetic treatment and surgical removal of bone from the prominent premaxilla may improve the situation, it is frequently impossible to reduce the discrepancy completely and the patient will retain a Class II division 1 incisal relationship with the overlap reduced to perhaps 5–10 mm. Any further reduction may be impossible because

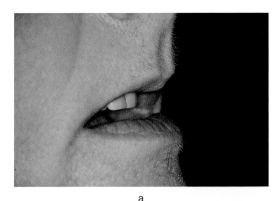

a

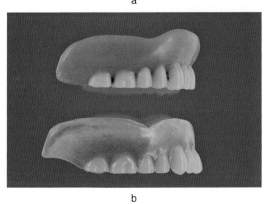

b

Figure 12.6 (a) Unsatisfactory relationship of upper teeth to the upper lip produced by the top denture in (b). (b) The lower of the two dentures is a replacement with the anterior teeth placed further labially to improve their relationship with the lip.

the amount of bone to be removed would totally eliminate the alveolar ridge anteriorly. In addition, it is important to realise that the alveolar bone provides the upper lip with some of its support. If too radical an approach is chosen, the loss of lip support may be such that the change in appearance is anything but acceptable.

Class II division 2

The deep vertical overlap mentioned in the Class II division 1 case also occurs commonly in Class II division 2 patients; the vertical over-

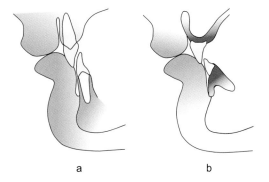

a   b

Figure 12.7 (a) Class II division 2 natural incisal relationship. (b) Artificial teeth placed in the same position as the natural ones; the crown length of both the upper and lower teeth has been reduced.

lap can be reduced either by shortening the crowns or by increasing the occlusal vertical dimension. For the reasons already stated, any increase in occlusal vertical dimension is virtually never a viable option.

The deep vertical overlap shown in Fig. 12.7 may be altered by reducing the crown length of the upper artificial teeth. However, the patient with this type of natural incisal relationship rarely complains about the appearance of the teeth and so a change in incisal level is unlikely to be accepted. Fortunately, the situation regarding the lower teeth is not so critical and it is usually possible to reduce the crown length without detriment to appearance.

Class III

Two extremes of skeletal pattern are recognised.

In the first the maxilla is small and the Frankfort-mandibular plane angle is large (Fig. 12.8). The prognosis for retention of an upper denture is often poor because of the small denture-bearing area. If the upper anterior teeth are moved labially to establish a Class I incisal relationship, the force of the upper lip on the labial face of the denture may be so great as to tip the balance between adequate stability and complete failure. Also the tipping forces

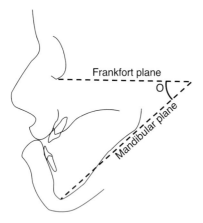

Figure 12.8 A lateral skull tracing from a patient with a skeletal Class III relationship and a large Frankfort-mandibular plane angle.

generated during incision may be too great for the patient to control the denture successfully during mastication. At best, it is usually advisable to create no more than an edge-to-edge incisal relationship, although on occasion a less ambitious reverse horizontal overlap will have to be accepted if a stable upper denture is to be produced.

In the second, the maxilla has developed normally, the mandible is large and the Frankfort-mandibular plane angle is small. Because of a favourable palatal shape and size, the prognosis for retention of an upper denture is usually good and thus greater latitude may be present for positioning the artificial teeth.

Anterior open bite

The act of swallowing involves the production of an anterior oral seal, which is normally made by the lips meeting and the tongue remaining within the dental arches. However, in some people the seal is made by the tongue thrusting between the upper and lower anterior teeth and contacting the lips. In the majority of cases, this behavioural pattern is adaptive. For example, if the upper incisors are unduly protrusive, the lower lip finds it extremely hard to move

around this dental barrier and meet the upper lip; therefore, the anterior oral seal is made more economically by the tongue meeting the lower lip. If the dental barrier is removed by orthodontic or prosthetic treatment so that the lips are able to come together, the tongue gives up its adaptive thrust and returns to more normal function.

There remains a very small number of people, calculated as 0.6% of the population, where the tongue thrust appears to be the result of an innate neuromuscular behavioural pattern (Tulley 1969). This so-called endogenous tongue thrust is frequently associated with a severe lisp and is resistant to treatment. If artificial teeth are positioned in a Class I relationship, a dental barrier will have been erected against the tongue as it continues to protrude. The outcome of such treatment will be instability of both upper and lower dentures, the likelihood of a sore tongue and a complete inability of the patient to adapt to such a foreign incisal arrangement. An example of a typical patient is shown in Fig. 12.9.

Prevention of failure

Treatment failure due to an inappropriate relationship of the dentures to the surrounding musculature can be prevented if particular care is taken in the assessment of the patient, in identifying and recording the optimum position of the denture teeth and in subsequent laboratory procedures.

Assessment of the patient

The task of assessing the edentulous patient and deciding upon the classification of the previous natural incisal relationship becomes more difficult the longer the patient has been edentulous. The reasons are as follows:

• The patient's own fading memory of the relationship of the natural teeth.

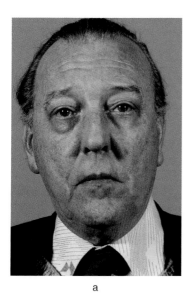

a

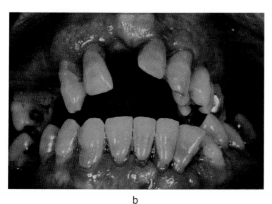

b

Figure 12.9 (a) This dentate patient has a large lower face height. Considerable muscular effort is required to bring the lips together. (b) The anterior oral seal is made between the tongue and the lower lip, resulting in the anterior open occlusion shown here.

- Resorption of the alveolar bone leads to loss of support for the lips and cheeks and consequent changes in the facial features upon which the clinician depends for vital clues.
- An alteration in the jaw relationship following loss of teeth will occur through change in mandibular posture. Loss of tooth support allows the mandible to move closer to the

maxilla and assume a more protrusive position which might falsely suggest a skeletal Class III relationship (Fig. 12.10).

- Increased activity of the lower portion of the orbicularis oris and mentalis muscles occurs in long-term denture wearers. This change in muscle activity may cloud the clinician's judgement when assessing the patient.

Nevertheless, in spite of these difficulties, orthodontic knowledge does allow the clinician to seek for clues in the edentulous patient:

Class I

Patients in this group have competent lips, a skeletal Class I jaw relationship and an obtuse labiomental groove.

Class II division 1

A patient who possesses a Class II division 1 incisal relationship superimposed upon a skeletal Class II base is relatively easy to diagnose. Typical features to observe are a retrusive mandible, an oval face, an acute labiomental groove and frequently a small lower face height (Fig. 12.11).

Class II division 2

A patient with a Class II division 2 incisal relationship possesses certain features which are distinctive in the dentate patient and may still be clearly seen in the edentulous state (Fig. 12.12). These features include a small lower face height, an acute labiomental groove, a small Frankfort-mandibular plane angle, a prominent mental region of the mandible, a square gonial angle and prominent zygoma. It is common for this type of patient to have a less marked skeletal discrepancy than is sometimes seen in the Class II division 1 subject. It is necessary to stress, however, that these features are not

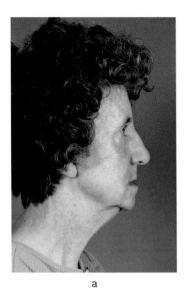
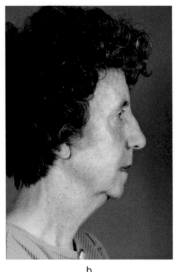

a   b

Figure 12.10 (a) A patient in occlusion wearing her old dentures which have become badly worn. She appears to have a skeletal Class III jaw relationship. (b) The true jaw relationship once the occlusal vertical dimension has been restored with new dentures. The patient, in fact, possesses a skeletal Class II jaw relationship.

necessarily diagnostic outside the UK. For example, such a facial structure is commonly seen in Scandinavia and is not associated with a Class II division 2 incisal relationship.

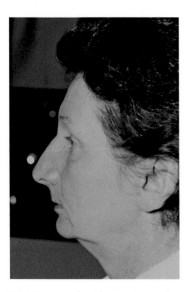

Figure 12.11 An edentulous patient. The retrusive mandible, small lower face height and acute labiomental groove point to the fact that the patient probably possessed a Class II division 1 natural incisal relationship.

Class III

An edentulous patient who possesses a Class III occlusal relationship on one of the two skeletal Class III base types is perhaps the easiest to diagnose. In the first type there may be evidence of the large lower face height, the obtuse Frankfort-mandibular plane angle and the overall length of the face (Fig. 12.13). The second type with a normal maxilla and overdeveloped mandible is also readily recognised.

Anterior open bite

In the dentate subject possessing an anterior open bite associated with an endogenous tongue thrust, circumoral muscular activity is seen during swallowing and there is often a characteristic lisp. Neither of these diagnostic clues is reliable in the edentulous patient, because the absence of teeth leads to indistinct speech while the absence of lip support results in abnormal muscular behaviour during swallowing. However, a combination of these factors may point the way to the correct assessment. Without doubt, this small group of

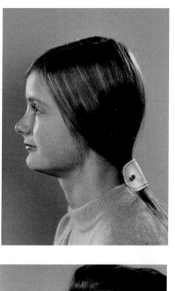
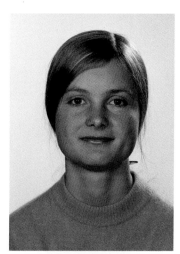
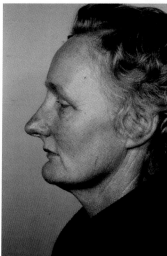
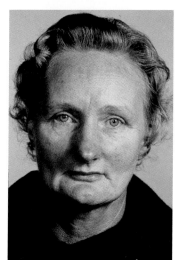

Figure 12.12 The upper pictures are of a dentate subject possessing a Class II division 2 incisal relationship and illustrate the characteristic facial features described in the text. The similar features of the edentulous woman shown in the lower pictures suggest that she once possessed a Class II division 2 natural incisal relationship.

patients creates considerable problems in assessment and diagnosis.

Reliable information on the degree of lip competence is more likely to be obtained if the patient is encouraged to relax completely and is then assessed from a distance. If the patient is seemingly unobserved, there is more likelihood of natural lip activity being encouraged.

Adjusting the record rims

Remembering that one of the objectives of recording the occlusion is to show the dental technician where the artificial teeth are to be placed, it is vital that the record rims are shaped so that they reproduce the incisal relationship appropriate for the particular patient. In

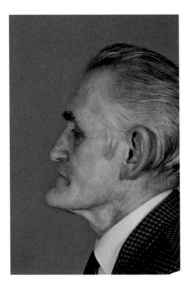

Figure 12.13 An edentulous patient. The combination of large lower face height, obtuse Frankfort-mandibular plane angle and obtuse labiomental groove indicate that he possesses a skeletal Class III jaw relationship.

patients where only a horizontal overlap is required, the procedure is relatively simple.

Complications arise in the skeletal Class III patient if the clinician underestimates the required occlusal vertical dimension. The relative protrusion of the mandible becomes more pronounced as the mandible approaches the maxilla with the result that the production of an acceptable incisal relationship becomes increasingly difficult. Thus, the possibility of positioning the labial segment in front of the neutral zone is increased (Fig. 12.14).

For a skeletal Class II patient, a horizontal overlap is automatically produced if the routine objectives of recording the occlusion are satisfied, namely the rims being shaped to provide satisfactory lip support and positioned in the neutral zone to achieve stability. However, difficulties arise where a marked vertical overlap is required. If the incisal level of each rim is adjusted to produce a pleasing appearance and the same height maintained over the entire occlusal surface, it is likely that the occlusal vertical dimension will be excessive. The reasons for this become apparent when considering the occlusal plane of the natural dentition shown in Fig. 12.15, where it can be seen that the vertical overlap is the product of a particularly steep curve in the occlusal plane. If this curve is reproduced on the record block, then it is possible to provide the dental technician with the exact

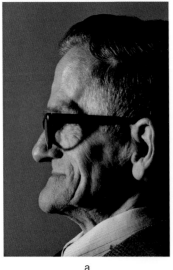

a

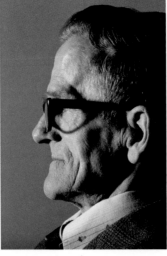

b

Figure 12.14 Effect of change in occlusal vertical dimension on a skeletal Class III jaw relationship. (a) A reduction in occlusal vertical dimension accentuating the Class III jaw relationship. (b) Restoration of the occlusal vertical dimension allowing a more acceptable incisal relationship to be produced.

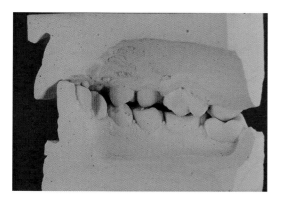

Figure 12.15   A sagittal section through casts of a Class II division 1 incisal relationship. The vertical overlap is the result of a steeply curved occlusal plane.

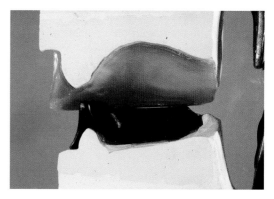

Figure 12.16   Recording the jaw relationship for a patient who possessed a Class II division 1 incisal relationship. Correct incisal levels and the degree of vertical overlap are produced by creating a step on the lower rim.

information on incisal relationship and height of occlusal plane. One method of achieving this is described in the following section.

Adjusting the rims for a Class II division 1 incisal relationship

First, the upper rim is carved labially and incisally to indicate the correct position for the anterior teeth. Palatally, the rim is reduced in thickness to correspond to the size of the denture teeth. The lower rim is then shaped to the neutral zone and to the correct incisal height. The height of the lower rim in the buccal region is reduced so that the correct occlusal vertical dimension is established. When the patient closes together on the rims, the lower labial segment will fit in behind the upper one and so establish the required vertical overlap (Fig. 12.16). In some instances, it will be necessary to reduce the height of the upper buccal segments as well, in order to gain adequate freeway space.

At this stage, a somewhat artificial step has been created between labial and buccal segments of each rim. This abrupt step is softened when the rim is replaced by the artificial teeth, but the overall curvature of the occlusal plane, as found in the natural dentition, is retained.

Positioning lower anterior teeth

Placing the lower anterior teeth in the neutral zone is crucial, especially if there has been considerable resorption of the mandible and the mentalis muscle is particularly active. As a general rule, the necks of the artificial teeth should be placed close to the crest of the residual ridge, otherwise it is likely that the muscle activity of the lower lip will displace the denture. Having made this point, it should also be mentioned that it is frequently possible to give the incisors a slight labial tilt. Such a proclination can help to establish a favourable incisal relationship, while ensuring that the incisors remain in a position of muscle balance between the lower lip and the tongue.

Recording the neutral zone

So far, the descriptions of recording the neutral zone in this chapter and in Chapter 11 have been restricted to the conventional method whereby the wax record rim is shaped so that it lies within the neutral zone and is thus stable. For the vast majority of patients, this technique is perfectly satisfactory.

There are, however, a few patients for whom a functional recording of the neutral zone is indicated. These patients may give a history of numerous unstable lower dentures and on examination the clinician may anticipate that it is going to be difficult to identify the neutral zone by simply carving the record rims. There may be instances where the intraoral anatomy is so altered – for example, as a result of surgery – that many of the usual anatomical landmarks no longer exist. In other cases it may be the amount and strength of activity of the oral musculature which suggests that a functional recording of the neutral zone would be helpful. In such cases the clinical technique is as follows.

At the stage of recording the occlusion, the upper rim is shaped carefully so that it sup-

ports the muscles of the cheeks and upper lip and fulfils all the criteria listed on pp. 155–158. The lower rim is trimmed so that a recording of the correct jaw relationship can be made. This stage can be accomplished quickly if the occlusal contact is restricted to a limited area in the premolar-molar region as described on p. 161. After the casts have been articulated, the upper trial denture is constructed.

A lower base is made in cold-curing acrylic resin. Molar pillars on the base are made to occlude with the upper denture at the correct occlusal vertical dimension. A thin spine, which will help to support the recording material, can be added to the rest of the base and left clear of occlusal contact (Fig. 12.17a). In exceptional cases the molar pillars and the spine can get

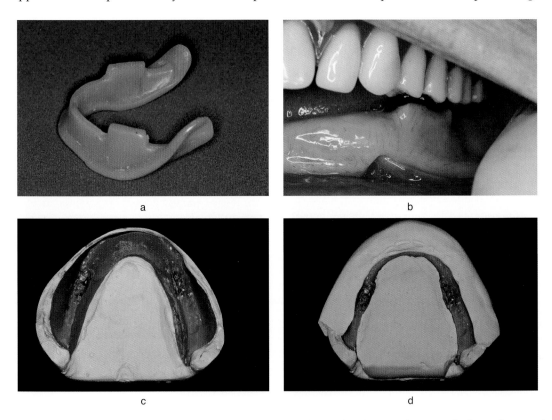

a

b

c

d

Figure 12.17 (a) Lower base for neutral zone impression. (b) Occlusal contact between the lower base and the upper trial denture checked before the addition of the impression material. (c) Neutral zone impression which has been moulded by the muscles of the lips, cheeks and tongue. (d) Buccal and lingual indices in silicone putty.

in the way of the investing muscles and therefore affect the recording. In such cases a simple acrylic base is produced, and molar pillars are created intra-orally using a chairside reline material. During its plastic phase this material will be shaped by the muscles into the neutral zone. Once it has set the clinician can adjust the height of the pillars to the required occlusal vertical dimension.

At the stage of recording the position of the neutral zone, checks are made of the upper trial denture and of the occlusal contact with the molar pillars (Fig. 12.17b). A mouldable material, with an extended setting time of several minutes, is applied to the lower base which is then reinserted in the mouth. The bulk of the added material must be carefully judged so that the rim produced does not exceed the anticipated thickness of the finished denture. The patient is instructed to alternately sip water and talk. In this way, the surrounding muscles shape the recording material (Fig. 12.17c).

When the material has set, the recording of the denture space is returned to the laboratory where it is seated on the master cast and indices are constructed around the buccal and lingual surfaces (Fig. 12.17d). The dental technician now has a recording of the denture space enabling the artificial teeth to be positioned within its boundaries.

The benefit of a lower denture shaped by the neutral zone impression technique has been shown in a study measuring the magnitude of force needed to lift the denture away from its surrounding musculature. A larger force was required to remove the 'neutral zone' denture than the conventional denture (Miller et al. 1998). For some patients this enhanced retentive ability of the tongue acting through the specially shaped polished surface may make the difference between success and failure.

Care in the dental laboratory

It is, of course, essential that the dental technician accurately follows the blueprint of the record blocks or neutral zone recording when setting up the trial dentures. This is best achieved if the artificial teeth are set into the rim with only a small portion of the rim being cut away each time. The remaining rim acts as a guide to the overall arch shape.

A postscript – pre-extraction records

Having read this chapter, the reader may conclude that the designing of complete dentures is to a large extent a matter of deduction and guesswork. This is in fact true when one is faced with an edentulous patient and no record of the previous natural dentition. However, the amount of guesswork can be considerably reduced if pre-extraction records of the natural dentition are available. Many methods of obtaining pre-extraction records have been described. Certainly, good-quality photographs and occluded casts of the natural dentition provide information about the incisal relationship. However, the casts do not indicate the all-important relationship of the teeth to the underlying jaws and the surrounding musculature. In rare cases a lateral cephalogram radiograph may be available showing the true underlying skeletal pattern. However, in the majority of cases, such information can be obtained only by the recording rims being shaped in the mouth.

The best method of transmitting the characteristics of the natural dentition through to the artificial one is undoubtedly by means of immediate dentures. The patient should be advised that these will always be a valuable source of information to a clinician for the construction of replacement dentures and therefore should never be discarded.

It can be argued that if all edentulous patients possessed their original immediate dentures, the number of prosthetic problems would be reduced considerably. For although immediate dentures will cease to fit the mouth accurately after a few years, and post-extraction changes in the jaws and muscles will result in a shifting of the neutral zone, the clinician still has evidence of tooth shape, tooth position and incisal relationship – without doubt information that can be invaluable in achieving a successful outcome.

Communication with the dental technician

Both the clinician and the dental technician should have a clear understanding of the principles which lie behind the provision of dentures with the correct incisal relationship and relationship to the neutral zone.

The record rims should be shaped accurately so as to provide an accurate blueprint for the dental technician.

It is essential to reinforce this blueprint by means of a written prescription.

Quality control and enhancement

The following themes might be considered when instituting a review of performance in a series of patients:

- In what percentage of patients' records is there a clear indication that an assessment of the appropriate incisal relationship has been made?
- In what percentage of cases has the dental technician been given a clear prescription of the incisal relationship and neutral zone?

- When comparing old dentures with the replacements, in how many instances has a significant change been made to the incisal relationship? In how many cases has the change resulted in an improvement in appearance, stability and function?

References and additional reading

Berry, D.C. & Wilkie, J.K. (1964) Muscle activity in the edentulous mouth. *British Dental Journal*, 116, 441–7.

Foster, T.D. & Walpole Day, A.J. (1974) A survey of malocclusion and the need for orthodontic treatment in a Shropshire school population. *British Journal of Orthodontics*, 1, 73–8.

Liddelow, K.P. (1964) Oral muscular behaviour. *Dental Practitioner and Dental Record*, 15, 109–13.

Miller, W.P., Monteith, B. & Heath, M.R. (1998) The effect of variation of the lingual shape of mandibular complete dentures on lingual resistance to lifting forces. *Gerodontology*, 15, 113–19.

Murphy, W.M. (1964) Pre-extraction records in full denture construction. *British Dental Journal*, 116, 391–5.

Neill, D.J. & Glaysher, J.K.L. (1982) Identifying the denture space. *Journal of Oral Rehabilitation*, 9, 259–77.

Richardson, A. (1965) The pattern of alveolar bone resorption following extraction of anterior teeth. *Dental Practitioner and Dental Record*, 16, 77–80.

Tallgren, A. (1963) An electromyographic study of the behaviour of certain facial and jaw muscles in long-term complete denture wearers. *Odontologisk Tidskrift*, 71, 425–44.

Tulley, W.J. (1969) A critical appraisal of tongue-thrusting. *American Journal of Orthodontics*, 55, 640–50.

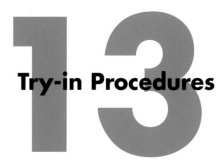

Try-in Procedures

Trial dentures are constructed by setting up denture teeth on shellac or acrylic resin (temporary or permanent) bases. This stage is used to check the accuracy of the registration stage and to assess the appearance of the dentures so that any appropriate modifications can be carried out. This clinical stage may be regarded as the 'dress rehearsal'.

The trial dentures should be examined first on the articulator and then in the mouth.

Assessment on the articulator

An efficient and reliable examination of the trial dentures is more likely to be achieved if the operator inspects each of the denture surfaces in turn, checking the aspects listed below.

General appearance

The trial dentures as supplied from the dental laboratory should be neat, clean and tidy. It is important to ensure that all requests included in the prescription completed at the previous clinical stage have been taken through to the trial dentures.

Impression surface

Fit

The bases of the trial dentures should be accurately adapted to the casts such that there is no movement when finger pressure is applied to the occlusal surfaces. If the trial dentures are on permanent acrylic bases the impression surfaces should be checked for any sharp projections, roughness or excessive extension into undercuts.

Extension

The border regions of the dentures should be shaped to conform to the depth and width of the sulci on the casts. In the upper jaw, the base should normally be extended posteriorly to the post-dam cut or formed in the cast, and in the lower jaw over the pear-shaped pads.

Relief chamber

If a relief chamber has been requested, a check should be made that it is present and of the

Prosthetic Treatment of the Edentulous Patient, Fifth Edition, © R.M. Basker, J.C. Davenport and J.M. Thomason
Published 2011 by Blackwell Publishing Ltd.

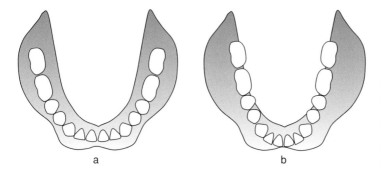

a   b

Figure 13.1 Occlusal view of two lower dentures: (a) the teeth follow the crest of the ridge; (b) marked discrepancies between the position of the teeth and the crest of the ridge are present, suggesting that the teeth will not be in the neutral zone.

required size and shape. If it has been left with sharp margins these will need to be rounded.

Polished surface

Position of the lower teeth

The teeth on a lower denture should normally be positioned to conform fairly closely to the crest of the mandibular ridge. If there are gross discrepancies between the position of the teeth and the ridge (Fig. 13.1), the teeth may not be in the neutral zone (p. 65) and could become the cause of instability in the mouth. However, this is not invariably the case, so final judgement on this aspect must be delayed until the dentures have been examined in the mouth.

Position of the upper teeth

If a biometric approach is being adopted in the design of the upper denture (Chapter 10), the position of the teeth and the polished surfaces should be checked in relation to the palatal gingival vestige and incisive papilla. The trial denture can also be compared with the record rim if this is still available, or with the positions of the teeth on the existing denture if this has been used as a reference.

Inclination of the polished surfaces

The buccal and lingual aspects of the polished surfaces should converge occlusally so that pressure from the surrounding muscles of the cheeks, lips and tongue contributes to retention rather than displacement (Fig. 4.3). The exception to this rule is found in the upper anterior region where the labial surface of the flange often faces upwards and outwards (Fig. 12.6b).

Surface contour

The polished surface of the denture should normally be smooth for optimum comfort and to facilitate plaque removal. This is particularly important around the necks of the teeth. Where the requirements of appearance make it desirable the polished surface may be contoured and stippled to simulate the mucosal surface. This is usually only indicated for the upper labial flange.

Comparison with previous dentures

If the patient already has dentures, they should be compared with the trial dentures to see whether any planned similarities or changes, such as arch shape or arrangement of the anterior teeth, have been reproduced correctly.

Occlusal surface

There should normally be bilateral even contact in the intercuspal position. Opposing cusped teeth should interdigitate accurately. Where an average movement or semi-adjustable articulator has been used excursions should be checked to see if balanced articulation is present.

Assessment in the mouth

The dentures should first be assessed individually for:

- physical retention;
- stability;
- extension of the denture bases;
- relationship to the neutral zone.

Details of the clinical procedures are described in Chapter 7. The dentures should then be assessed together for:

- evenness of occlusal contact;
- occlusal vertical dimension;
- appearance.

Physical retention

If the prognosis for retention in the upper jaw is good, dislodgement should be expected to be difficult. In the case of the lower denture, retention is often poor because of the relatively small denture-bearing area and the difficulty in obtaining an efficient border seal. If the physical retention of an upper trial denture is not as good as would be expected from the anatomical conditions existing in a particular patient, the cause should be identified and, if found to be a fault in the denture, must be corrected. Denture faults may include the absence of a border seal resulting from:

- under-extension;
- inadequate width of flange;
- ineffective seal at the posterior border;
- poor fit of the denture base.

Stability

Movement of either denture of more than 2 mm suggests lack of stability of the denture. A

judgement then needs to be made as to whether this is due to:

- lack of fit of the denture; or
- displaceability, or unfavourable shape, of the denture-bearing tissues.

Extension of the denture bases

The accuracy with which the denture borders conform to the depth and width of the sulci must be determined. The all-important posterior extension of the dentures over the pear-shaped pads in the lower jaw and to the junction of the hard and soft palate in the upper jaw must also be checked.

If marked over-extension of the denture flanges is present, stretching of the sulcus tissues will occur when the denture is inserted into the mouth and their subsequent elastic recoil will cause dislodgement of the denture. Therefore, if the denture is displaced immediately after being seated, over-extension should be suspected. A small degree of over-extension may cause dislodgement of the denture when the clinician gently manipulates the lips and cheeks or when the patient raises the tongue. The exact location of such an error can be determined only by carrying out a careful intra-oral examination. When over-extension is present in areas where the visibility is good, displacement of the sulcus tissues will be seen as the denture is seated. However, in the lingual pouches, visibility is poor, so the clinician will have to make an assessment based on the behaviour of the lower denture as the tongue is moved. Correction of over-extension is by reducing the depth of the offending flange. If this is not carried out, the finished dentures will traumatise the mucosa in that area and will be unstable because of the large displacing forces exerted by the soft tissues.

The presence of under-extension is determined primarily by intra-oral examination, when the depth of the sulcus will be seen to be greater than that of the denture flange. In

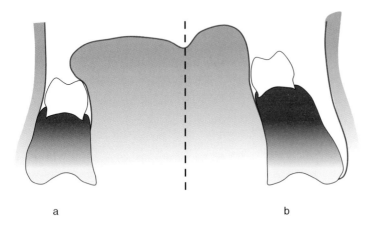

Figure 13.2 The relationship of the lower posterior teeth to the cheeks and tongue: (a) correct – buccal surfaces of the teeth are in close proximity to the buccal mucosa; the level of the occlusal plane allows the tongue to rest on the occlusal surfaces; (b) incorrect.

a

b

the case of the upper denture, however, a preliminary indication of under-extension will be given by the existence of poor physical retention. Correction of any under-extension will usually entail taking a new impression in the trial denture. Failure to do this will result in reduced physical retention of the finished dentures and inadequate distribution of load to the tissues.

Relationship to the neutral zone

The positioning of teeth in the neutral zone is of particular importance in the case of the lower denture because the physical retention is relatively weak. Identification of the neutral zone will have been attempted while shaping the record block at the earlier visit and now the trial denture must be checked to see if that assessment was correct and has been transferred accurately to the denture. When the lower denture is inserted, it should remain in place when the mouth is half open and the tongue is positioned so that its tip lies just behind the lower anterior teeth. The tongue must not be allowed to adopt the retracted 'defensive tongue' posture otherwise it will not be possible to make the required assessment. A useful 'rule of thumb' is that the lower denture will usually be stable if narrow teeth are used and

are placed as far buccally, or labially, as possible without displacing the cheek and lip tissues. By this means, maximum tongue room is provided within the limits dictated by the lips and cheeks (Fig. 13.2a). If there is space between the buccal surfaces of the posterior teeth and the mucosa of the cheek (Fig. 13.2b), it is almost certain that there is inadequate tongue space.

If displacement of the denture does occur, the cause must be identified and the denture modified to correct the instability. An area where this difficulty commonly arises is the lower anterior region where the lip may exert excessive pressure, causing the denture to move upwards and distally. Correction of this type of fault should be carried out at the chairside so that the effect of the alterations can be assessed in the patient's mouth. The offending teeth may be reset in the correct relationship to the soft tissues or they may be removed and replaced with a wax rim which is shaped with a wax knife until a stable denture is produced. The dental technician is then asked to reset the teeth in the position indicated by the rim.

If the dentures being constructed are replacements for dentures which have given good service in the past, it may usually be assumed that the relationship of the old denture to the cheeks, lips and tongue is satisfactory and that consequently this relationship should be copied in the trial dentures. Both old and new dentures should be compared in the mouth to see whether this relationship has been faithfully reproduced.

While assessing the position of the lower teeth relative to the soft tissues, the height of the occlusal plane in relation to the tongue should be noted. When the tongue is relaxed, it should be able to rest on the occlusal surfaces of the teeth – a situation which favours retention of the lower denture (Fig. 13.2a).

Occlusal vertical dimension

Assessment of the occlusal vertical dimension

Measurement
The lower trial denture should be inserted and the rest vertical dimension measured. Then, after inserting the upper denture and measuring the rest and occlusal vertical dimensions, an initial impression can be gained of the adequacy or otherwise of the freeway space. If a negative freeway space is suspected then it is worth reassessing the rest vertical dimension, this time without the lower denture.

Facial appearance
The initial impression regarding the freeway space should be backed up by an assessment of the patient's appearance. If the patient's facial proportions and contact between upper and lower lips appear to be appropriate when the teeth are occluded, it suggests that the occlusal vertical dimension is correct. This assessment can be broadened by asking the patient to occlude and then to relax the mandible several times while the clinician assesses the freeway space by observing the amount of mandibular movement. Changes in facial proportions, lip posture and jaw relations during these movements will also help the observer to decide whether the occlusal vertical dimension is acceptable.

Speech
Finally, the patient should be asked to speak while wearing the trial dentures. The teeth do not normally contact during speech but approach most closely when the 'S' sound is made. The separation is known as the closest speaking distance and is usually about 1 mm. If the occlusal vertical dimension of the trial dentures is excessive, the space may be absent; correspondingly, it will be increased if the occlusal vertical dimension is too small. This assessment can be made by asking the patient to count out loud from 'sixty' to 'seventy'.

Correction of the occlusal vertical dimension

Occlusal vertical dimension too small
When the freeway space is too large, it is corrected by adding the appropriate thickness of wax to the occlusal surfaces of the posterior teeth on one of the dentures, adjusting the wax to produce an even occlusion at the desired occlusal vertical dimension and then re-recording the jaw relationship in the retruded contact position.

Occlusal vertical dimension too large
When the freeway space is too small, or absent altogether, teeth will have to be removed from one of the dentures and be replaced with a wax rim before the new recording can be made. The decision as to which denture should be reduced in height will depend on how much more freeway space needs to be created, the relationship that the corrected height of occlusal plane would have to the tongue (Fig. 13.2) and the effect any change in height would have on appearance. It is often sufficient to remove just the posterior teeth for this purpose, but it may also be necessary to remove the anterior teeth where the horizontal overlap is such that further closure would be prevented by anterior tooth contact.

Evenness of occlusal contact

When a shellac or temporary acrylic base has been used, there may be some looseness of the upper trial denture which may make it impossible to carry out an accurate assessment of the occlusion in patients, especially where anatomical factors are unfavourable. In these circumstances, application of a denture fixative to the impression surface can provide a solution. This should, though, be done only if all other causes of instability have been eliminated.

A bowl of cold water should be available at the chair side so that frequent chilling of the trial dentures can be carried out. If the dentures are left in the mouth for more than a few minutes at a time, softening and distortion of the wax will occur.

Retruded contact position

The occlusion should first be checked with the mandible in the retruded contact position. The patient closes slowly so that the clinician can observe the *initial* occlusal contact. This first contact should not be on one or 2 teeth but should be a widespread and even contact around the arch. The *final* occlusal relationship is not so reliable for assessment, as the early contact of one or 2 teeth may have been masked by compression of the mucosa beneath the denture, tipping of the denture or posturing of the mandible.

Lateral and protrusive positions

These positions will already have been examined on the articulator. If further assessment is carried out in the mouth the patient must be strongly advised to only use very light tooth contact, as the excursive movements can readily displace the denture teeth from the wax.

Methods of occlusal assessment

Visual

If a relatively large occlusal discrepancy is present, the clinician will be able to see this without any difficulty. However, the existence of smaller faults may be deduced from evidence such as slight tipping or lateral movement of the dentures as they occlude.

Patient perception

The patient should be asked if the dentures are contacting evenly. Many patients are able to detect occlusal unevenness which is so slight that it could be overlooked by the clinician.

Articulating paper

The use of articulating paper is not indicated at this stage because of the following reasons:

- Teeth are readily displaced from the wax by the pressure required to make the paper mark the teeth.
- Direct visual checking of the occlusion together with the patient's comments are usually sufficient to allow the clinician to answer the key question – 'Are there any errors in the occlusion large enough to require re-recording of the jaw relationship, or are they so small that their correction is best left until the dentures are processed and the teeth are firmly anchored in the acrylic bases?'

Correction of occlusal faults

Both vertical and horizontal discrepancies in the occlusion may occur.

Vertical occlusal discrepancy

A vertical occlusal discrepancy may take the form of a unilateral, anterior or posterior open occlusion. If this type of fault is present, the retruded position should be re-recorded after modifying one or both of the dentures to produce an even occlusion at the correct occlusal vertical dimension. There are several ways in which this may be achieved, the choice of method depending on the occlusal vertical dimension of the trial dentures (Fig. 13.3). Before carrying out the modifications, the clinician should determine whether or not the

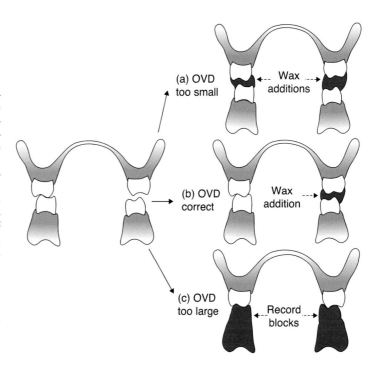

Figure 13.3 Methods of correcting a unilateral open occlusion at the try-in stage: (a) if the occlusal vertical dimension is too small, an appropriate thickness of wax is added to the upper or lower denture on both sides of the dental arch; (b) if the occlusal vertical dimension is correct, wax is added to the side with the open occlusion to produce even bilateral occlusal contact; and (c) if the occlusal vertical dimension is too large, the teeth on one of the dentures are removed and replaced with a wax rim reduced in height by an appropriate amount. Final recording of the retruded contact position may be made in each case using a suitable registration material placed on both sides of the arch.

orientation of the occlusal plane of the upper denture is correct in lateral and anteroposterior planes; if it is, the alterations will be carried out on the lower denture. If the plane is wrong, the upper denture will also have to be modified by resetting the anterior teeth, or replacing the teeth with a wax rim, to indicate to the dental technician the correct position of the occlusal plane.

Horizontal occlusal discrepancy

An occlusal discrepancy in the horizontal plane may be detected by observing that the upper and lower centre lines are not coincident, that the posterior tooth relationship is not symmetrical, or that the horizontal overlap is not the same in the mouth as it is on the articulator. A new recording of the retruded contact position should be obtained after the teeth from one of the dentures have been removed and replaced with a wax rim. If the teeth are not removed, there is a danger that the cusps will guide the

mandible back into the incorrect intercuspal position.

Appearance

The appearance must be assessed by both clinician and patient.

The clinician's assessment

At the try-in stage, the clinician must re-assess the information concerning the appearance of the dentures which was acquired at the appointment for recording occlusion. This includes the following:

- Shade of the teeth
- Mould of the teeth
- Size of the teeth
- Orientation and level of the occlusal plane
- Position of the centre line
- Degree of lip support

A check on basic aspects of the trial dentures, such as orientation of the occlusal plane and position of the centre line, can best be made if the upper lip is reflected so that a clear view of the maxillary teeth is obtained. However, this method of examination is not appropriate when assessing the overall aesthetic effect. To make this latter judgement, the teeth should be observed during function by the clinician engaging the patient in conversation and, if possible, encouraging the patient to smile naturally. This functional assessment is very important because dentures which have a pleasant appearance in repose may suddenly become glaringly unsuitable as soon as the patient's lips move in speech.

The patient's assessment

The patient must be given ample opportunity to see the dentures in situ and form an opinion regarding their appearance. This stage is of paramount importance and is not uncommonly allotted too little time. It is, of course, essential that the patient's requirements regarding the appearance of the dentures should be discussed fully, not only at the try-in stage but also during the preceding stages of the course of treatment. The clinician's role in these discussions should be that of an adviser who ensures that the patient is in possession of all the information required to make a sensible decision. For example, some patients will request that their dentures have anterior teeth which are small, white and even – a combination which will almost guarantee that the dentition is easily recognised as being an artificial one. However, these patients will often change their minds if given the opportunity at the try-in stage of seeing the improvement that even a small amount of alteration can make.

If a patient has strongly held views about how the dentures should look, the clinician should take great care not to be too persuasive so that the patient accepts an arrangement of anterior teeth which conflicts with these views.

If this happens, the patient is likely to be dissatisfied with the finished dentures and could, with complete justification, request that they be remade.

Sometimes it is difficult for a patient to form a clear opinion regarding the appearance of the dentures in the relatively strange surroundings of the dental surgery. If a friend or relative is available to offer an opinion, this can be of considerable help to the patient, particularly if the clinician leaves the room so that they are able to discuss the appearance in an uninhibited manner. In the absence of a friend, discussing the appearance with the dental nurse can be very beneficial.

It is preferable for the patient to assess the appearance of the dentures by looking at them in a wall mirror at a normal viewing distance, rather than using a hand mirror which may be held too close to the face and give an unrealistic view. In exceptional cases, where there is particular difficulty in determining what an acceptable appearance is, it may even be necessary to permit the patient to take the trial dentures home for a short time provided the fragile nature of the trial dentures is made quite clear.

Achieving a natural appearance

The final appearance is created by:

- detailed arrangement of the anterior teeth;
- shaping the gingival margins;
- grinding the incisal edges where necessary.

If the arrangement of the anterior teeth requires correction, the modifications should ideally be carried out at the chair side, so that the altered dentures can be tried in the mouth and the effectiveness of the changes assessed by both the clinician and the patient. If the dental technician does need to be involved it is of immense value for him or her to be present in the surgery to see the situation directly rather than relying on written or telephoned instructions.

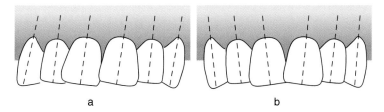

a   b

Figure 13.4   (a) Imbalance produced by inclining the vertical axes of the anterior teeth in the same direction. (b) The improvement in appearance produced by counterbalancing the inclination of the axes on one side of the mouth with those on the other.

The clinician should attempt to create the illusion of natural teeth when finalising the appearance. In order to carry out this visual deception successfully, the appearance of the dentures should be appropriate for the patient in question and also appropriate for the population from which the patient comes. If these requirements are fulfilled, the teeth will appear to 'belong' to the patient and the deception will be complete.

Introducing irregularity

It should be remembered that the prevalence of irregularity or crowding of natural teeth is high. Therefore, if dentures are constructed with a 'perfect' arrangement, the risk of the resulting appearance seeming artificial is considerable. As a general rule, imperfection in the anterior tooth arrangement is a basic requirement in creating the illusion of natural teeth. Complete symmetry should be avoided: for example, the anterior teeth should not be placed so that the incisal edges are all at the same level. Some form of crowding, which may vary in degree from minimal irregularity to marked overlapping of the teeth, should usually be incorporated into the anterior tooth arrangement. When producing irregularity, care should be taken to ensure that a general impression of balance is maintained even though the two sides of the dental arch may not be identical. For example, if the centre line of the teeth is some distance from the midline of the face, or if the incisal level is not horizontal, a sense of im-

balance will result and the appearance will be poor. The vertical axes of the anterior teeth can be varied, but if the inclination of these axes on one side of the mouth does not approximately balance that on the other, an unsatisfactory appearance will result (Fig. 13.4).

Incisal relationship

The method of determining an incisal relationship which is appropriate for an edentulous patient's skeletal relationship has been discussed in Chapter 12. If a patient is provided with dentures which have an inappropriate incisal relationship, for example, a Class I incisal relationship on a marked skeletal Class II base, there is a risk that, in addition to problems with stability, the dentures will appear incongruous and the aesthetic result will be poor.

Age

Changes in the shape of the crowns of natural teeth commonly occur as a result of increasing age. These alterations in crown shape are produced by incisal wear and gingival recession. Anterior teeth on dentures can therefore be given a definitely youthful, or aged, appearance by incisal grinding where appropriate and correct shaping of the gingival margins (Fig. 13.5). If a 'young' dental appearance is provided for an older patient, or vice versa, it will be only too apparent that the patient is wearing dentures.

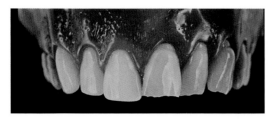

Figure 13.5 Use of incisal grinding and gingival contouring to convert a youthful appearance UR3-UR1 to an aged one UL1-UL3.

Sex

When determining the appearance of dentures, the sex of the patient should also be taken into account. Although there is no evidence that the form and arrangement of natural teeth are related to the sex of the individual, there is a view that artificial teeth can be arranged to create either a so-called 'feminine' or 'masculine' appearance (Fig. 13.6) (Hyde et al. 1999). Masculinity can be suggested by increasing the irregularity of the arrangement and by using squarish moulds with obvious surface character while, conversely, a more even arrangement of rounded, smooth-surfaced anterior teeth will impart a feminine quality to the appearance. Rotation of the incisors in a vertical plane may

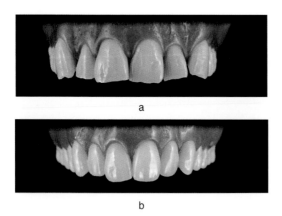

Figure 13.6 (a) An example of a 'masculine' anterior tooth arrangement. (b) An example of a 'feminine' anterior tooth arrangement.

Table 13.1 Features that can help to determine the 'sex' of dentures.

Male	Female
Large teeth	Small teeth
Square moulds	Rounded moulds
Characterised labial surface	Smooth surface
Irregularity	Even arrangement
Distal margins labially	Distal margins palatally
Significant wear of incisal edges	Minimal wear of incisal edges
Diastemas	Closed contact points
Prominent canines	Canines not prominent

also help to 'sex' the dentures; moving the distal margins labially will increase the vigour and masculinity of the appearance and vice versa.

Features that help to determine the 'sex' of dentures are summarised in Table 13.1.

Arrangement of the lower anterior teeth

Once the upper anterior teeth have been adjusted, consideration should be given to the lower teeth. These, in some patients, will not make such an important contribution to the appearance; nevertheless, they should not be ignored. In many patients, they will be displayed more during function than the upper teeth and therefore may be a dominant factor in determining the patient's dental appearance. Again, the same general rules regarding perfection and evenness of tooth arrangement which have been discussed previously should be applied.

Labial flange

In some patients, the upper labial flange will be visible during speech and smiling. If this is the case, a natural appearance will be achieved only if the acrylic flange is contoured to resemble natural gum, and if the surface of the flange is slightly irregular or stippled to break up any reflections (Fig. 13.5). If melanotic pigmentation of the mucosa is present, a pale pink flange will seem out of place. The technician should therefore be requested to tint the labial flange during processing.

Denture marking

Markers in dentures can be of immense value for the identification of the following:

- Dentures – in dental laboratories, hospitals and care homes.
- Individuals – following loss of consciousness, memory or life.

Identification of dentures in dental laboratories

This is important in dental laboratories where large numbers of dentures are being processed. This procedure is widely practised by dental technicians and does not require instructions from the clinician.

Identification of dentures in hospitals and care homes

The ability to identify dentures is of great value in hospitals and care homes because older and confused patients, and sometimes staff, not infrequently misplace the dentures (Michaeli et al. 2007). Losses are particularly regrettable because the dentures may be virtually irreplaceable as a result of an older person's difficulty in adapting to new dentures of different design. And yet, surveys into the marking of dentures in care homes showed that this had been done in only 35–47% of cases (Bengtsson et al. 1996; Stenberg & Borrman 1998). In a more recent study, whereas over 80% of prosthodontic specialists believed that the marking of dentures was a worthwhile procedure, yet just over half actually carried it out routinely; none of the care homes included in the study followed suit (Murray et al. 2007).

An identification mark allows a misplaced denture and its owner to be reunited. The following steps should be taken routinely to reduce the considerable number of dentures which are actually lost:

- The care programme for the patient should record whether the patient possesses dentures, whether they are usually worn and whether they are with the patient rather than being looked after by relatives.
- There should be an understanding within the care team that dentures are normally in one of two places – either in the patient's mouth or in a clearly labelled denture pot. If not, a search must be made urgently as the precious dentures could easily have been wrapped up in dirty linen or be languishing in a waste-paper basket.

Identification of individuals

Dentures can be marked to allow identification of patients following loss of consciousness, memory or life. For this system to be fully effective, the marker needs to be indestructible and to incorporate a code which is universally acceptable. As the latter requirement has not been fulfilled at the present time, such markers are not widely used in general dental practice. However, they are routinely used in the Armed Forces and are regulated by law in Sweden, Iceland and in many states in the USA (Borrman et al. 1999). Requirements for denture markers used for this purpose include that they are:

- Biologically inert
- Inexpensive
- Widely available
- Easy to inscribe
- Retrievable after an accident
- Able to survive elevated temperatures
- Visually acceptable to the patient (Richmond & Pretty 2009)

Identification marks fall into two broad categories, surface markers and inclusion markers.

Surface markers

Scribing the cast

Marks may be produced on the impression surface of the denture by scribing the cast before processing the denture. The irregularities produced on the denture surface are clinically undesirable and therefore should be reserved for identifying dentures in laboratories after processing. The marks should be removed before delivering the denture to the patient.

Pen or pencil

Marks on a denture can be made by writing with either a spirit-based pen or a fine pencil. However, pencil marks require protection with a polymer varnish. Both techniques offer relatively short-term benefits. Exposure of spirit pen marks to hypochlorite cleaners can result in rapid fading. Also, there can be a rapid loss of definition of both pencil and spirit pen marks if an abrasive cleaner is used. Thus, unless the marks are checked at regular intervals and renewed as necessary, the methods are perhaps suitable only for the identification of dentures belonging to patients admitted to hospital for a short stay.

Inclusion markers

Names can be written or typed on metallic markers, such as the stainless steel strip of the Swedish ID-band, which has become an international standard and FDI-accepted denture marking system (Thomas et al. 1995). Alternative non-metallic materials that have been used include tissue paper and ceramic materials. More recently, embedded radio frequency identification microchips have been described (Richmond & Pretty 2009).

Inclusion markers can either incorporated into a denture at the time of processing (Fig. 13.7) or inserted into the processed denture by cutting a recess, inserting the marker and covering with clear cold-curing acrylic resin. They

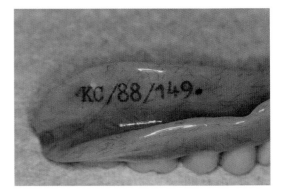

Figure 13.7 Inclusion marker inserted into lingual surface at time of processing.

should be placed posteriorly in the lingual or palatal areas of the dentures. In this position, the stresses induced by the markers are unlikely to cause significant weakening of the dentures. Furthermore, the markers are less likely to be destroyed in the event of the patient's death by burning.

If identification marks of the inclusion type are required, the appropriate request must be made to the technician when the trial dentures are sent for processing.

Communication with the dental technician

The following topics might need to be included in the clinician's prescription to the laboratory:

- Confirmation that all items sent from the clinic to the laboratory have been disinfected.
- It must be made quite clear whether the dentures are to be processed, modified and then processed or modified and returned to the clinician for a further trial stage. If there are any lingering doubts, or there has been significant adjustment to the occlusion or the position of the teeth, a further trial stage is recommended. It is better to be safe than to be sorry.

- If the original recording of the jaw relationship was wrong, it will be necessary for the technician to re-articulate one or both casts and to reset a number of teeth. Very clear instructions must be given on the necessary procedures. A retry will be required.
- The use of the split-cast technique (p. 205) to correct any errors in occlusion resulting from processing.
- The elimination of unwanted undercuts, or the addition of a palatal relief when indicated, if instructions regarding these have not yet been given. (The post-dam should already have been carved into the cast where necessary by the clinician, p. 153.)
- Any special finish, such as stippling, to be applied to the surface of the labial flanges, if this has not already been produced on the wax-work of the trial denture.
- The shade of acrylic resin to be used if the standard shade would be unsightly. The provision of a diagram of any stains to be incorporated into the pink resin to simulate areas of melanotic pigmentation if this is required.
- The provision of some form of identification marker to be incorporated into the dentures should be considered.

Quality control and enhancement

At the conclusion of the try-in stage, and before the dentures are returned to the dental technician for processing, the clinician needs to have had positive answers to the following:

- Are the dentures retentive and stable?
- Is the occlusion balanced?
- Is there adequate freeway space?
- Is the patient happy with the appearance?
- Has the original treatment plan been fulfilled with respect to the design of the dentures?

Topics which might be investigated in an assessment of a series of patients include the following:

- In how many cases was the dental technician provided with appropriate information at the conclusion of the trial stage?
- In what proportion of cases was a second try-in procedure required? What were the reasons for this? Could the number of these occasions have been reduced?

References and additional reading

Bengtsson, A., Olsson, T., Rene, N., Carllson, G.E., Dahlbom, U. & Borrman, H. (1996) Frequency of edentulism and identification marking of removable dentures in long-term units. *Journal of Oral Rehabilitation*, 23, 520–3.

Borrman, H.I., DiZinno, J.A., Wasen, J. & Rene, N. (1999) On denture marking. *Journal of Forensic Odonto-Stomatology*, 17, 20–6.

Deb, A.K. & Heath, M.R. (1979) Marking dentures in geriatric institutions – the relevance and appropriate methods. *British Dental Journal*, 146, 282–4.

De Van, M.M. (1957) The appearance phase of denture construction. *Dental Clinics of North America*, 1, 255–68.

Engelmeyer, R.L. (1996) Complete denture aesthetics. *Dental Clinics of North America*, 40, 71–84.

Frush, J.P. & Fisher, R.D. (1958) Dynesthetic interpretation of dentogenic concept. *Journal of Prosthetic Dentistry*, 8, 558–81.

Harrison, A. (1986) A simple denture marking system. *British Dental Journal*, 160, 89–91.

Heath, J.R. (1987) Denture identification – a simple approach. *Journal of Oral Rehabilitation*, 14, 147–63.

Hyde, T.P., McCord, F., Macfarlane, T. & Smith, J. (1999) Gender aesthetics in the natural dentition. *European Journal of Prosthodontics and Restorative Dentistry*, 7, 27–30.

Lombardi, R.E. (1973) The principles of visual perception and their clinical application to denture aesthetics. *Journal of Prosthetic Dentistry*, 29, 358–82.

Michaeli, L., Davis, D.M. & Foxton, R. (2007) Denture loss: an 8-month study in a community dental setting. *Gerodontology*, 24, 117–20.

Murray, C.A., Boyd, P.T., Young, B.C., Dhar, S., Dickson, M. & Currie, J.N.W. (2007) A survey of denture identification marking within the United Kingdom. *British Dental Journal*, 203, E24.

Oliver, B. (1989) A new inclusion denture marking system. *Quintessence International*, 20, 21–5.

Richmond, R. & Pretty, I.A. (2009) A range of post-mortem assault experiments conducted on a variety of denture labels used for the purpose of identification of edentulous individuals. *Journal of Forensic Sciences*, 54, 411–4.

Schwarz, W.D. (1963) Improving full denture appearance. *Dental Practitioner and Dental Record*, 8, 319–27.

Stenberg, I. & Borrman, H.I. (1998) Dental condition and identification marking of dentures in homes for the elderly in Göteborg, Sweden. *Journal of Forensic Odonto-Stomatology*, 16, 35–7.

Thomas, C.J., Mori, T., Miyakawa, O. & Chung, H.G. (1995) In search of a suitable denture marker. *Journal of Forensic Odonto-Stomatology*, 13, 9–13.

Wright, S.M. (1974) Prosthetic reproduction of gingival pigmentation. *British Dental Journal*, 136, 367–72.

Fitting Complete Dentures

Objectives of this clinical stage

The overall objective when fitting complete dentures is to ensure that the patient is given the best possible start with the new prostheses. This may be achieved by checking that:

- there is no pain when the dentures are inserted and removed from the mouth, or when the teeth are brought into occlusal contact;
- the teeth meet evenly;
- the dentures stay in place when inserted and during normal opening of the mouth;
- the patient understands:
  - how to control the dentures;
  - what to expect of them;
  - how to clean them.

As a result of this preparation the patient should be reasonably confident when meeting family and friends. It should be remembered that to achieve this satisfactory outcome with a patient who has not worn dentures previously will require very careful advice and instruction by the clinician.

The main changes in the dentures since the try-in stage are in the impression and occlusal surfaces. This chapter will focus on the assessment and correction of these two surfaces.

Assessment and correction of the impression surface

Before inserting the new dentures for the first time, the impression surface must be carefully checked for any potential causes of pain. If found these must be eliminated to ensure patient comfort and also to avoid the adoption of abnormal paths of closure of the mandible, which may be followed to avoid occlusal pressure at the site of discomfort.

The common causes of pain arising from the impression surface of a denture are shown in Fig. 14.1:

- *Acrylic nodules and spicules*. These are produced by acrylic resin being processed into indentations or porosity in the cast. These areas of roughness can be detected by observation of the dried denture surface and by

Prosthetic Treatment of the Edentulous Patient, Fifth Edition, © R.M. Basker, J.C. Davenport and J.M. Thomason
Published 2011 by Blackwell Publishing Ltd.

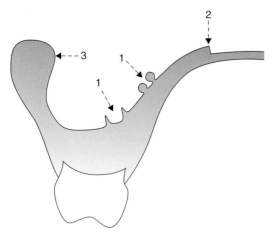

Figure 14.1 Common causes of pain arising from the impression surface of a denture are indicated by numbers (1) surface roughness associated with sharp projections and acrylic nodules; (2) sharp edge of relief chamber; (3) overextension into bony undercuts.

passing a gauze napkin or cotton wool roll over the surface so that the threads catch on the offending areas. They should be carefully removed with a stone without modifying the fit of the denture.

- *Sharp acrylic margins.* Sharp edges can be caused by the presence of a tin-foil relief on the cast and can be identified by direct observation. Bevelling of these edges should be carried out.
- *An undercut flange.* A good indication of whether or not an undercut flange is likely to cause pain or mucosal injury can often be obtained by a careful visual inspection of the impression surface. A disclosing material, such as soft wax or silicone rubber, can then be used to locate the offending area precisely. A thin, even layer of the disclosing material is applied to the suspect area and the denture is gently inserted until the patient just begins to experience slight discomfort, and is then removed. The location of the undercut producing the discomfort is shown up as an area of acrylic from which the disclosing material has been displaced.

Retention and stability

The retention and stability of new dentures should be carefully evaluated at the fit stage. This may be achieved as follows.

Retention

The dentures are inserted and, after a short interval during which the denture becomes enveloped by a saliva film, they should normally stay in place during moderate opening of the mouth. The upper denture should offer resistance when pulled downwards by finger and thumb gripping the incisors. The lower denture, however, will not normally offer significant resistance to attempted displacement because it has a relatively inefficient border seal.

Stability

Neither denture should rock when finger pressure is applied alternately to either side of the occlusal surfaces in the first molar region. Horizontal displacement should not result in a shift of the centre line of more than 2 mm.

Further discussion of retention and stability can be found in Chapters 4 and 13.

Assessment of the occlusal surface

The occlusion of the dentures is checked once completion of the adjustments mentioned above have ensured that:

- each denture can be inserted and removed from the mouth without discomfort;
- firm pressure can be applied to the occlusal surface without eliciting pain.

Before discussing the methods of occlusal adjustment the possible causes of occlusal error arising from the laboratory processing of the dentures will be considered.

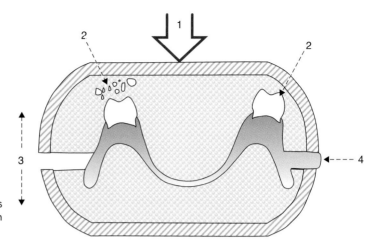

Figure 14.2 Laboratory causes of occlusal error (for a description of the causes, see the text).

Laboratory occlusal errors

Causes of errors

Poor laboratory technique (Fig. 14.2) can result in the movement of individual teeth or in an increase in occlusal vertical dimension of the denture.

(1) Excessive packing pressures resulting in the artificial teeth being forced into the investing plaster. This can occur:
  - If the acrylic resin has reached an advanced dough stage and thus offers increased resistance to closure of the flask. Excessive pressure will then be needed to bring the two halves of the flask together.
  - If the two halves of the flask are closed too quickly, resulting in a rapid build-up of pressure in the flask.
(2) Normal packing pressures breaking the investing plaster and causing movement of the teeth when the layer of investing plaster is weakened as a result of:
  - porosity in the mix;
  - the use of an incorrect powder–water ratio;
  - an inadequate thickness of plaster between the walls of the flask and the denture.

(3) If pressure on the flask is released during the curing cycle, the two halves are likely to separate, thus increasing the occlusal vertical dimension of the completed denture.
(4) Separation of the two halves of the flask by a layer of excess resin which should have been removed during trial closure of the flask. This 'flash' results in an increased occlusal vertical dimension of the denture.

In spite of taking all due precautions to prevent the errors just described, small occlusal inaccuracies invariably occur. It has been shown that a processed denture exhibits an average increase in height of 0.5 mm and a shift in tooth contact towards the posterior region. These errors can be corrected in the laboratory if a split-cast mounting technique is used.

Correction of errors

Laboratory occlusal errors can be effectively corrected by using the split-cast technique. This technique involves replacing the processed dentures, still on their casts, back on to the articulator in exactly the same jaw relationship as when the trial dentures were produced (Figs. 14.3–14.5). Any deflective occlusal contacts resulting from displacement of individual teeth

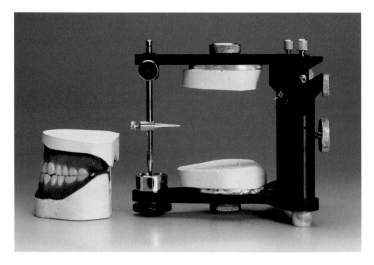

Figure 14.3 Split-cast mounting technique (1). The trial dentures had been mounted on an average movement articulator. Before the master casts were plastered to the articulator, location grooves were cut into each cast. A film of petroleum jelly was applied to the location grooves and to the peripheral areas of each cast; as a result, the master casts were readily detached from the topping plaster before processing.

can then readily be seen. An overall increase in occlusal vertical dimension will be indicated by the incisal pin failing to make contact with the incisal table.

There is evidence to show that if complete dentures are processed by injection moulding rather than the more common compression-moulding technique there is significantly less incisal pin opening and generally fewer occlusal inaccuracies (Nogueira et al. 1999).

Clinical occlusal errors

If all appropriate precautions have been taken while processing the dentures, any remaining occlusal errors detected when the dentures are placed in the mouth are likely to be primarily of clinical origin and to have passed undetected at the trial stage.

The objectives of adjusting the occlusion on the finished dentures are to achieve:

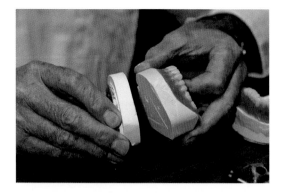

Figure 14.4 Split-cast mounting technique (2). In the laboratory, the denture, still seated on the cast, has been removed from the investing plaster after processing. It can now be relocated onto the topping plaster via the locating grooves.

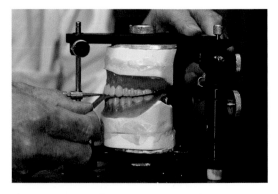

Figure 14.5 Split-cast mounting technique (3). In the laboratory, the master casts, on which the dentures are still seated, have been accurately relocated on the topping plaster and secured with sticky wax. The occlusion can now be refined.

- occlusal balance in the intercuspal position;
- a balanced articulation.

Occlusal errors can be identified and subsequently corrected by occlusal adjustment with or without remounting the dentures on an articulator.

Occlusal adjustment without remounting the dentures on an articulator

In general, small occlusal discrepancies in the absence of a horizontal slide can be corrected effectively by chair side adjustment following a thorough intra-oral assessment using the methods described in the following.

Identification of occlusal errors

(i) *Visual assessment.* Visual assessment of occlusal contact relationships of the dentures by the clinician can be an effective way of recognising obvious deflective occlusal contacts and slides which occur after the initial contact. It is essential that the clinician bases an assessment of the occlusion on the initial contact of the dentures rather than on the final occlusal relationship, as the latter can be the product of the dentures tipping and of mucosal displacement.

(ii) *Feedback from mucosal mechanoreceptors.* A usually reliable guide to identifying occlusal imbalance in dentures is the patient's sensory nervous system, as the mechanoreceptors in the oral mucosa are capable of fine pressure discrimination. They are generally able to detect the presence of a deflective occlusal contact, but may not precisely identify the specific site that should be adjusted. This will usually require the use of articulating paper.

(iii) *Articulating paper.* When searching for deflective contacts with articulating paper, using the technique described in the next section, it should be remembered that ar-

ticulating paper marks can be very misleading. False marks can readily be created because of the following reasons:

- Even thin articulating paper may fill the space between non-occluding teeth and mark areas of the occlusal surfaces that are not actually contacting.
- Mucosal displacement and tipping of the dentures can bring non-occluding teeth into contact with the articulating paper.
- The vertical overlap of teeth associated with cusp/fossa relationships and vertical overlap of anterior teeth can 'crimp' the articulating paper and produce false marks (Fig. 14.6).

Correction of occlusal errors

This may be undertaken as a two-stage process:

(i) *Produce a balanced occlusion in the muscular position.*

- When the dentures have been made comfortable, the patient is encouraged to relax and is then instructed to open and close without making occlusal contact. In this way, the pattern of jaw movement is largely determined by sensory input from the temporomandibular joint receptors and from the muscle spindles in the muscles of mastication.
- Sensory input from the mechanoreceptors in the denture-bearing mucosa is then introduced by asking the patient to continue opening and closing in a relaxed manner but to make initial, light contact on the teeth and to report on the location of that contact. It is essential that the patient refrains from heavy contact; this ensures that the joint sensory input prevails and thus prevents alteration to the path of closure of the mandible. In addition, it should be remembered that heavy contact is likely to compress the underlying mucosa, or tip

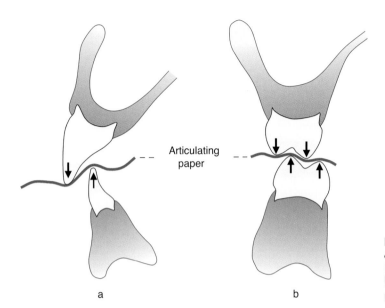

Articulating paper

Figure 14.6 Articulating paper can mark the teeth that are not in contact when it is 'crimped' by a deep vertical overlap or by posterior teeth with cusps.

a

b

the dentures, and so mask the presence of the deflective contact.

The majority of patients are able to offer such comments as 'The dentures are meeting on the left side first of all', or 'I am meeting on the back teeth only'. This discrimination comes from stimulation of the mechanoreceptors in the denture-bearing mucosa. It is the clinician's task to interpret this evidence, and with the assistance of additional tests eliminate the deflective contacts.

- A piece of thin horseshoe-shaped articulating paper is inserted between the teeth and the patient is asked to repeat the jaw movements. A single strip of articulating paper should not be placed on only one side of the dental arch as this is likely to induce jaw movement to that side.
- Instructing the patient how to occlude onto the articulating paper needs to be carried out with care. The request to 'bite together' is not advisable as it encourages protrusion of the mandible towards an edge-to-edge incisal relation-

ship and consequently an incorrect result. On the other hand, 'close on your back teeth' will encourage a normal closure pattern. Once the desired position has been obtained the patient is requested to tap the teeth together several times in that position in order to mark the occlusal surfaces.

- Adjustment of the occlusal surfaces should be made only on those markings made by the articulating paper which coincide with the patient's comments. The process is repeated until the patient reports that the teeth meet evenly.

(ii) *Produce a balanced articulation.* Having established a balanced occlusion in the muscular position, the clinician should normally check that there is an area of balanced articulation 1–2 mm around this position. Articulating paper is again used to mark interfering contacts requiring adjustment. With a horseshoe of articulating paper between the teeth the patient closes into intercuspal position and then slides the mandible into the lateral or protrusive position being assessed.

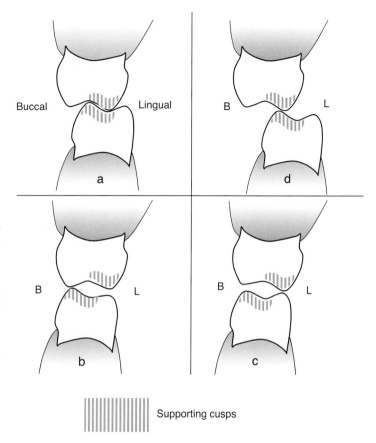

Figure 14.7 (a) Contact between supporting cusps maintains the occlusal vertical dimension and occlusal balance in tooth position. (b) Deflective contact between buccal cusps on the working side in lateral occlusion is corrected by grinding the buccal upper cusp. (c) Deflective contact between lingual cusps on the working side in lateral occlusion is corrected by grinding the lingual lower cusps. (d) Deflective contact on the balancing side is corrected by reducing the interfering contact on one or other of the supporting cusps.

The occlusal vertical dimension and occlusal balance in intercuspal and muscular position normally depend on contact between the palatal upper cusps and the buccal lower cusps of the posterior teeth (Fig. 14.7a). These cusps are therefore known as supporting cusps.

Having established even occlusal contact in muscular position, further adjustment of these supporting cusps should be avoided wherever possible. Thus, if, in a lateral occlusal position, a deflective contact is detected on the working side between a buccal upper and buccal lower cusp, it is the buccal upper cusp (BU) that should be reduced. Similarly, if interference is observed on the working side in lateral occlusion between a palatal upper and lingual lower cusp, it is the lingual lower cusp (LL) that should be reduced (Figs. 14.7b and 14.7c). This approach to correcting the occlusion on the working side is known as the BULL rule.

However, this rule cannot be applied to the correction of deflective contacts on the balancing side, because here both upper and lower supporting cusps are in opposition (Fig. 14.7d). It is usually possible in this situation to reduce the interfering contact without eliminating the supporting contact. If this is not possible, it is necessary to adjust one of the offending cusps and to accept loss of supporting contact in this area. Overall balance in muscular position will not be lost as a result.

Occlusal adjustment with remounting of the dentures on an articulator – the check record

Adjusting an occlusal discrepancy that is large enough to be visible clinically can be a time-consuming and rather inaccurate exercise if attempted in the manner just described. This is especially so if the error produces an antero-posterior or lateral slide after the initial occlusal contact. It is therefore recommended that the check record procedure, in which the dentures are remounted on an articulator, is used for anything other than relatively minor occlusal corrections. There is, in fact, evidence to suggest that it is advantageous to undertake a check record as a routine procedure on the grounds that its use results in fewer post-insertion complaints of discomfort (Firtell et al. 1987).

When a satisfactory occlusion has been achieved in this way it should be recognised that the situation does not remain stable indefinitely. Post-insertion changes in the masticatory system such as mucosal displacement, neuromuscular adjustment, bone resorption and wear of the acrylic teeth tend to result in a gradual deterioration of the occlusion (see Chapter 15). When such a deterioration is recognised a repeat check record is likely to be the most effective way of correcting it, as long as the post-insertion change has not been so dramatic that there is gross occlusal wear and a significant loss in occlusal vertical dimension.

A laboratory check record will usually require an additional appointment for the patient as it is unusual for the dental laboratory to be on the surgery premises. This inconvenience acts as a disincentive to the use of the technique and is the reason why a chair side check record was devised. Stages of the check record procedure are illustrated in Fig. 14.8.

Both techniques are described below.

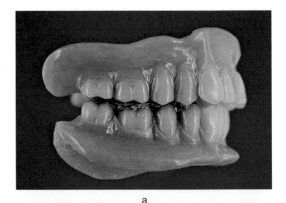

a

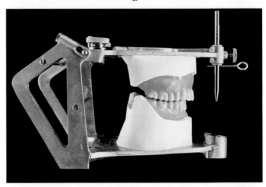

b

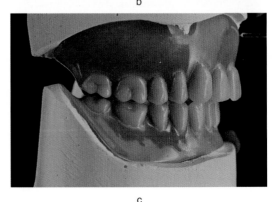

c

Figure 14.8 Stages of the check record procedure: (a) a recording of the jaw relationship with the mandible in the retruded position and with the dentures out of occlusion; (b) the dentures are articulated, the occlusal record removed, the incisal pin raised and occlusal contact made; (c) view of the dentures on the articulator to show an occlusal error.

Recording the jaw relationship

After the denture bases have been made comfortable, a recording is made of the jaw relationship with the mandible in the retruded position and with the dentures just out of occlusion. This procedure, described below, ensures that normal jaw closure and the relationship of the dentures to the supporting tissues are not influenced by uneven occlusal contact:

(i) A wax containing fine metal particles is useful as a recording material. The softened wax is placed on the posterior teeth of one of the dentures, care being taken to confine it to the occlusal surface. If an excessive amount of material is used, sensory nerve endings in the tongue and cheek mucosa are stimulated and the sensory input may influence jaw movement adversely.

(ii) After initial closure in the retruded position, the dentures are removed and the wax is inspected to ensure that there has been no penetration of the wax by the artificial teeth.

(iii) Once an apparently satisfactory record has been obtained the wax is chilled and then trimmed using a sharp blade to minimise the chance of distortion. Buccal excess is removed because it obscures the contact relationship of opposing teeth with the wax record, making a visual check on accuracy impossible.

(iv) Occlusal excess is removed until only the indentations made by the tips of the opposing cusps are visible. This is necessary because deep occlusal indentations increase the likelihood of denture displacement and mandibular deviation.

(v) Once the excess wax has been removed, a definitive intra-oral check on the accuracy of the record can be made.

(vi) Accuracy is crucial to the success of the procedure and therefore it is a common practice to verify the accuracy of the all-important record before committing oneself to the occlusal adjustment. This involves obtaining more than one record and then only proceeding with mounting the dentures on an articulator and their subsequent occlusal correction if the records agree.

If the dentures are mounted on an average-movement articulator without using a face bow, the relationship of the upper denture to the articulator's hinge axis conforms to the average value for the relationship of the maxilla to the condylar axis. However, if the clinician wishes to record this latter relationship more accurately for a particular patient a facebow record is obtained and used to mount the upper denture on the articulator; this is commonly undertaken on a semi-adjustable articulator, but can be done equally effectively on those average movement articulators able to accept a face bow.

Articulating the dentures

The task of mounting the dentures on an articulator is conventionally carried out by the dental technician using routine laboratory procedures. However, the time required to mount the dentures on the articulator may act as a disincentive to the use of the check record procedure, particularly if there is no dental technician on the premises. The process can be speeded up considerably if the laboratory is requested to return the finished dentures with the upper denture already on a plaster-holding cast on the articulator. It is then a quick and simple matter for the clinician to mount the lower denture against the upper when the check record has been obtained. Of course, this variation is possible only at the stage of fitting the dentures. If the check record is to be undertaken at a later visit, when the articulator is no longer available, one of the other techniques will have to be used.

The time required for the laboratory remounting of the dentures on an articulator can be reduced to about 10 minutes by using

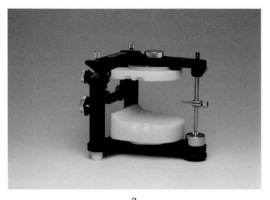

a

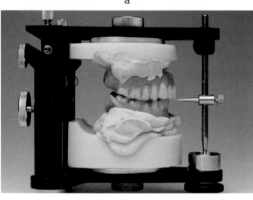

b

Figure 14.9 (a) Acrylic mounting platforms attached to an average-movement articulator to allow a rapid check record procedure at the chairside. (b) The jaw relationship having been recorded, the dentures are fixed to the acrylic mounting platforms with impression plaster. When the plaster has set the procedure for adjusting the occlusion follows the stages described already.

an instrument which has special acrylic platforms fixed to the upper and lower arms. These platforms have small locating notches cut into them and provide convenient tables onto which quick-setting impression plaster can be poured (Oliver & Basker 1994). The stages of the mounting procedure are shown in Fig. 14.9.

Adjusting the occlusion

Before starting the occlusal adjustment, the inter-occlusal wax record is removed, the incisal pin raised and the articulator closed un-

til initial tooth contact is made. The occlusion is then adjusted until even occlusal contact is obtained.

If there is a gross error in the jaw relationship, it may be necessary to remove the artificial teeth and set up new ones in the correct position. In such a situation, the trial stage should normally be repeated. When the jaw relationship is at last correct, the new teeth can be attached to the denture base with cold-curing acrylic resin.

Advice to the patient

The ultimate success of new dentures depends to a large extent upon the quality of advice offered by the clinician. Sensible advice put over in a clear manner gives confidence to the new denture wearer, ensures that the patient starts off on the right footing and increases patient satisfaction. It is often more effective to stress particular points by the spoken rather than the written word. Thus, the clinician should spend time in explaining the intricacies of denture wearing. This advice must be supplemented with printed instructions, which will act as a reminder for the patient.

With regard to advice on cleaning dentures, especially when given to older patients, verbal information alone is unlikely to result in any more than a short-term improvement. Long-term change in behaviour is likely to occur only if verbal information is subsequently followed up by practice and reinforcement (Burnett et al. 1993).

Although advice to the patient is considered in this chapter on fitting dentures, it is important to explain the relevant points repeatedly during the earlier stages of treatment so that only reinforcement of this information is required when the dentures are inserted. Information must be remembered and assimilated if it is to be effective. If new dentures have just been placed in the mouth, the patient is wondering how to control them, how to cope with the new sensation and possibly what to do with the sudden outpouring of saliva. The patient is therefore too preoccupied to fully appreciate what is being explained by the clinician. This thought is even more relevant if the patient is older and cannot readily assimilate new information. If, however, the basic information has already been given, repetition at the stage of fitting the dentures can help to reinforce the earlier message. For some older patients it may be particularly helpful to give the advice to the carer.

The advice given to the patient may be considered under the following headings.

Limitations of dentures

When the patient was examined initially, an assessment of the prognosis for denture treatment should have been made. It is of the utmost importance that if anatomical and, perhaps, adaptive problems indicate the possibility of future difficulties with dentures, the patient is informed of this at the outset. It is crucial that realistic expectations of dentures are created in the patient before treatment is actually started. If the information is first given after the dentures have been fitted and when complaints have already been made, it is likely that the patient will believe that the valid explanation is, in fact, an excuse for inadequate clinical work.

Controlling dentures

It should be explained to patients that once the dentures have been fitted, new muscular behaviour must be developed in order to control them. It is helpful to reassure patients that although it takes time the required skills are usually acquired in due course and that it is important not to be discouraged by any early difficulties. It has been reported that although approximately 60% of experienced denture wearers were able to eat and speak satisfactorily within a week of the replacement dentures being fitted, a further 20% of these patients required up to 1 month to become proficient (Bergman & Carlsson 1972). A few patients take even longer.

The clinician can facilitate the learning process by giving appropriate advice. Simple tasks should be mastered before advancing to more complex skills. Thus, the patient should be advised to take small mouthfuls of non-sticky food and to chew on both sides of the mouth at once during the initial stages. Such well-known phrases as 'learn to walk before you run' and 'practice makes perfect' convey the sense admirably. For first-time denture wearers and significantly older people, there may be benefit in their being advised to commence with soft food for the first 2–3 days followed by the gradual introduction of more challenging foods (Cleary et al. 1997).

Appearance

If the new dentures make an obvious change to the appearance of the patient, as for example when restoring a loss of vertical dimension, it is very important to warn the patient in advance that friends and relatives may look twice and even pass a remark on a change in appearance. Unless this warning is given, there is a risk that the patient will interpret a chance remark or a second glance as realisation by the friend that new dentures have been provided. Whereas most people are more than happy that new clothes or new hairstyles are admired, they may be particularly sensitive to new dentures being recognised. As there is a danger that such recognition may bias the patient against the dentures, it is wise to remind him or her of the original aims of the treatment and that the much-needed improvement in appearance may be noticed. The patient should be encouraged to appreciate that friends and relatives, as well as the patient, may require a period of adaptation to the new dentures.

Initial sensations

It is wise to reassure the patient regarding the immediate changes that may be noticed when the dentures are inserted. For example, some inexperienced denture wearers salivate excessively and thus find it extremely difficult to speak. Reassurance that this outpouring usually settles down within several hours and that the strange sensations disappear within a few days helps to boost morale.

Soreness

In spite of all the care that is taken throughout all the stages of treatment, it is not unusual for the patient to experience some soreness during the first few days of wearing new dentures. Helpful advice can be given as follows:

- If the discomfort is minimal and of short duration the patient should be advised that the dentures should continue to be worn and that adjustments will be made at the recall visit.
- If the discomfort is considerable and persistent the patient may need to discontinue wearing the new dentures and revert to the old ones before the recall appointment. It is important to make it clear to the patient that if it is at all possible the new dentures should be reinserted a few hours before the recall appointment so that the area of trauma can be accurately pin-pointed and appropriate treatment provided.

Wearing dentures at night

If new dentures are worn at night for at least the first two weeks after they have been fitted, the continuous stimulation of the mechanoreceptors in the oral mucosa helps to speed up adaptation. After this initial period of adaptation has been successfully completed, the dentures should ideally be left out at night because it has been shown that coverage of the denture-bearing mucosa day and night has the following significant disadvantages:

- Preventing cleaning of the mucosa by the tongue and saliva.

- Stimulating the growth of denture plaque.
- Prolonging the exposure of the mucosa to denture plaque.
- Not accommodating an extended period of immersion of the dentures in a cleanser.
- Creating the possibility for parafunctional clenching and grinding of the teeth during sleep thus traumatising the denture-bearing mucosa.

If the dentures are not worn at night, the mucosa is allowed a rest period to recover from the day's activity. This is especially relevant for those patients with a thin atrophic mucosa and with a reduced ability to repair tissue, features commonly found in the older patient. However, the clinician's advice to leave the dentures out at night is frequently ignored because, as has been said, 'To leave the dentures in a glass in the bathroom or at the bedside all night is an unattractive thought to most people, even if they sleep alone, or with partners whose capacity for simple domestic pleasures and skills has fallen off'. Advice to take dentures out just before sleep rather than leaving them out at night is a subtle variation which can prove more acceptable to some patients. Alternatively, advice that the dentures are removed for a period when patients are by themselves during the day may be more acceptable.

Cleaning dentures – its importance

A variety of deposits form on dentures, such as:

- Microbial plaque
- Calculus
- Food debris

These deposits may be responsible for a number of problems:

- Denture stomatitis (p. 111).
- Angular stomatitis (p. 119).
- Unpleasant tastes and odours.
- Unsightly appearance because of staining.

- Accelerated deterioration of some denture materials such as short-term and long-term soft lining materials.
- Systemic disease and the infection of others, e.g. carers, by organisms such as methicillin-resistant *Staphylococcus aureus* (MRSA) (Glass et al. 2001). Fortunately immersion denture cleansers have been shown to be effective against MRSA (Lee et al. 2009; Maeda et al. 2007; Murakami et al. 2002).

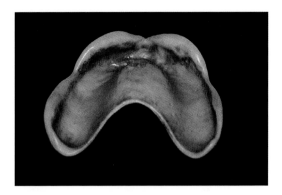

Figure 14.10 Microbial plaque stained by disclosing solution applied to the impression surface.

The effective cleaning of dentures is therefore of great importance to the patient's general well-being and oral health and, potentially, also to their carers or contacts.

The importance of giving advice on the cleaning of dentures cannot be over-emphasised. Unfortunately, there is evidence that a high proportion of patients appear not to have been given such instruction (Jagger & Harrison 1995).

Brushing will remove the majority of the plaque and will tend to disrupt the remainder, thus facilitating its subsequent penetration by an immersion cleanser. The objective of soaking dentures in an immersion cleanser is to remove any plaque left behind on the denture surface as a result of difficulty in brushing inaccessible areas or because of a patient's visual impairment or lack of manual dexterity.

Brushing

When new dentures are fitted, the patient should be advised to carefully brush them regularly using soap, water and a soft nylon tooth brush the head of which is small enough to reach into all areas of the denture surface. Many commercially available denture brushes have heads which are too large to reach into all the nooks and crannies of the denture surface. Also their bristles are often so stiff that they cannot conform satisfactorily to the contours of the denture and can also cause significant abrasion of the acrylic resin.

Older patients with arthritic hands can find it difficult to hold and manipulate a conventional toothbrush. For such patients there are brushes with handles designed for easy gripping or simple modifications that can be made to the handle of a conventional toothbrush.

The importance of removing all deposits, not just the more obvious stains and food particles, should be emphasised. Disclosing solutions may be used by the patient at home to indicate when complete removal of denture plaque has been achieved. Food dyes are suitable for this purpose as long as their correct use has been explained. If the clinician needs to reinforce denture hygiene procedures and motivate the patient at a later stage, a commercial disclosing agent may be used (Fig. 14.10).

Some patients prefer to brush their dentures with a paste rather than with soap and water. Both conventional toothpastes and pastes designed specifically for dentures are used by patients. The former have been shown to be more abrasive for acrylic resin than the latter (Freitas-Pontes et al. 2009). Overzealous brushing of the denture with a stiff brush and an abrasive paste can cause marked abrasion of the acrylic resin, both of the denture base and of the teeth (Fig. 14.11). This can result in a significant deterioration in the appearance and fit of the dentures. Studies have shown that pastes

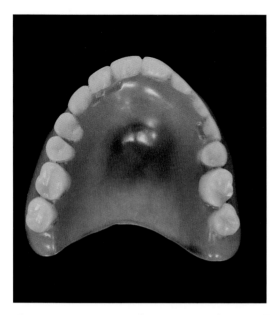

Figure 14.11 Denture showing severe abrasion of the acrylic resin as a result of over-enthusiastic brushing.

containing dicalcium phosphate are less abrasive than those containing calcium carbonate, but that the amount of wear that occurs even with the latter group of pastes is insignificant provided that the brushing load is not excessive (Murray et al. 1986a,b).

Immersion

Patients should be advised to regularly supplement the careful brushing of their dentures with periodic soaking in an immersion cleanser. Combining these two cleaning methods has been shown to be a particularly effective strategy for denture plaque control (Paranhos et al. 2007)

There has been some concern that immersion cleansers might damage materials used in the construction or maintenance of dentures. Most of the adverse changes reported have occurred in soft linings or chair side relining materials and usually take the form of increased roughness and colour change (Benting et al.

2005; Handa et al. 2008; Haywood et al. 2003; Jin et al. 2003; Mese 2007). However, these changes are usually slight and are unlikely to be significant clinically.

It should also be remembered that if immersion cleansers are not used and the denture plaque control is not therefore maintained at a high level, rapid degradation of soft linings can occur as a result of microbial invasion of the material.

Types of cleanser

There are several different types of liquid cleansers into which a denture can be immersed:

- Bleaches – e.g. sodium hypochlorite.
- Effervescent solutions – e.g. alkaline peroxides, perborates and persulphates.
- Acid cleansers.

Hypochlorite cleansers

Although investigations into the relative effectiveness of the various denture cleansers for removing denture plaque have produced some conflicting results in the case of the effervescent cleansers, there is widespread agreement as to the effectiveness of the hypochlorite preparations (Lima et al. 2006). These cleansers are not only effective disinfectants, but unlike some others, good at removing non-viable organisms and other organic deposits from the denture surface. They are not effective for the removal of calculus. Immersion of the dentures in a hypochlorite cleanser for periods in excess of 6 hours will result in removal of plaque and heavy staining. Bleaching of the acrylic resin has not been reported but corrosion of cobalt-chromium has been seen when hypochlorite cleansers have been used. These cleansers may cause some loss of colour of acrylic and silicone soft lining materials but neither softness nor elasticity of the linings is affected significantly (Davenport et al. 1986). In addition, microbial invasion, a common cause of soft lining failure, is prevented. Some of the commonly used short-term soft lining materials are compatible with hypochlorite cleansers; in fact, the regular use of such a cleanser can extend the useful life of a tissue conditioner from a few days to several months.

Effervescent cleansers

These may take the form of alkaline peroxides, perborates or persulphates. They are the most widely used type of immersion cleanser. Their cleaning action is largely due to the formation of small bubbles which dislodge loosely attached material from the denture surface. They are not particularly effective cleansers and there is evidence that their ability to remove microbial plaque is limited. They are safe, pleasant to use and do not damage acrylic resin or the metals used in denture construction. However, it has been demonstrated that they are capable of causing rapid deterioration of certain short-term soft lining materials (Harrison et al. 1989). Severe bleaching of acrylic resin resulting in a white denture has been reported; however, this has been shown to occur because the manufacturer's recommendations for use of the cleanser have not been followed and excessively hot water has been added to the cleaning agent (Crawford et al. 1986; Robinson et al. 1987).

Acid cleansers

One type of acid cleanser contains sulphamic acid. Immersion in this solution helps to control the formation of calculus on dentures. The compatibility of this agent with the commonly used denture materials, including the metals, appears to be good.

Another type of acid cleanser contains 5% hydrochloric acid. This cleanser is applied to the denture surface to wet the calculus and soften it so that it can be removed by brushing. Care is necessary as damage to clothing can result if the solution is spilled accidentally.

Corrosion of stainless steel or cobalt-chromium palates can occur if there is frequent and prolonged contact with the acid.

Other denture cleaning methods

Enzymes

There are a number of commercial preparations for cleaning dentures that contain enzymes, but they have not been proven to be effective (Hashiguchi et al. 2009; Lima et al. 2006).

Ultrasonic cleansers

Ultrasonication has been found to be as effective as immersion in denture cleansers for reducing the population of *Candida albicans* on acrylic resin plates in vitro (Arita et al. 2005; Hashiguchi et al. 2009).

Microwave exposure

This has been found to be effective when used in conjunction with an immersion cleanser (Goodson et al. 2003). Even when used on its own, microwave exposure is still likely to kill microorganisms on the denture; however, it will not remove the residual film of organic matter.

Recall procedures

When the dentures are fitted, it should be stressed that a recall visit within the next few days is necessary. To help boost the patient's confidence, it is useful to make the points that small problems may be experienced, that these are part and parcel of the adaptation process and that where appropriate these will be dealt with at the recall appointment.

To reduce the risk of mucosal damage and bone resorption, a check should be made every year. It is important that the patient is not under the mistaken belief that once the artificial substitute for the natural teeth has been provided there will be no further problems, and no need for further maintenance. Treatment carried out at subsequent visits is discussed in the next chapter.

Quality control and enhancement

- At the stage of fitting the dentures keep a record of the amount of occlusal adjustment that was found to be necessary and the method used to make the adjustment.

The effectiveness of this stage of treatment can also be assessed at the first recall appointment. The following topics might be part of a clinical audit undertaken on a series of patients. Patients can be asked at recall:

- 'After the dentures had been fitted at the last visit, did you then find that you had worries which had not been dealt with by the advice and instructions given to you?' 'What were those worries?'
- 'Did you feel confident with your new dentures when you left the surgery at the last visit?' If the answer is negative, find out what the problem was.

References and additional reading

Altman, M.D., Yost, K.G. & Pitts, G. (1979) A spectrofluorometric protein assay of plaque on dentures and of denture cleaning efficiency. *Journal of Prosthetic Dentistry*, 42, 502–6.

Ambjornsen, E. & Rise, J. (1985) The effect of verbal information and demonstration on denture hygiene in elderly people. *Acta Odontologica Scandinavica*, 43, 19–24.

Arita, M., Nagayoshi, M., Fukuizumi, T., Okinaga, T., Masumi, S., Morikawa, M., Kakinoki, Y. & Nishihara, T. (2005) Microbicidal efficacy of ozonated water against *Candida albicans* adhering to acrylic resin denture plates. *Oral Microbiology & Immunology*, 20, 206–10.

Benting, D., Pesun, I. & Hodges, J. (2005) Compliance of resilient denture liners immersed in effer-

vescent denture cleansers. *Journal of Prosthodontics*, 14, 175–83.

Bergman, B. & Carlsson, G.E. (1972) Review of 54 complete denture wearers. Patients' opinions 1 year after treatment. *Acta Odontologica Scandinavica*, 30, 399–414.

Budtz-Jørgensen, E. (1979) Materials and methods for cleaning dentures. *Journal of Prosthetic Dentistry*, 42, 619–23.

Burnett, C.A., Calwell, E. & Clifford, T.J. (1993) Effect of verbal and written education on denture wearing and cleansing habits. *European Journal of Prosthodontics and Restorative Dentistry*, 2, 79–83.

Cleary, T.J., Hutter, L., Blunt-Emerson, M. & Hutton, J.E. (1997) The effect of diet on the bearing mucosa during adjustment to new complete dentures: a pilot study. *Journal of Prosthetic Dentistry*, 78, 479–85.

Crawford, C.A., Lloyd, C.M., Newton, J.P. & Yemm, R. (1986) Denture bleaching: a laboratory simulation of patients' cleaning procedures. *Journal of Dentistry*, 14, 258–61.

Davenport, J.C. (1972) The denture surface. *British Dental Journal*, 133, 101–5.

Davenport, J.C., Wilson, H.J. & Basker, R.M. (1978) The compatibility of tissue conditioners with denture cleaners and chlorhexidine. *Journal of Dentistry*, 6, 239–46.

Davenport, J.C., Wilson, H.J. & Spence, D. (1986) The compatibility of soft lining materials and denture cleansers. *British Dental Journal*, 161, 13–17.

Firtell, D.N., Finzen, F.C. & Holmes, J.B. (1987) The effect of clinical remount procedures on the comfort and success of complete dentures. *Journal of Prosthetic Dentistry*, 57, 53–7.

Freitas-Pontes, K., Silva-Lovato, C. & Paranhos, H. (2009) Mass loss of four commercially available heat-polymerised acrylic resins after toothbrushing with three different dentifrices. *Journal of Applied Oral Science*, 17, 116–21.

Glass, R., Goodson, L., Bullard, J. & Conrad, R. (2001) Comparison of the effectiveness of several denture sanitizing systems. *Compendium of Continuing Education in Dentistry*, 22, 1093–6.

Goodson, L, Glass, R., Bullard, J. & Conrad, R. (2003) A statistical comparison of denture sanitation using a commercially available denture cleanser with and without microwaving. *General Dentistry*, 51, 148–51.

Guckes, A.D., Smith, D.E. & Swoope, C.C. (1978) Counselling and related factors influencing satisfaction with dentures. *Journal of Prosthetic Dentistry*, 39, 259–67.

Handa, R., Jagger, D. & Vowles, R. (2008) Denture cleansers, soft lining materials and water temperature: what is the effect? *Primary Dental Care*, 15, 53–8.

Harrison, A., Basker, R.M. & Smith, I. (1989) The compatibility of temporary soft materials with immersion denture cleansers. *International Journal of Prosthodontics*, 2, 254–8.

Hashiguchi, M., Nishi, Y., Kanie, T., Ban, S. & Nagaoka, E. (2009) Bactericidal efficacy of glycine-type amphoteric surfactant as a denture cleanser and its influence on properties of denture base resins. *Dental Materials Journal*, 28, 307–14.

Haywood, J., Wood, D., Gilchrist, A., Basker, R. & Watson, C. (2003) A comparison of three hard chairside denture reline materials. Part II. Changes in colour and hardness following immersion in three commonly used denture cleansers. *European Journal of Prosthodontics and restorative Dentistry*, 11, 165–9.

Hutchins, D.W. & Parker, W.A. (1973) A clinical evaluation of the ability of denture cleaning solutions to remove dental plaque from prosthetic devices. *New York State Dental Journal*, 39, 363–7.

Jagger, D.C. & Harrison, A. (1995) Denture cleansing – the best approach. *British Dental Journal*, 178, 413–17.

Jin, C., Nikawa, H., Makihira, S., Hamada, T., Furukawa, M. & Murata, H. (2003). Changes in surface roughness and color stability of soft denture lining materials caused by denture cleansers. *Journal of Oral Rehabilitation*, 30, 125–30.

Lee, D., Howlett, J., Pratten, J., Mordan, N., McDonald, A., Wilson, M. & Ready, D. (2009) Susceptibility of MRSA biofilms to denture-cleansing agents. *FEMS Microbiology Letters*, 291, 241–6.

Lima, E., Moura, J., Del Bel Cury, A., Garcia, R. & Cury, J. (2006) Effect of enzymatic and NaOCl treatments on acrylic roughness and on biofilm accumulation. *Journal of Oral Rehabilitation*, 33, 356–62.

Maeda, Y., Kenny, F., Coulter, W., Loughrey, A., Nagano, Y., Goldsmith, C., Millar, B., Dooley, J., James, S., Lowery, C., Rooney, P., Matsuda, M. & Moore, J. (2007) Bactericidal activity of denture-cleaning formulations against planktonic health care–associated and community-associated methicillin resistant *Staphylococcus aureus*. *American Journal of Infection Control*, 35, 619–22.

Mese, A. (2007) Effect of denture cleansers on the hardness of heat- or auto-cured acrylic- or silicone-based soft denture liners. *American Journal of Dentistry*, 20, 411–5.

Murakami, H., Mizuguchi, M., Hattori, M., Ito, Y., Kawai, T. & Hasegawa, J. (2002) Effect of denture cleanser using ozone against methicillin resistant *Staphylococcus aureus* and *E coli* T1 phage. *Dental Materials Journal*, 21, 53–60.

Murray, I.D., McCabe, J.F. & Storer, R. (1986a) Abrasivity of denture cleaning pastes in vitro and in situ. *British Dental Journal*, 161, 137–41.

Murray, I.D., McCabe, J.F. & Storer, R. (1986b) The relationship between the abrasivity and cleaning power of the dentifrice-type denture cleaners. *British Dental Journal*, 161, 205–8.

Nogueira, S.S., Ogle, R.E. & Davis, E.L. (1999) Comparison of accuracy between compression- and injection-molded complete dentures. *Journal of Prosthetic Dentistry*, 82, 291–300.

Oliver, O. & Basker, R.M. (1994) Check records – a chairside mounting procedure. *Quintessence International*, 25, 763–6.

Paranhos, H., Silva-Lovato, C., Souza, R., Cruz, P., Freitas, K. & Peracini, A. (2007) Effect of mechanical and chemical methods on denture biofilm accumulation. *Journal of Oral Rehabilitation*, 34, 606–12.

Robinson, J.G., McCabe, J.F. & Storer, R. (1987) Denture bases: the effects of various treatments on clarity, strength and structure. *Journal of Dentistry*, 15, 159–65.

15 Recall Procedures

In this chapter, we stress the importance of planning a programme of recall appointments after fitting complete dentures, to ensure that the tissues are not being damaged and that the dentures are functioning efficiently and comfortably. A recall visit also gives the patient an opportunity to seek advice over any concerns.

Short-term and long-term recalls are considered separately.

Short-term recall

The first recall appointment should be no longer than 1 week after fitting the dentures. At this visit it is necessary to obtain a careful history of any complaint, such as pain or looseness of the dentures, and to undertake a thorough examination.

The patient's complaints

The clinician should routinely enquire about the patient's progress during the first week of denture wearing. This is important because the more timid patient may need positive en-couragement before being willing to comment about a matter of concern. Of course, there are other patients who require no such invitation and will have already composed a list of difficulties. However, even then the routine enquiry about progress is likely to be welcomed as an example of a caring 'after-sales service'.

Whatever the type of patient response, advice and explanation by the clinician may be all that are needed to overcome certain denture problems, particularly if the patient is an inexperienced denture wearer. Other problems will require intervention to modify the dentures.

Problems with the dentures may be caused by faults that passed unnoticed at the fit stage, or by changes occurring in the mouth since that time. There can also be persistent difficulties caused by insurmountable hurdles related to unfavourable anatomy, unrealistically high patient expectations, or lack of adequate denture control skills.

The more common complaints are:

- Discomfort
- Looseness

Prosthetic Treatment of the Edentulous Patient, Fifth Edition, © R.M. Basker, J.C. Davenport and J.M. Thomason
Published 2011 by Blackwell Publishing Ltd.

- Appearance
- Speech

The first two problems occur most frequently. The last two are dealt with elsewhere in the book.

Discomfort

Examples of injury to the mucosa which arise from faults on the impression surface include mucosal damage in the sulcus due to over-extension, and on the most bulbous part of a ridge where the denture base has been inadequately relieved from a bony undercut. Where there is a clear relationship between mucosal damage and the impression surface, appropriate correction of the denture should be undertaken. It may be tempting to assume that all mucosal damage is directly related to faults in the impression surface. However, such an assumption would be fraught with danger as the damage could be equally due to faults in the occlusion causing movement of the denture or concentrations of occlusal pressure. It is important to appreciate that the occlusal error causing a problem may be some distance from the site of inflammation (Fig. 15.1). It is also important to remember that when there is a complaint of discomfort an assessment of the occlusion must always be made before any adjustment of the impression surface is carried out.

Looseness

Looseness of the dentures may occur because the patient has not, as yet, learned to control the new shapes in the mouth, rather than being due to denture faults or anatomical shortcomings. Thus, a check must be made on the patient's progress in adapting to the new dentures. Bearing in mind that 20% of experienced denture wearers require up to a month in which to become proficient with their new dentures (Bergman & Carlsson 1972), it is likely that a significant number of patients will benefit from the offer of further advice, reassurance and follow-up.

Routine checks and treatment

Checks that should always be made at the recall appointment when carrying out an examination of the patient's mouth and dentures are:

- Occlusion
- Tissue health
- Denture cleanliness

Occlusion

It must be remembered that because new dentures are seated on a surface which is compressible and liable to change, the initial few days of function may have caused an alteration in the occlusion. Such an alteration is a potent cause of

Figure 15.1 (a) A posterior premature contact, resulting in forward movement of the lower denture (dotted arrow), produces inflammation of the mucosa on the lingual aspect of the alveolar ridge in the anterior region. (b) Lateral displacement of the lower denture produces inflammation of the mucosa in areas closely related to the occlusal error.

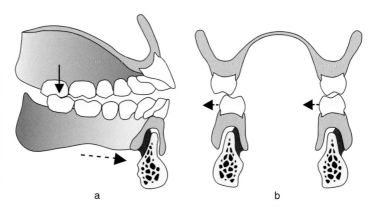

a   b

mucosal injury, and it can also lead to problems with the masticatory muscles. Patients attempt to adapt to an uneven occlusion by altering the normal pattern of mandibular movement. Such an attempt is liable to produce muscular disorders which, in the short term, may pass unnoticed by the patient, but in the longer term can give rise to significant discomfort. Methods of carrying out occlusal adjustment are described in Chapter 14.

Tissue health

Even if the patient expresses complete satisfaction and reports perfect comfort, it is essential to carry out a thorough examination to check on tissue health. This is because occasionally there may be mucosal injury, even frank ulceration, without the patient apparently being aware of it. The absence of a complaint under such circumstances may be due to a high pain threshold or a desire to please. With the information gleaned from the history and an examination, a diagnosis of any problem should be established and appropriate treatment decided upon.

The impression surface of the denture should never be adjusted in an empirical manner. Once any occlusal faults have been eliminated, a further check of the impression surface should be made using a pressure-disclosing medium. If this sequence is not carried out, it is difficult to judge whether an area of inflammation is due either to an impression surface defect or to an occlusal error. Pressure-disclosing media suitable for this purpose include silicone rubber materials formulated for the purpose, pressure-disclosing paste or wax and low viscosity alginate.

If the mucosal damage has been diagnosed as being due to a fault with the impression surface and is localised, a disclosing material is applied to the impression surface of the denture in the suspect area. The denture is then seated firmly for a few seconds and on removal any pressure points are indicated by the pink denture base showing through the material. Ad-

justment of the impression surface can then be carried out in a relatively precise manner.

If the mucosal damage is more generalised, an alternative technique which is simple, quick and revealing is to obtain a wash impression over the whole of the impression surface using a low viscosity mix of alginate or silicone rubber. The set impression gives a clear picture of pressure points and base extension. Any pressure points can be marked with a pencil before the material is removed allowing their precise correction. If adhesive has not been applied to the denture beforehand, the impression can then be quickly and cleanly removed from the denture after the adjustments have been completed.

Denture cleanliness

A check on denture plaque control can be made by direct visual inspection assisted where necessary by the use of a disclosing solution. If there are significant deposits it is essential to discover what cleaning technique the patient is using. Reinforcement of advice at this stage may prevent the development of denture-induced stomatitis, angular stomatitis, staining of the dentures and mouth odour. If there have been significant problems at the first recall appointment, a further appointment for short-term review should be made to check on progress. The clinician can also ensure that any modification to the dentures has been successful. The patient should be advised about the importance of a review in a year's time for reasons that will become apparent in the next section of this chapter. Thereafter reviews at intervals of 2–3 years will usually be appropriate.

Long-term recall

All the checks carried out for the short-term recall should also be completed at long-term recall appointments. However, the following points will be discussed further.

Mucosal changes

In Chapter 7 the need to carry out periodic checks with respect to oral cancer was stressed (Craig & Johnson 2000; Conway et al. 2002). In 2007, in the UK, there were 5325 new cases and 1841 deaths, with an increased prevalence in deprived communities (Chadwick 2009). It should be emphasised that the typical edentulous patient falls into a risk group, as a retrospective study of patients with oral cancer showed that 59% were edentulous, tended to be older than 60 years, were tobacco and alcohol users, had a lower socioeconomic status and had a somewhat negative attitude to recall appointments (Guggenheimer & Hoffman 1994; Craig & Johnson 2000).

Bone resorption

The long-term changes in shape of the residual ridges and the consequent effect on dentures have been studied extensively. A continuing reduction in height of the alveolar ridges over a period of 25 years has been observed. There appears to be a marked reduction in the first year of denture wearing and in the next few years a continuing loss averaging 1 mm each year. Over periods of time, the loss in height of the anterior lower ridge is four times that of the upper (Tallgren 1972; Douglass et al. 1993). As the lower denture covers a much smaller area, the functional stress transmitted to the underlying tissues is greater than that to the upper tissues; thus, it is likely that the greater loss of mandibular bone is due to the physiological limit of this tissue being exceeded. The resorption of bone brings in its wake a loss of both occlusal vertical dimension and rest vertical dimension. The former dimension is reduced to a greater extent and thus the freeway space is increased.

Occlusal changes

The progressive loss of fit of dentures, resulting from resorption of bone, also leads to de-

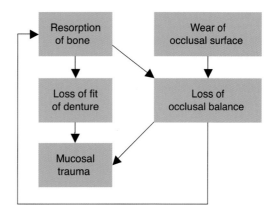

Figure 15.2 Cycle of tissue damage resulting from lack of denture maintenance.

terioration in occlusal balance. In the case of dentures with acrylic teeth this occlusal deterioration can be aggravated by occlusal wear. The combination of loss of fit and occlusal imbalance encourages mucosal inflammation and further bone resorption, thus establishing a vicious cycle (Fig. 15.2). It is clearly important, if oral health and function are to be maintained, that this cycle is broken by regular denture review and effective maintenance.

Adaptation of the patient

The progressive long-term deterioration of dentures that has been described is not invariably associated with a complaint. This is because adaptive changes can occur and a tolerance can develop which allows patients to continue wearing the dentures. Thus, a considerable amount of tissue damage can go unnoticed. Whereas successful adaptation to new dentures is a prerequisite for success, a patient who tolerates slowly developing faults beyond a certain point will store up troubles for the future. In addition to the likelihood of tissue damage, reduction in rest vertical dimension and the adoption of abnormal mandibular postures create problems for both the clinician and the patient when replacement dentures are eventually required (Chapter 8).

Dental health surveys

Deterioration in both the dentures and the health of the mouth is the result of patients not seeking regular denture maintenance. The size of the problem has been highlighted by national surveys of adult dental health which reported that, whereas 40% of complete denture wearers reported problems with eating, drinking, speaking and appearance, only 13% planned to seek advice (Walker & Cooper 2000). It appears that the longer patients have been edentulous the less inclined they are to seek treatment. In an earlier survey it was reported that a third of the edentulous population had had their current dentures for over 20 years and a quarter of them had not visited a dental clinician for more than 20 years (Todd & Lader 1991). Clearly, many patients do not have a realistic perception of what is required to maintain their dentures and mouth in good condition.

Having made these comments, which almost suggest a laissez-faire attitude amongst complete denture wearers, it is worth making the point that people who express satisfaction with old dentures, even though they are ill-fitting, can in fact appreciate the benefits of new dentures. This is suggested by the fact that patients reported that chewing with their new dentures was more enjoyable than with their old ones and that they had discovered they had a greater food choice (Garrett et al. 1996).

Long-term recall schedule

The importance of the clinician convincing the patient of the need to seek regular denture maintenance is obvious in the light of this discussion. It should be explained that the first long-term recall appointment should be made no more than a year after the dentures were first fitted. Thereafter, an appointment every 2 or 3 years to check on tissue health and quality of the dentures is a realistic arrangement, on the mutual understanding that the patient will attend sooner if problems develop

in the meantime. The clinician should make the point that the dentures have a limited life and should stress to the patient the potential dangers of wearing dentures that have become inadequate.

At this stage it is worth sounding a warning note. The clinician can be faced with a dilemma if, at review, it is apparent that a denture fault has developed but there is no concern expressed by the patient, nor any signs of tissue damage. The clinician has to decide whether or not to correct the deficiency. In the absence of both signs and symptoms, it will often be foolhardy to tamper with well-accepted dentures just because a minor shortcoming has developed. Absence of current signs and symptoms is not the only consideration, however, as the clinician needs to consider whether the presence of the problem, even though undetected by the patient, is likely to give rise to significant difficulties in the future.

Treatment required at long-term recall appointments will be one, or a combination, of the following:

- Adjustment of the impression surface
- Correction of denture base extension
- Occlusal adjustment with or without a check record
- Reline or rebase of the dentures
- Construction of replacement dentures.

Relining and rebasing will now be considered in more detail, and the other procedures in the list having already been considered in previous chapters.

Clinical procedures for relining or rebasing

Relining

In simple terms, a reline involves a straightforward substitution of the layer of impression material within the denture by a layer of new acrylic resin (Fig. 15.3a). Such a method is

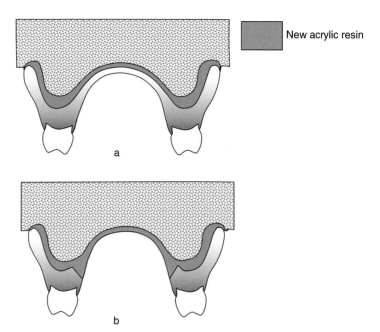

New acrylic resin

Figure 15.3 Cross section through upper dentures that have been (a) relined and (b) rebased.

quite satisfactory for a lower denture but will increase the thickness of the palate of an upper denture, the degree of increase depending upon the impression material used. The more viscous zinc oxide-eugenol impression pastes are likely to produce an unacceptable thickness, while minimal change will occur with light-bodied silicone impression materials.

Rebasing

Rebasing entails the replacement of most of the original acrylic base of the denture with heat-curing acrylic resin (Fig. 15.3b). A rebasing technique does not suffer from the disadvantage just mentioned and is thus preferred by many for correcting the impression surface of an upper denture. Certainly, a rebase should be undertaken when the existing denture base material has deteriorated or when there is a history of previous fractures of the palate. Whatever laboratory technique is requested, the basic principles of the clinical method remain the same.

Diagnosis and treatment planning

It is apparent that as the reline/rebase alters the impression surface of a denture, it will be of benefit only when a patient's complaint can be attributed to a defect in that surface. The common history a patient gives is one of recent looseness following a period of trouble-free denture wearing. If the complaint of looseness is the result of defects in the other surfaces, such as an unbalanced occlusion, it is quite useless to reline/rebase the denture.

Preparatory procedures

Three routine preparatory procedures are carried out whatever reline/rebase technique is followed:

(i) The occlusion must be balanced to ensure that, when the impression is taken, uneven contact does not bring about a bodily shift or tilt of the denture when the patient is asked to occlude.

(ii) Any over- or under-extension of the borders must be corrected.

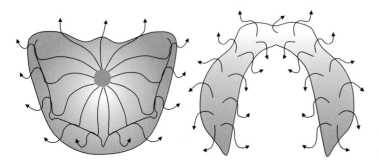

Figure 15.4 Escape routes for excess impression material.

(iii) Undercuts within the impression surface of the denture must be eliminated so that the technician can remove the denture from the cast.

Impression procedures

When an impression is taken within an existing denture, care must be taken to ensure that the jaw relationship in the horizontal plane is not altered. This is achieved by taking great care in seating the denture and checking the accuracy of this by getting the patient to occlude in the intercuspal position. Inevitably, the occlusal vertical dimension is increased slightly by the thickness of the impression material. Unless there has been a corresponding reduction in occlusal vertical dimension during the life of the dentures this increase should be kept to a minimum. It is usual, therefore, to choose an impression material which can be reduced to a thin film as the denture is seated and is accurate in thin section. Low viscosity silicone elastomers and zinc oxide-eugenol impression pastes are good examples of materials of this type. The more fluid silicone will produce the least change in occlusal vertical dimension. When an impression is taken within a lower denture, excess material in the middle of the impression surface has only a short distance to travel before it escapes at the periphery. Thus, the force needed to extrude the material and seat the denture is small, and the risk of displacing the underlying tissues or of altering the occlusal relationship is minimal. The sit-

uation is obviously somewhat different in the upper jaw as the excess material has a longer and more circuitous route to follow (Fig. 15.4). Greater force is therefore needed to seat the upper denture, bringing with it the potential complication of undue displacement of the mucosa with consequent reduction in retention of the relined/rebased denture. Also, unless great care is taken, the denture may not be seated correctly in the antero-posterior plane; too much impression material may be left under the labial flange resulting in the relined/rebased denture being positioned too far anteriorly. This brings with it inevitable occlusal and aesthetic complications. Creating a series of small perforations in the palate of the denture will facilitate the escape of excess impression material and reduce the chance of the above problems occurring.

Intra-oral reline

It will be appreciated that the above procedures require the patient to be without the denture for a period of time while the laboratory work is being completed. If this approach is unacceptable for any reason it is possible to carry out a reline as a one-stage chair side procedure. These materials are discussed further in Chapter 16.

References and additional reading

Bergman, B. & Carlsson, G.E. (1972) Review of 54 complete denture wearers. Patients' opinions 1 year after treatment. *Acta Odontologica Scandinavica*, 30, 399–414.

Bergman, B., Carlsson, G.E. & Ericson, S. (1971) Effect of differences in habitual use of complete dentures on underlying tissues. *Scandinavian Journal of Dental Research*, 79, 449–60.

Chadwick, B. (2009) Oral cancer annual evidence update. *NHS Evidence – oral health NICE*, www.evidence.nhs.uk

Conway, D.l, Macpherson, L.M.D., Gibson, J. & Binnie, V.I. (2002) Oral cancer: prevention and detection in primary dental healthcare. *Primary Dental Care*, 9, 119–23.

Craig, G. & Johnson, N. (ed) (2000) *Opportunisitic oral cancer screening – a management strategy for dental practice*. British Dental Association, London.

Douglass, J.B., Meader, L., Kaplan, A. & Ellinger, C.W. (1993) Cephalometric evaluation of the changes in patients wearing complete dentures. A 20-year study. *Journal of Prosthetic Dentistry*, 69, 270–5.

Garrett, N.R., Kapur, K.K. & Perez, P. (1996) Effects of improvements of poorly fitting dentures and new dentures on patient satisfaction. *Journal of Prosthetic Dentistry*, 76, 403–13.

Guggenheimer, J. & Hoffman, R.D. (1994) The importance of screening edentulous patients for oral cancer. *Journal of Prosthetic Dentistry*, 72, 141–3.

Jackson, R.A. & Ralph, W.J. (1980) Continuing changes in the contour of the maxillary residual alveolar ridge. *Journal of Oral Rehabilitation*, 7, 245–8.

Shaffer, F.W. & Filler, W.H. (1971) Relining complete dentures with minimum occlusal error. *Journal of Prosthetic Dentistry*, 25, 366–70.

Sheppard, I.M., Schwartz, L.R. & Sheppard, S.M. (1971) Oral status of edentulous and complete denture-wearing patients. *Journal of the American Dental Association*, 83, 614–20.

Sheppard, I.M., Schwartz, L.R. & Sheppard, S.M. (1972) Survey of the oral status of complete denture patients. *Journal of Prosthetic Dentistry*, 28, 121–6.

Tallgren, A. (1972) The continuing reduction of the residual alveolar ridges in complete denture wearers: a mixed-longitudinal study covering 25 years. *Journal of Prosthetic Dentistry*, 27, 120–32.

Todd, J.E. & Lader, D. (1991) *Adult Dental Health 1988 United Kingdom*. HMSO, London.

Walker, A. & Cooper, I. (eds) (2000) *Adult Dental Health Survey – Oral Health in the United Kingdom 1998*. The Stationery Office, London.

Yusof, Z.Y., Netuveli, G., Ramli, A.S. & Sheiham, A. (2006) Is opportunistic oral cancer screening by dentists feasible? An analysis of the patterns of dental attendance of a nationally representative sample over 10 years. *Oral Health and Preventive Dentistry*, 4, 165–71.

Some Clinical Problems and Solutions

16

The topics that will be covered in this chapter are:

- Pain and instability
- Lack of saliva
- Hard and soft materials for modifying the impression surface of dentures
- The flabby ridge
- Denture breakages
- Gagging
- The burning mouth syndrome
- Disturbance of speech

Pain and instability

The most common problems associated with complete dentures are pain and instability of the dentures (Lechner et al. 1995). Many of the causes have been described in earlier chapters but to give a simplified picture they are summarised in Table 16.1. The most likely main complaints have been indicated in each case. However, it should be remembered that there is considerable overlap between the two columns,

as any cause of instability may additionally give rise to a complaint of pain. It should also be stressed that there may be more than one cause of a complaint.

Persistent pain

This problem is more often seen in the lower jaw where the area available for distribution of the occlusal load is relatively small. As noted in Table 16.1, there are many possible causes of this complaint, which may be attributed to the denture design and to the patient.

A diagnostic flow chart is shown in Fig. 16.1. The clinician may find it helpful to base the history and examination on this chart in order to arrive at a diagnosis. An example of the diagnostic process is presented in Table 16.2.

Discomfort can arise from overloading of the mucosa as a result of clenching or grinding the teeth. These occlusal habits are caused by increased activity of the masticatory muscles produced during stressful situations. Clues to such a diagnosis come from the absence of errors in

Prosthetic Treatment of the Edentulous Patient, Fifth Edition, © R.M. Basker, J.C. Davenport and J.M. Thomason
Published 2011 by Blackwell Publishing Ltd.

Table 16.1 Summary of the causes of pain (P) and looseness (L)

CAUSE	COMPLAINT	
DENTURE FAULTS		
Impression surface		
Inaccurate fit	P	L
Over-extension	P	L
Under-extension	P	L
Flange width inadequate for facial seal		L
Post-dam absent		L
Relief chamber absent but required	P	L
Roughness	P	
Cast damaged before processing	P	
Extension into bony undercuts	P	
Polished surface		
Denture not in neutral zone		L
Shape unfavourable for muscle control		L
Occlusal surface		
Occlusion unbalanced	P	L
Cuspal interference	P	L
Occlusal plane too high		L
Inadequate freeway space	P	
Occlusal table too wide	P	L
PATIENT FACTORS		
Bruxism/parafunction	P	
Low pain tolerance	P	
Poor neuromuscular control		
Slow rate of adaptation (e.g. elderly patient)		L
Neuromuscular disorders (e.g. Parkinsonism)		L
Mucosa		
Flabby		L
Atrophic	P	
Bone		
Sharp spicules	P	
Prominences (mylohyoid ridges, tori, genial tubercles)	P	
Advanced resorption		L
Mental foramen near crest of ridge	P	
Pathology within the bone	P	
Saliva		
Deficient or absent	P	L
Systemic disease		
Iron-deficiency anaemia	P	

denture design together with evidence of shiny wear facets on the occlusal surface of the teeth. It is helpful to ask the patient, 'When you are not eating are your upper and lower teeth nor-mally in contact or out of contact?' It is not un-usual for such patients to reply that their teeth are usually together and for them to assume that this is quite normal.

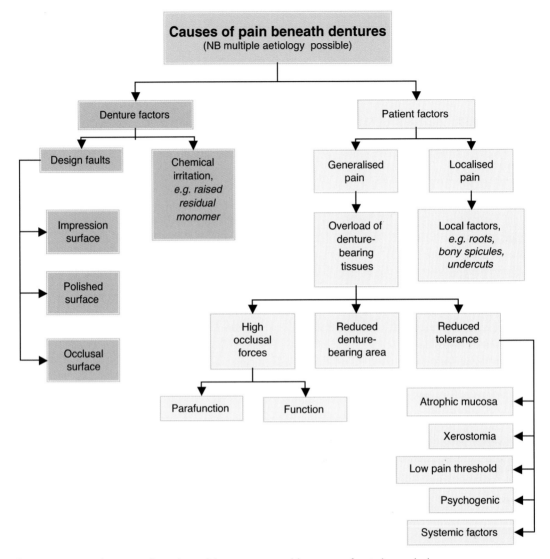

Figure 16.1 A diagnostic flow chart of the various possible causes of pain beneath dentures.

In treating parafunction, the patient must be made aware of the problem and should be told that teeth should be out of contact for most of the time. It is important to reassure the patient, describe the link between stress, parafunction and pain under dentures and point out that there is no sinister change in the oral mucosa. The importance of conscious relaxation should be emphasised and the patient should be strongly encouraged to leave both dentures, or at least the lower denture, out at night.

Lack of saliva

Functions of saliva

Saliva possesses the following functions in the edentulous patient (Lewis, 2009):

Table 16.2 The history taking and possible significance of the patient's answers are presented for an elderly person complaining of persistent pain in the lower denture-bearing area. The objective of the table is to stress that (1) many denture problems are multifactorial; (2) a seemingly simple complaint may have wider ramifications – especially with older patients; (3) a correct diagnosis is unlikely to be established unless a properly structured history and examination are undertaken.

CLINICIAN'S QUESTIONS	SUMMARY OF ANSWERS	SIGNIFICANCE
COMPLAINT		
'What's your problem?'	'I can't eat with my dentures'	A common answer reflecting a common concern, but it tells us little.
'Why do you have difficulty in eating?'	'Because my lower gum hurts'	We now know that pain rather than instability of the denture is the problem.
'How long have you had the problem?'	'For about 1 year'	
'How long have you had this set of dentures?'	'For the same time'	This could suggest that a DENTURE FAULT is contributing to the problem, or it could be a coincidence.
'Where is the pain?'	'All round the lower gum'	
'What's the pain like?'	'A continuing soreness – severe at times'	
'How often do you get the pain?'	'All day, every day'	
'Does anything make it better or worse?'	'Worse after eating. Better if the lower denture is removed. I now always leave it out at night'	Answers to the last four questions paint a picture of tissue overload. A DENTURE FAULT is one possibility.
'When you wore the lower denture at night, how was the lower gum when you woke in the morning?'	'Very sore'	The timing suggests the possibility of PARAFUNCTION.
'When you are wearing the dentures (and not eating) are your upper and lower teeth usually apart or together?'	'Usually together'	Suggests LACK OF FREEWAY SPACE and/or PARAFUNCTION.
PAST DENTAL HISTORY		
'How long have you been wearing complete dentures?'	'About 10 years'	
'How many sets have you had in that time?'	'Three'	
'Tell me about them'	First set was fitted immediately after the teeth were taken out. One year later a further set made. Worn successfully for eight years. Third set are the troublesome ones.	Suggests DENTURE FAULT with the latest prostheses. But could be due to deterioration of the supporting TISSUES. It is important to examine the successful dentures and compare them with the most recent ones to clarify this.

(Continued)

Table 16.2   (*Continued*)

CLINICIAN'S QUESTIONS	SUMMARY OF ANSWERS	SIGNIFICANCE
'Why did you decide to seek replacements for the successful set?'	'The teeth were worn down and my face was beginning to look old'.	There might have been an INCREASE IN OVD in the troublesome dentures which cannot be tolerated.
MEDICAL HISTORY		
A full history is taken including a question on current medication.	'I'm taking an anti-depressant and a diuretic'.	DRY MOUTH is a possible contributory factor to the oral complaint.
'For how long have you been taking these tablets?'	'One year'	
SOCIAL HISTORY		
'Why were you prescribed the anti-depressant tablets?'	'Last year my wife was found to have Alzheimer's. I have had to rearrange my life to look after her. I retired early'.	It is possible that worry and anxiety (and a degree of frustration) have led to PARAFUNCTION.

Comment: The history has revealed a number of possible causes of the persistent pain. The diagnosis can be established only after a careful examination of the patient, the mouth and the various sets of dentures in order to confirm or eliminate the various possibilities. The point should be made that unless a full history is obtained some of the possible causes might never be identified. The provision of new dentures would do little to resolve the problem if the persistent pain was due to a dry mouth and/or parafunction.

- *Denture retention* – saliva is an essential component in the physical retention of complete dentures.
- *Lubrication* – the glycoproteins in saliva facilitate movement of the soft tissues during speech, mastication and the swallowing of food.
- *Cleansing* – saliva physically washes food and other debris from the soft tissues and from the polished surfaces of prostheses.
- *Taste* – flavours are perceived only when substances are in solution in saliva or other fluids.
- *Digestion* – digestion begins during mastication when salivary amylase starts to break down glucose.
- *Antimicrobial* – there are antimicrobial components, such as antibodies, in saliva which help to maintain a normal balance of the oral flora.

Problems of reduced salivary flow

A reduction or absence of saliva, known as xerostomia, is responsible for a range of symptoms resulting from an interference with some or all of the functions of saliva listed above. As a result, a general and significant reduction in the quality of life can result. Reduced retention of dentures can be a particular problem for edentulous patients. However, the literature is inconclusive about whether or not treating the hyposalivation has a beneficial effect on denture retention (Turner et al. 2008). There may also be an increased susceptibility to denture trauma resulting in complaints of pain and in some cases the burning mouth syndrome, discussed later in this chapter (Soh et al. 2007). A complaint of dry mouth can occur in the absence of the clinical signs of dryness ('symptomatic xerostomia'). Under such circumstances the physical retention of the dentures would not be expected to be diminished.

Aetiology of reduced salivary flow

Old age *per se* probably does not result in reduced salivary flow rates (Scott & Baum 1990). The condition is more common in females than in males (Flink et al. 2008) and is relatively common in middle-aged and older people, the main candidates for complete dentures, with up to a third of adults complaining of a dry mouth (Locker 1995; Field et al. 2001; Marton et al. 2008; Johansson et al. 2009). This relatively high prevalence of xerostomia is likely to be due to the fact that older individuals are more likely to be suffering from systemic disease or to be taking drugs that can reduce salivary flow (von Bultzingslowen et al. 2007).

The most common causes of dry mouth (Niedermeier et al. 2000; Field et al. 2001; Guggenheimer & Moore, 2003) are:

- *Adverse effects of drug therapy* – over 500 medications have been implicated in xerostomia, e.g. tricyclic antidepressants, beta-blockers, diuretics, recreational drugs such as ecstasy.
- *Auto-immune disease (Sjögren's syndrome)* – this affects 1-3% of the UK population, particularly middle-aged females.
- *Poorly controlled diabetes* – reduced salivary flow results from raised blood sugar, and increased micturition which can lead to dehydration.
- *Radiotherapy* – an increasing number of patients with malignant disease of the head and neck receive radiotherapy as part of their treatment. Salivary tissue is very sensitive to radiation and so, in spite of strategies to limit exposure of the salivary glands reduction in salivary flow often follows.
- *Other causes* – these include depression, chronic anxiety, dehydration, mouth breathing and smoking.

Management of dry mouth

In clinical xerostomia there are intra-oral signs of dryness such as a dry, atrophic mucosa and lack of saliva pooling in the floor of the mouth. The clinician can check the dryness of the buccal mucosa simply and quickly during the examination of the patient by carrying out the 'mirror test'. For this the clinician lightly presses the face of the mirror against the buccal mucosa and then tries to remove it. If the mirror comes away easily the mucosa is still covered by a substantial film of saliva; if the mucosa adheres to the mirror then it is dry. Referral to the patient's general medical practitioner or to a specialist in oral medicine is likely to be necessary if a more thorough investigation is indicated.

Measures for managing xerostomia may be local or systemic

Local measures

- *Artificial saliva.* In cases where the salivary flow rate cannot be improved, limited relief may sometimes be obtained by the use of artificial saliva (Ship et al. 2007; Oh et al. 2008). These preparations are usually based on either carboxymethylcellulose or mucin. But it should be remembered that as the mucin preparations are of animal origin, they may not be acceptable to vegetarians or to some religious groups. Some patients with dry mouth find that frequent sips of water or milk are equally, or even more, effective than artificial saliva in alleviating their symptoms.
- *Denture and oral hygiene.* It is very important for a denture patient with a dry mouth to maintain an excellent level of denture hygiene. The likelihood of the proliferation of *Candida albicans* and other microorganisms is increased in xerostomia and therefore unless denture hygiene is maintained at a high level the denture is likely to be rapidly colonised by the microorganism, increas-

ing the likelihood of oral disease (Almstahl et al. 2008; Leung et al. 2008). Motivation and instruction of the patient, followed by monitoring the quality of denture hygiene, are essential.

- *Denture retention.* In cases where an intractable dry mouth gives rise to a persistent problem of loose dentures a denture adhesive will usually provide some improvement in denture function.

Systemic measures

- *Treatment of an underlying disease.* It might be possible, for example, to change an existing xerostomic drug to one less liable to reduce salivary flow. Also if the patient is diabetic, an improved glycaemic control will alleviate the xerostomia.
- *Increasing fluid intake.* As there is a relationship between fluid intake and secretory performance, it is essential that the patient is kept well hydrated.
- *Sialogogues.* Pilocarpine can stimulate salivary flow where some functional salivary tissue remains, particularly in drug-related xerostomia, but it commonly has unpleasant side effects such as increased sweating. The dry mouth may also be occasionally alleviated by sialogogues such as chewing gum or glycerine and lemon mouthwash.

Hard and soft materials for modifying the impression surface of dentures

In a chapter dealing with problems and solutions it is logical to consider materials which can be used to modify the impression surface of a denture to overcome some of these problems; these materials can be either applied by the clinician at the chair side or constructed by the dental technician in the laboratory.

The materials may be classified as follows:

- Hard materials
- Short-term soft lining materials
- Long-term soft lining materials

Hard materials

Recent years have seen the development of a group of useful materials, frequently described as chair side reline materials, which can be used to modify the impression surface of an existing denture.

Composition

Commonly these materials consist of a powder containing polyethylmethacrylate together with a liquid monomer, butylmethacrylate. The important point to make is that monomeric methylmethacrylate, a tissue irritant, is avoided. Many of the products include a bonding agent to enhance the adhesion of the material to the existing denture polymer (Mutluay, 2005). The available materials vary in working time, setting time and viscosity.

Clinical applications

These materials can be immensely useful for relining dentures. As they can be used at the chair side a 'one-stop' reline technique can be employed. This has great benefits in the following situations:

- *A laboratory reline would require the patient to be without any denture for an inconvenient length of time.* This is likely to include patients who only have one set of dentures that they can wear and who find being without dentures for any period of time socially unacceptable. In particular, immediate denture patients usually fall into this category. The materials can be used to improve the fit of an immediate denture that has become loose as a consequence of bone resorption. This hard material is usually added after initial healing of the residual ridge has occurred. In the early days following the extraction of teeth it is more likely that a short-term soft lining material will be used (see below). The great advantage in changing from the short-term soft lining material to the hard material after the initial healing period is that the latter can be trimmed and polished for a high-quality finish and is much more durable. The 'one-stop' reline technique can also be very useful when treating older patients, particularly when a domiciliary service is being provided.

- *A reline is required, but it is not necessary for it to last for much longer than a year.* After this period of time the hard chair side relining material is likely to have deteriorated to the point when replacement is required. Again, the immediate denture patient is likely to fall into this category, as after a year the chair side reline will usually need replacing by a permanent rebase or by a replacement denture.
- *Where a direct technique is indicated.* A chair side reline is a direct technique that does not involve the intermediate stages of impression taking, cast pouring and laboratory processing. There are therefore fewer opportunities for errors to creep into the process and consequently there is the potential for greater accuracy.

Clinical performance

Clinical trials have shown that the best of this group of materials are convenient to use and provide immediate improvement of fit and comfort. Over a period of time there is a loss of material, especially at the borders of the denture; this loss is more apparent in the lower denture. However, the loss does not appear to cause marked deterioration of fit or comfort (Hayward et al. 2003). The better materials

should be regarded as having a working life of about one year. The surface can be cleaned in the normal manner and there is relatively little discolouration (Hayward et al. 2003).

Short-term soft lining materials

Composition

Most materials are supplied in a powder/liquid form. An alternative presentation is in a ready-to-use sheet form which can be found in one product available to the dental profession and in several 'over the counter' products available directly to the general public. The method of self-treatment is to be discouraged, except as an emergency measure, as it is not based on a sound clinical diagnosis and can result in severe tissue destruction. It is essential that traumatised tissue is examined by the clinician and that rational, rather than empirical, treatment is prescribed. The composition of the powder/liquid types is as follows:

- *Powder* – polyethylmethacrylate, or copolymers of polyethyl/methylmethacrylate.
- *Liquid* – a mixture of an aromatic ester, such as dibutyl phthalate, which acts as a plasticiser, and ethyl alcohol.

The setting process

After the powder and liquid have been mixed, the ethyl alcohol causes swelling of the polymer particles and permits penetration by the ester so that a gel is formed. This is a physical change; there is no chemical reaction. The presence of ethyl alcohol is necessary to initiate this process and the amount present in the liquid is related to the particle size and molecular weight of the polymer; the higher the alcohol content, the shorter the gelling time (Murata et al. 1994). If particle size and molecular weight are low, then the ethyl alcohol content can be kept to a minimum. This state of affairs is desirable as large amounts of ethyl alcohol produce an unpleasant taste and sensation in the mouth.

Some materials suffer from dimensional change as a consequence of water absorption and solubility of the material (Murata et al. 2001). The ethyl alcohol and plasticiser are leached out reducing the flow of the material with time and causing the material to harden and shrink. The more ethyl alcohol there is in the formulation, the quicker is the rate of hardening. The rate can also be accelerated by dietary solvents found in fatty foods and foods containing alcohol (Jepson et al. 2000).

Clinical applications

Short-term soft lining materials are placed in existing dentures for the following reasons:

- *Tissue conditioning*. For tissue conditioning, the material is applied for a period of a few days to the impression surface of a denture when the denture-bearing mucosa is traumatised and inflamed. The tissue conditioner acts as a cushion absorbing the occlusal loads, improving their distribution to the supporting tissues and encouraging healing of the inflamed mucosa.
- *Temporary soft reline*. A short-term soft lining material can be used to improve the fit and comfort of a denture, typically an immediate restoration.
- *Diagnosis*. A short-term soft lining material can be used as a diagnostic aid where the clinician wishes to check the reaction of the patient and the tissues to an improvement in fit of a denture. If the patient is happy with the change made by the short-term lining material, the clinician has first-hand evidence of the degree of improvement that can be expected if a long-term soft reline is to be inserted. An important advantage of this approach is that the information has been obtained by a reversible procedure. If the pa-

tient is unhappy the lining can be removed and the denture returned to its original state.
- *Functional impression*. A short-term soft lining material can be used as a functional impression material applied to the impression surface of a denture for the purpose of securing an impression under functional stresses.
- *Recording the neutral zone*. The ability of these materials to be moulded by the oral musculature over an extended period of several minutes allows them to be used to record the neutral zone (p. 185).

It is probably true to say that these products are used less as functional impression materials than as tissue conditioners and temporary soft lining materials.

Relevant properties

The properties of soft lining materials which are of particular clinical relevance are:

- *Softness*. This property of the set material alters with time. The longer the powder/liquid types are left in the mouth, the harder they become. However, those with a low alcohol content remain softer for longer and are thus more effective as tissue conditioners.
- *Viscoelasticity*. The current range of available materials varies considerably with respect to viscoelastic behaviour and each material can be modified in this respect by altering the powder/liquid ratio, although the scope for doing this is limited. The gelling material should have sufficient flow to allow it to adapt accurately to the mucosal surface, but should not flow so readily that most of it is squeezed out when the patient occludes on the dentures. Those materials with a low alcohol content exhibit plastic behaviour for the first few hours after mixing. Elasticity increases as the materials age, but some of the powder/liquid materials are elastic from the

start and are therefore unsuitable as functional impression materials.

- *Dimensional stability*. Those materials with a low alcohol content exhibit good dimensional stability for the first few hours after mixing. Thus they are the materials of choice if a functional impression is being obtained (see below). It is apparent that these properties vary from brand to brand, and the clinical importance of each varies with the particular use to which the material is being put. Therefore it is important for the clinician to be able to select the best material for the job in hand. This topic is discussed further in the next section 'Clinical implications'.

Clinical applications

Tissue conditioning

A material used for this purpose should ideally be soft and elastic so that it provides a good cushioning effect.

If a tissue conditioner is applied to the impression surface of an old denture, it will help to resolve inflammation of the denture-bearing tissues. However, as the inflammation is reduced the traumatised mucosa will alter in shape so that the lining ceases to be accurately adapted to the mucosa, thus slowing the rate of healing. Of course, if the material remains soft and elastic, its deformation by relatively small forces in the mouth will adapt it to the tissues while it is under load. Nevertheless, it is a wise practice to replace the tissue conditioner with new material after a few days to ensure that the traumatised tissue reverts to a healthy state as rapidly as possible.

If one of the less viscous products is chosen, it is particularly important to instruct the patient to close on the dentures with the lightest possible contact while the material gels so that a thickness of at least 2 mm is maintained. Needless to say, it is essential to check that the freeway space of the dentures allows a lining of this thickness to be inserted.

It must be emphasised that a course of tissue conditioning will not be effective unless other traumatic factors, such as an unbalanced occlusion, under-extension and overextension of the base are corrected before applying the conditioning material to the impression surface.

Functional impression

A material used for this purpose should ideally:

- Exhibit plastic flow – so that it can be moulded to the denture-bearing tissues during function.
- Be dimensionally stable after the impression-taking period – so that it retains its shape while the cast is poured.

As many of the materials available for functional impressions exhibit elastic recovery even after several hours, there is the danger that in the time interval between removing the denture from the mouth and pouring the cast, the impression will change shape. The following regimen is suggested as the best way of minimising this potential problem:

(i) The impression surface and borders of the denture are inspected. Where there is obvious over- or under-extension the borders are adjusted so that a gap of 1–2 mm is created between the acrylic border and the functional depth of the sulcus. This size of gap allows the functional impression material to be moulded by the sulcus tissues and at the same time provides adequate support for the impression when the cast is made.

(ii) If an undercut ridge is present, it is wise to remove between 2 and 3 mm of the impression surface of the denture in the region of the undercut. This allows for an increased thickness of functional impression material so that the shape of the tissue undercut is recorded more accurately.

(iii) The impression surface of the denture is cleaned and dried to ensure good adhesion. The functional impression material is mixed according to the manufacturer's instructions and placed in the denture. After the denture is inserted into the mouth, the patient is instructed to close gently together so that the normal occlusal relationship is maintained. Natural movements of the tongue, cheek and lip musculature are encouraged to achieve border moulding of the impression.

(iv) Once the material has gelled sufficiently for there to be little risk of it distorting, the denture is removed with care and excessive impression material is cut away from the polished surfaces with a scalpel, taking care to maintain the full border shape.

The functional impression material is applied to the denture approximately 1 hour before the patient is due to have a meal and the patient is asked to return to the surgery after that meal. If the patient's report is favourable and the impression is satisfactory a cast is poured immediately. In this way, the risk of elastic recovery is reduced to a minimum, and a more accurate cast can be obtained (Murata et al. 2001). Attention to detail will lead to good results being obtained from this most useful technique.

Temporary soft lining

When a short-term soft lining material is used as a temporary reline to improve the fit of a denture it is essentially acting simply as a space-filler. Ideally the material should gel within a reasonably short time and be elastic so that it remains within the denture and can be inserted and removed over undercuts without resulting in significant permanent deformation. The available materials vary in their softness. If the lining is to be inserted into an immediate denture soon after the extraction of teeth, a relatively soft type should be selected as it will be more comfortable for the patient. On the other hand, if a reasonable amount of healing has occurred, a harder material can be chosen.

Cleaning

Beneath the surface the short-term soft lining materials are porous. If cleaning is ineffective plaque readily penetrates the lining which then takes on the unsavoury appearance of what has aptly been described as 'an infected sponge'. Any tissue conditioning effect is rapidly lost and mucosal inflammation is aggravated as a result. Thus it is essential when using these materials to give the patient detailed instructions on how to keep them clean.

A brush should not be used on the lining as it is likely to damage the surface. Frequent swabbing and rinsing of the lining should be carried out together with daily soaking in a compatible immersion cleanser. Studies have shown that certain immersion denture cleanser/short-term lining combinations are compatible while others can be very damaging to the surface of the lining (Harrison et al. 1989). Alkaline hypochlorite cleansers, which are particularly efficient at removing plaque, are compatible with most of the soft materials and should normally be the type of cleanser recommended. Patients should be informed which specific cleansers will damage their particular lining and warned not to use them.

Long-term soft lining materials

Long-term soft lining materials distribute stress more evenly under dentures than do the hard denture base materials. They also absorb impacts that can arise from masticatory function (Kawano et al. 1997a). They can therefore be said to have a shock-absorbing or cushioning effect. Consequently it has been shown that the addition of a long-term soft lining to a complete lower denture improves the ability to bite and chew and provides general improvement in comfort when compared with hard relines

(Bhat & Wright 2001; Kimoto, 2004; Mutluay et al. 2008); the lining has also been shown to improve masticatory performance (Hayakawa 2000). Heat-cured silicone materials seem to be particularly beneficial in these respects.

Indications for use

- Persistent pain under a denture
- Thin atrophic mucosa
- Parafunction

It is useful to consider the first three indications together, as a complaint of persistent pain may be due to the poor quality of the denture-bearing mucosa or to the patient's inability to regulate gripping or grinding habits. The whole problem may be exacerbated by gross resorption of the mandible which results in the normal masticatory forces being distributed over a reduced area. It is important to make two points: first, the problem is almost always found in the lower jaw and, second, it is essential to ensure that all existing denture faults have been eliminated before deciding to proceed with a long-term soft lining:

- *Replacing an existing denture which has a soft lining.* Once a patient has successfully worn a lower denture with a soft lining and has got used to its 'feel' it is often wise to repeat the prescription. If this is not done and the new denture is made with a hard base the patient may have problems in adapting to it and reject the prosthesis as a result.
- *Sharp bony ridges or spicules.* The pattern of resorption of the mandible may result in sharp ridges or spicules of bone on which the denture-bearing mucosa, in essence, becomes impaled. The problem might be overcome, at least in the short term, by surgically smoothing the bone. However, there are often occasions where poor health or a strong preference by the patient to avoid surgery, are contraindications to this approach. There is also the danger that surgical interference

with the mandible will speed up resorption of the bone, resulting in further destruction of the denture-bearing area. An alternative, conservative approach is to provide a soft lining, which often provides an acceptable level of comfort under these circumstances.

- *Superficially placed mental nerve.* Another consequence of advanced resorption of the mandible is that the mental foramen and mental nerve may become superficially placed within the denture-bearing area so that the nerve is traumatised during function. This typically gives rise to a complaint of a severe, sharp, stabbing pain from the area of the mental foramen which is brought on by biting. A soft lining restricted to the problem area may provide relief. However, it is not uncommon to find that a superficial mental nerve requires greater pressure relief than can be provided by a soft lining. If this is the case it may be necessary to cut the denture away in the area of the nerve to eliminate pressure on the nerve altogether.

Types of long-term soft lining materials

Soft linings are made either of silicone rubber or soft acrylic. The silicone materials may be cold-curing or heat-curing. The soft acrylics are heat-curing; cold-curing soft acrylics have a very limited lifespan and are best thought of as temporary soft linings.

Cold-curing silicone rubber materials

One of the most important variations in composition is the percentage of filler content. As the content increases, so does the level of water sorption with resultant worsening of dimensional stability. The rupture properties of these materials can be poor so that the soft lining is liable to tear and to become detached from the denture base. In isolated instances, the commonly used catalyst, dibutyltin dilaurate has been found to be a mucosal irritant. The abrasion resistance of these materials is poor.

Heat-curing silicone rubber materials

In contrast to the cold-curing silicones, the water absorption of these materials is low. As a result, the dimensional stability is improved and accuracy of fit is little affected by the oral environment. Improvements in rupture properties and adhesion to the denture base complete the picture of superiority.

Acrylic resin materials

Most of the materials use polyethylmethacrylate or polybutylmethacrylate as the basic polymer. The materials are heavily plasticised to create softness.

A comparison of silicone and acrylic long-term soft lining materials

The following properties are of particular clinical importance:

- *Elasticity.* As shown in Fig. 16.2, silicone rubber materials react quite differently from soft acrylic resins when a load is applied through a penetrometer. The heat-curing silicone material responds almost immediately to the application and removal of a load; it is elastic in nature. In contrast, the heat-curing soft acrylic material shows a more gradual response; it is viscoelastic (McCabe et al. 1996). The elastic nature of the silicone soft lining material is responsible for its ability to absorb shock more effectively than the acrylic lining and is no doubt the reason why it has been shown to be better at enhancing masticatory performance.
- *Ageing.* The properties of some long-term soft lining materials alter dramatically with age and with immersion in water. Whereas the softness and elastic behaviour of heat-curing silicone materials have been shown to remain stable with time (Dootz et al. 1993; Jepson et al. 1993; Kawano et al. 1997a) soft acrylic materials become harder with time and with immersion in water as a conse-

quence of the plasticiser leaching out into the liquid medium.
- *Bonding.* Heat-curing silicone and heat-curing soft acrylic materials have similar bond strengths to the hard denture base polymer, whereas some cold-curing silicone soft liners have lower values. This problem of low bond strength appears to be restricted to those materials with a high filler content. Of particular significance is the fact that higher bond strengths are found if the soft lining is processed against polymerised polymethylmethacrylate than against the unpolymerised material. In practice this means that it is better to add a soft lining to an existing hard denture base than to process both materials at the same time (Kawano et al. 1997b).

Further practical considerations

Durability

There has been a reluctance to prescribe soft linings because of the belief that their clinical life is too short. It is possible that such a viewpoint stems from the observed hardening of soft acrylic materials and the debonding of heavily filled cold-curing silicone materials. Evidence from clinical surveys supports the long-term benefit of a heat-curing silicone soft lining. In one of the surveys (Wright 1994), a number of linings had been in situ for up to 8 years. Patients sought replacement dentures, not because of problems with the soft linings but because the acrylic teeth had worn down. Another survey (Jepson et al. 1994) showed that the survival time of a heat-curing silicone soft lining was better than a heat-curing soft acrylic resin. This last study also showed that survival time was related to thickness of the lining but that there was no benefit in increasing the thickness beyond 2 mm.

Midline fracture

A frequently reported complication is fracture of the lower denture. As the soft lining must be

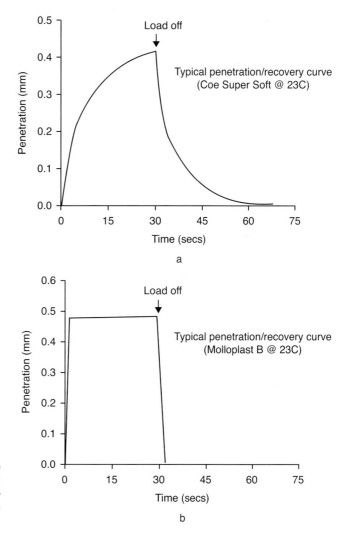

Figure 16.2 Penetration/recovery curves showing: (a) the gradual response of a heat-curing soft acrylic lining material; (b) the rapid response of a heat-curing silicone soft lining material to the application and removal of a load.

at least 2 mm thick if its beneficial properties are to be fully effective, a corresponding reduction in the thickness of the hard acrylic resin of the denture base is necessary to make room for the lining, which weakens the denture. Finite element analysis of lower dentures has shown the presence of high stress concentrations lingually in the lower canine areas and also around the area of the labial notch (Shim & Watts 2000). To reduce the risk of fracture a strengthener in the form of a cobalt-chromium lingual plate may be added to the denture (Fig. 16.3).

Cleaning

Some soft lining materials suffer from high levels of water sorption. When the lining is placed in the mouth it absorbs saliva and can be invaded by oral microorganisms. It is perhaps this set of circumstances that has led to the belief that soft linings may cause infections of the oral mucosa. Whilst soft linings do not actively support the growth of yeasts such as *Candida albicans* they do permit it and can in fact encourage it due to the ready availability of nutrients and to the difficulty of cleaning the surface of

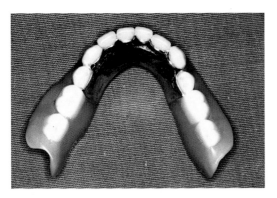

Figure 16.3 A lower denture with a cobalt-chromium lingual plate strengthener.

the lining (Wright et al. 1998). Effective cleaning is more difficult if the surface of the lining is rough. With respect to the retention of *Candida albicans* a rough silicone lining is worse than a rough soft acrylic lining (Verran & Maryan 1997).

It is therefore essential to achieve a smooth surface to the lining (see below), and to give the patient detailed instructions on how best to clean the lining (Davenport et al. 1986). This information should stress that the manufacturer's recommendation with respect to temperature of the water used with denture cleansers should be followed; if not, there is a risk that there may be a detrimental effect on colour of the lining and creation of surface roughness (Handa et al. 2008).

Dietary advice, such as avoiding frequent intake of carbohydrates to restrict the supply of nutrients to the microorganisms, may also be of value. A sodium hypochlorite denture cleanser is effective in eliminating *Candida albicans* and *Staphylococcus aureus* from the lining (Baysan et al. 1998; Yilmaz et al. 2005; Ferriera et al. 2009), while not adversely affecting the mechanical properties of the lining itself. However, it will cause some loss of colour and might cause corrosion of a metal lingual plate strengthener. Microwave irradiation has been shown to inhibit colonisation by *Candida albi-*

cans (Buergers et al. 2008) but should not be used if the denture has a metal lingual plate.

Adjustment
Long-term soft linings can be difficult to adjust unless the burs and stones designed specifically for trimming these materials are used. After any reshaping has been completed it is important to leave as smooth a surface as possible.

The flabby ridge

The flabby ridge is most frequently seen in the anterior maxillary region and has been reported in up to a quarter of edentulous patients (Carlsson, 1998). The bone is grossly resorbed, sometimes up to the level of the anterior nasal spine, and is partly replaced by fibrous tissue. As a result of this mobile fibrous tissue, the support for a complete denture is poor in the affected region leading to instability of the prosthesis. Both function and appearance can be heavily compromised.

Aetiology

It has long been believed that the condition, sometimes called the 'combination syndrome', is the result of wearing a maxillary complete denture opposed only by lower natural anterior teeth. This unfavourable relationship encourages tipping of the denture, overloading of the anterior maxillary ridge and rapid resorption of alveolar bone (Lynch & Allen 2006). However, an assessment of controlled studies does not reveal strong evidence to support this conclusion (Carlsson 1998). This is probably not surprising when the many factors that influence bone metabolism are considered. Nevertheless it is probably wise to keep such patients under regular review to ensure that damage to the ridge is not occurring.

Management

Approaches to treatment

Surgical
- Excision of the fibrous tissue to try and create a firm foundation for the prosthesis.
- Osseo-integrated implants with, or without bone grafting.

There are frequently contraindications to the surgical approach:

- The patients are often older, or have a medical history, or a preference which makes surgery inappropriate.
- Removal of the fibrous tissue will reduce the extent and volume of the denture bearing area. This can reduce denture retention and will require replacement of the excised tissue with denture-base material making the prosthesis bulky and heavy.
- There will usually be too little alveolar bone left for the placing of implants, so to adopt this approach is likely to require further surgical intervention in the form of bone grafting.

It is the opinion of the authors that in the vast majority of cases a satisfactory denture can be made without resorting to surgery.

Non-surgical
A key aspect in the non-surgical management of the flabby ridge is the choice of impression technique employed:

- To employ a mucodisplacive impression technique which compresses the flabby tissue in order to try and obtain maximum support from it or,
- To use a mucostatic impression technique with the aim of achieving maximum retention.

There is little published evidence in the literature that one approach produces better results

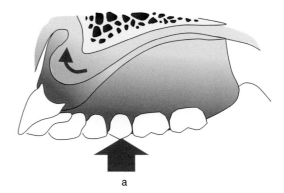

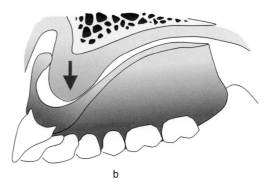

Figure 16.4   (a) Under occlusal pressure, the upper denture is seated and the flabby anterior ridge displaced. (b) When the teeth are apart, the flabby tissue recoils and displaces the denture downwards.

than the other. However, it is the authors' clinical experience that it is more effective to use a mucostatic impression technique which does not displace the flabby tissue. This is because, if the fibrous tissue is distorted by a mucodisplacive impression, the denture will fit only when seated by occlusal pressure (Fig. 16.4). When the teeth move out of occlusion and the pressure is released the compressed tissues rebound and displace the denture.

If, however, the denture is constructed on a cast obtained from a mucostatic impression of the flabby ridge in its resting position, the denture maintains its contact with the tissues when the teeth are out of occlusion. Retention will therefore be optimal for the case in question. Support will be gained primarily from the hard palate and firm areas of the ridge rather than from the flabby tissue.

Recommended impression techniques for the flabby ridge are as follows:

- Preliminary impressions are taken in a stock tray using an alginate of low viscosity. This material will cause less tissue displacement than if impression compound were used, with the result that less modification of the special tray will subsequently be required.
- In many cases, it will be found that the traumatised denture-bearing mucosa is inflamed. Resolution of this inflammation should be achieved before the working impressions are taken. This might be achieved by leaving the dentures out for several days beforehand, or by a combination of appropriate modifications to the existing dentures such as occlusal adjustment or the application of a short-term soft lining material to the impression surface.
- Where the degree of mucosal displacement is only slight, a satisfactory result may be achieved by taking a working impression in a spaced tray using an impression material of low viscosity. Suitable impression materials for this purpose are low viscosity silicone rubber, alginate or impression plaster. If desired, pressure on the displaceable tissue can be further reduced by using a tray with perforations in the region covering the flabby ridge. A technique of this type has been described by Lynch and Allen (2006).
- Where the risk of displacement of the flabby ridge is high, a two-part impression technique can be very effective:
    (i) A preliminary impression is obtained as described above. The area of flabby tissue, determined by intra-oral palpation, should be marked out on the preliminary cast.
    (ii) A cold-curing acrylic resin special tray is constructed that is close-fitting in the

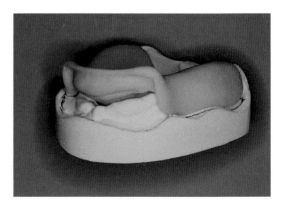

Figure 16.5   A close-fitting acrylic tray cut away to uncover the flabby anterior ridge. The tray is spaced from the mucosa along its anterior edge. The rim handle prevents the unset plaster falling into the mouth when the patient is supine.

firm denture-bearing area and leaves the flabby ridge uncovered (Fig. 16.5).

(iii) The tray is tried in the mouth, checked, and if necessary adjusted so that it is not displacing the flabby tissue. It is a major advantage of this type of tray that direct vision can be used to make absolutely certain that the tray does not displace the flabby ridge when it is fully seated. The borders of the tray are corrected in the normal way.

(iv) An impression is taken of the firm denture-bearing area using zinc oxide–eugenol impression paste or silicone rubber.

(v) If this first part of the impression proves to be satisfactory, it is replaced in the mouth, the patient is tipped back into the supine position and an impression of the flabby tissue, left uncovered by the tray, is obtained by applying a thin mix of impression plaster with a spatula, brush or syringe. As the impression plaster sets rigidly there is no need to support it on the labial aspect.

Once a satisfactory mucostatic impression has been obtained it is advisable to produce a heat-cured clear acrylic base from the master cast. This base is checked in the mouth to assess its accuracy and subsequently provides optimum retention and stability for the recording of the jaw relationship.

Denture breakages

Previous investigations into the size of the problem in the UK reveal that the National Health Service spent £7 million each year on denture repairs. This figure did not take into account the cost of repairs undertaken privately outside this government-financed scheme. Midline fracture of the complete upper denture accounted for 29% of all repair work in dental laboratories, whilst teeth debonded from complete dentures accounted for 33% (Darbar et al.1994; Jagger et al. 1999). These two common problems will now be considered.

Types of fracture

Fatigue of the acrylic resin

Fatigue fracture results from repeated flexing of the denture by forces too small to fracture it directly. Failure of the denture base is due to the progressive growth of a crack originating from a point on the surface where an abrupt change in the surface profile causes a localised concentration of stress many times that applied to the bulk of the denture. The crack often starts palatally to the upper central incisors, grows slowly at first but undergoes an enormously increased rate of growth just before the denture fractures. A failure of this type most commonly occurs in dentures that are about 3 years old.

Midline fracture due to fatigue is the commonest type of denture breakage and will be the primary focus of the discussion which follows.

Impact

Denture breakage might occur, for example, if the patient accidentally drops the denture while cleaning it. It might also result from an accident in which the patient receives a blow to the mouth.

Whenever possible, the cause, or causes, of the fracture must be identified before the denture is repaired or replaced. Unless this is done and the cause attended to, the denture is likely to fracture again within a short period of time.

Causes of fracture

Denture factors

Stress concentrators

Changes in the surface profile of the denture acting as stress concentrators include scratches, a median diastema and a deep frenal notch. Inclusions within the denture base such as porosity, plaster, dust, nylon filaments and relatively flexible metal mesh 'strengtheners' may predispose to fracture and also contribute to the rapid growth of the crack. Stress concentration can also develop around the pins of porcelain teeth.

Absence of a labial flange

An open-face denture is not as stiff as a flanged denture. Flexing will therefore be more marked and fatigue fracture more likely as a consequence. If this appears to be the primary cause of a fracture, and the anatomy of the anterior alveolus prevents the addition of a labial flange to the replacement denture, a metallic denture base is indicated.

Incomplete polymerisation of the acrylic resin

If the original curing cycle of the denture had not included a terminal heating period at 100°C, the maximum degree of polymerisation will not have been attained and the strength of the denture base will have been reduced from its normally expected value.

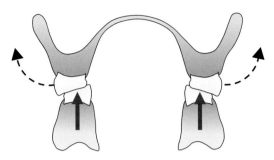

Figure 16.6 Wear of acrylic posterior teeth resulting in a wedge effect on the upper denture.

Previous repair

When a denture has fractured previously in the midline and has been repaired with cold-curing acrylic resin, a further fracture may occur because the cold-curing material is more susceptible to fatigue than the heat-cured resin. In addition, the original denture base material on either side of the fracture line will already be fatigued.

Shape of the teeth on the denture

When acrylic posterior teeth are set up with a normal buccal overjet, they may wear and produce the situation shown in Fig. 16.6, where a wedging action on the upper denture results from occlusion of the teeth. Locking of the occlusion also appears to predispose to midline fracture.

Poor fit

When resorption of the alveolar ridge has taken place beneath an upper denture, support will be provided primarily by the hard palate. As a result, flexing of the denture will occur when the teeth occlude. To correct this fault, the denture should be rebased after it has been repaired. By this process, the old highly stressed resin is replaced by stronger heat-curing resin.

Lack of adequate relief

If the mucosa overlying the crest of the ridge is more compressible than that covering the centre of the hard palate, flexing of the denture will occur when the teeth occlude. To compensate for this variation in mucosal compressibility, and to prevent the flexing, a palatal relief chamber should be incorporated in the denture (p. 162).

Patient factors

Anatomical factors

Certain features of the patient may give rise to denture factors, already discussed, which predispose to fracture. For example, a prominent labial frenum will require a deep notch in the flange resulting in stress concentration in that area.

High occlusal loads

These may occur in patients with powerful muscles of mastication, or whose natural lower teeth are still present, or who are bruxists.

Repairing a denture

An informative and comprehensive review of this subject has been published by Seo et al. (2007).

If a broken denture appears to be serviceable a repair would usually be attempted if only because the patient is likely to want the appearance restored as a matter of urgency. A repair can be effective, cheaper and, of course, quicker than remaking the denture.

An attempt should be made at the chair side to relocate the parts of the broken denture. If this can be achieved convincingly, the parts can then be secured by using either hard sticky wax or a cyanoacrylate adhesive before sending the denture to the laboratory for repair. A study by Goiato et al. (2009) has indicated that cyanoacrylate adhesive is more accurate than sticky wax for this purpose.

If, after the two pieces of the denture have been located accurately and securely, a lack of fit is diagnosed, one option is to reline or rebase the denture (p. 224). It is possible to take a wash impression at the patient's first visit rather than waiting for the repaired denture to be returned for an impression to be taken at a subsequent appointment.

A repair should have:

- adequate strength;
- dimensional stability;
- a good colour match with the original denture base.

Choice of repair material

The choice of repair material is not straightforward.

Cold-curing acrylic resin

This is the material most commonly used, but its transverse strength is relatively poor (about 60–65% of the strength of the original heat-curing base material) making a repeat fracture more likely.

Light-cured acrylic resins

These materials appear to be even weaker than cold-curing acrylic resin.

Microwave–cured acrylic resins

These resins have a transverse strength comparable to a heat-cured material, but the processing can distort the original denture base. There is little information in the literature on the clinical use of microwave-cured acrylic resins for denture repair.

Heat-cured acrylic resin

This has significantly better mechanical properties, but requires more complex laboratory procedures and higher costs.

Increasing the strength of repair

The strength of a repair can be increased by the following:

Choice of repair material

The best available repair material for the original denture base material should be selected.

For example, if time and cost do not rule it out, the use of a heat-cured material will give a superior repair to a cold-curing material.

The design of the repair surface

A common technique is for the fractured surfaces to be bevelled and slightly roughened to strengthen the bond between repair and original resin by increasing the bonding area.

Chemical treatment of the repair surface

The repair resin bonds more strongly to the repair surface if the latter is wetted with methyl methacrylate monomer, dichloromethane or ethyl acetone (Seo et al. 2007).

The use of reinforcements

These reinforcements include carbon, glass or aramid fibres, or metal wire (p. 249). Recent studies have indicated that when reinforcing, wires are air-abraded with alumina and treated with a metal conditioner to increase the adhesion of acrylic resin to them, and provided they are correctly positioned in the denture, they can be one of the most effective ways of strengthening cold-curing repair resin (Kostoulas et al. 2008; Shimizu et al. 2008).

Elimination of wax or saliva contamination

Careful technique is essential to avoid contamination of the repair surface by wax or saliva.

Replacing a broken denture with a stronger prosthesis

A repaired denture may be made stronger by altering its design or construction as indicated previously. However, when no such improvements are possible – yet fracture remains a problem, usually because of exceptionally high occlusal loading – a stronger denture base material is often indicated. Materials that may be used for this purpose are described briefly below.

Cobalt–chromium alloy

Although cobalt–chromium alloy provides a strong and well-fitting denture base it has certain disadvantages:

Weight

Upper dentures with cobalt–chromium palates tend to be heavier than those with acrylic bases; therefore, in cases where anatomical factors are unfavourable for retention, there is an increased likelihood that the denture will drop.

Lack of adjustability

Cobalt–chromium alloy as a denture base material is far less adjustable than acrylic resin. For example, if a post-dam (which is an integral part of the casting) requires modification, this can only be achieved to a very minor extent.

The problems of lack of adjustability and of increased weight can be minimised by restricting the cobalt-chromium component to a horseshoe-shaped palatal strengthener set into the acrylic base (Fig. 16.7). This design results in an impression surface of acrylic resin and thus preserves the advantage of adjustability.

If it is judged that greater strength is required than can be provided by a horseshoe strengthener, a more extensive metal base can

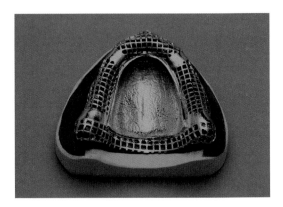

Figure 16.8 Cobalt–chromium palate with posterior mesh to which an acrylic post-dam will be attached.

be used and still retain the advantage of an adjustable post-dam if the design shown in Fig. 16.8 is employed. Acrylic resin, added to the mesh at the posterior border, becomes the material in contact with the mucosa; this material can be modified should the need arise. When constructing this type of denture base, the dental technician has to take great care to minimise the step between metal and acrylic at the finishing line. One way of achieving this is to dispense with the rather bulky spaced mesh altogether and to use a meta-resin for the post-dam region. This type of material adheres directly to cobalt–chromium alloy and therefore does not require the mechanical retention offered by the mesh.

Modified polymeric denture base materials

Polymeric materials can be modified and reinforced. Examples of polymer modification include the addition of elastomers or the creation of acrylic-elastomer copolymers. The elastomer absorbs the energy of impact and therefore provides protection for the acrylic resin. Such impact polymers are more expensive than conventional denture base polymers.

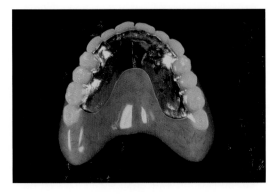

Figure 16.7 Upper denture with cobalt–chromium horseshoe-shaped strengthener.

Reinforcement of denture base materials

The following fibres have been used to reinforce and stiffen conventional denture base polymers. It is important that when reinforcing fibres are used they are positioned and shaped to achieve optimum performance. They may be conditioned to improve bonding to the denture base material. They should be positioned in the areas of maximum stress, at right angles to the anticipated line of fracture, and they should be fully enclosed within the denture base so that the fibres do not irritate the mucosa.

Carbon fibres

Techniques have been described by which conventional upper dentures are reinforced by the inclusion of carbon fibre inserts in the palate to reduce the flexibility of the denture base. This approach was reported to have reduced the incidence of fracture in a high-risk group of patients, but a disadvantage of the method is the black colour of the insert.

Ultra-high-modulus polyethylene fibres (UHMPE)

In recent years there have been reports of denture bases being reinforced with ultra-high-modulus polyethylene fibre (Karacaer et al. 2001). This material may be added either as a discrete woven insert into the denture base or as chopped fibre incorporated in the polymer powder before the resin is mixed (Braden et al. 1988; Gutteridge 1988). The fibre is transparent and its inclusion in the polymer as chopped fibre at a loading of 1% has resulted in an increase in impact strength exceeding that of commercially available 'high impact' resins. When the material is inserted as a woven mat, loadings of 20–30% are reported. Both approaches can be used when a new denture base is to be constructed, but the inclusion of a woven mat requires an additional technical stage.

Glass fibres

The inclusion of glass fibres into acrylic resin has been shown to improve fatigue resistance, flexural strength and impact strength (Kim et al. 2004). The fibres are produced either as a woven mat and inserted into the whole denture, or as individual fibres which are laid out in the region of a previous weakness. To obtain the full benefit, care must be taken to position the fibres correctly. Effective adhesion of the fibres to the surrounding denture base polymer is achieved by pre-impregnating the fibres with polymer before they are positioned (Narva et al. 2001; Kostoulas et al. 2008).

'Metal strengtheners'

Metal mesh is occasionally included in a denture as a 'so-called' strengthener, but has not been shown to effectively reinforce a denture base (Narva et al. 2001) and in fact might weaken it by acting as a stress concentrator. This finding conflicts with the more recent results for the effectiveness of wire strengtheners mentioned above. A possible explanation is that the wires are stiffer than the mesh and have been treated to create a good bond with the acrylic resin of the repair.

Debonding of teeth

Causes

Debonding of teeth from the denture base occurs more commonly on upper anterior teeth. In the presence of an existing weak bond the upward and outward force arising from contact by the lower anterior teeth causes bond failure.

The usual reasons for a weak bond between tooth and denture base are:

- The presence of tin-foil substitute on the ridge-lap surface of the tooth.
- The presence of residual wax on the same surface.
- The use of cross-linked teeth which are incompatible with the particular denture base polymer.

All the above factors prevent effective chemical union between the teeth and the denture base and the production of an acceptable interwoven polymer network (Cunningham & Bennington 1999; Takahashi et al. 2000).

Prevention

The literature is not unanimous about how best to achieve the maximum bond strength between teeth and denture base. The variable and sometimes conflicting results are possibly due to the different combinations of denture teeth and denture base polymers that were used in the studies. Of the various recommendations that have been made for minimising the risk of debonding the following have received fairly widespread support (Büyükyilmaz & Ruyter 1997; Cunningham & Bennington 1999; Takahashi et al. 2000; Dalal et al. 2009):

Selection of compatible artificial teeth and denture base polymer
This compatibility should be checked from information sheets provided with the products, or by seeking information from the manufacturers. Conventional denture teeth tend to achieve a higher bond strength than cross-linked teeth.

Removal of all traces of wax and tin-foil substitute from the teeth
The complete removal of wax before packing the mould is not consistently achieved with boiling water alone and so for optimum bond strength the use of a wax solvent is recommended (Cunningham & Bennington 1997).

Mechanical preparation of the teeth
Grinding and sandblasting the bonding surface of the teeth enhances the bond strength significantly (Chung et al. 2008). Small channels drilled into the palatal surface of the teeth will increase the area available for the curing denture base resin. However, it needs to be remembered that such recesses in the ridge-lap surface of the teeth can make complete wax removal

more difficult. Therefore particular care needs to be taken when removing the wax; otherwise, the adjustments can result in a weaker, rather than a stronger bond.

Chemical preparation of the teeth
Applying methyl methacrylate monomer (Barbosa et al. 2009), or a solvent such as dichloromethane or ethyl acetone to the ridge-lap surface of the teeth creates microscopic pores and channels which promote diffusion of the polymerisable materials and increase bond strength.

Use of a heat-curing denture base polymer
This material polymerises more slowly than a cold-curing material and ensures better penetration into the tooth substance. Medium or long curing cycles have been shown to result in higher tensile bond strengths between denture base material and acrylic teeth than the use of short curing cycles (Dalal et al. 2009).

Gagging

Gagging is a protective reflex to stop unwanted entry of substances into the mouth and oropharynx (Dickinson & Fiske 2005).

Aetiology of gagging

There are a number of causes of gagging that may be conveniently grouped together as follows.

Somatic
The term 'somatic' covers those situations where the reflex is triggered by tactile stimulation of the soft palate, posterior third of the tongue and fauces. Included in this group are numerous iatrogenic causes related to the design of dentures.

Some patients begin to gag when new dentures are inserted, but in most cases this reflex soon disappears as they adapt to the dentures.

However, the reflex may persist if there are faults with the dentures such as an excessive occlusal vertical dimension, or if the dentures are stimulating the sensitive areas of the soft palate and tongue directly. This stimulation may be caused by palatal over-extension, a posterior border which is too thick or poorly adapted, the teeth encroaching on tongue space or indeed by any factor producing denture instability. An upper denture whose posterior border is under-extended posteriorly can provoke gagging because as the edge of the denture terminates on relatively incompressible mucosa a satisfactory post-dam cannot be produced. This results in poor retention, which increases denture instability, stimulates the tongue and palate, and causes apprehension in the patient. When this diagnosis is established, it requires a very careful explanation by the clinician to convince the patient that to cure the problem it will be necessary to cover more, rather than less of the palate.

Psychogenic

Psychogenic causes may arise from sight, sound or thought. They include the sight of impression material being mixed or the sound of another patient gagging. The patient may be extremely apprehensive because of an unhappy first-hand experience of dental procedures or as a result of disturbing stories from friends. In rare instances, gagging may be a manifestation of a psychological disturbance which is not primarily related to the patient's dental treatment. It is within this group one finds the most severe problems.

Systemic

Less frequently, the causative factor may be systemic disease, particularly conditions affecting other regions of the gastrointestinal tract; for example, the link between gagging and alcoholism may be related to the persistent gastritis found in such patients. Persistent catarrh will prevent nose breathing and may contribute to the problem of gagging. A link between smok-ing and gagging has been described (Wright 1979).

Patient management

Assessment of the severity of the problem

A carefully taken history and an examination of the patient will reveal the patient's concerns and fears, what procedures have previously been tried and with what result. The findings will allow the clinician to gauge the severity of the problem and provide clues as to the cause. For example, a situation where a patient has been able to tolerate the clinical stages of denture construction but then has difficulty in wearing the finished dentures points to an iatrogenic cause which should be treated relatively simply by correcting the error in denture design. At the other extreme is the patient who gags as soon as a mouth mirror is brought up to the mouth.

Impressions

All but the most phlegmatic of individuals find impression taking unpleasant. However, gagging can usually be prevented by the following.

Reassurance and relaxation

It is very important that the clinician has a confident, relaxed and sympathetic chair side manner. It is essential that the anxious patient is reassured and encouraged to relax both physically and mentally. The dental nurse can also play a major role in creating an appropriate state of mind in the patient.

Position of the patient

The dental chair should be adjusted so that the patient is sitting comfortably in the upright position.

Breathing through the nose

Instructing the patient to breathe through the nose while the impression tray is being tried in

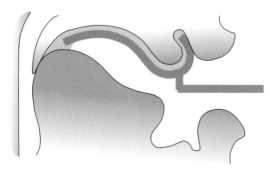

Figure 16.9   The tongue in its guarding position during the taking of an upper impression.

the mouth or the impression is being taken is one of the most helpful methods of preventing retching. During nasal breathing the soft palate remains stationary in a low position and makes contact with the tongue in its 'guarding' position, thus closing off the oral cavity from the nasopharynx (Fig. 16.9); this arrangement protects the nasopharynx from the perceived threat of the foreign body in the mouth. If the patient breathes through the mouth, the soft palate is raised and this protective feeling may well be lost.

A refinement of this technique is where the patient is instructed in a regime of controlled breathing which must be practised for 1 or 2 weeks before impression taking. Breathing should be slow, deep and even; the required steady rhythm can be ensured by asking the patient to link it mentally to a well-known tune.

Impression technique
Impression trays should be as well fitting as possible. As close-fitting special trays are less bulky than spaced trays, they are better tolerated and should be used whenever possible. When trying trays in the mouth, firm, positive, confident movements should be used. Most patients tolerate the lower impression better than the upper one, so if the lower impression is taken first, the success of the procedure is likely to reassure the patient. The impression material should be mixed or prepared out of sight of the patient and the amount placed in the tray kept to the minimum necessary to record the relevant structures. A saliva ejector should be used if copious amount of saliva collects in the floor of the mouth.

Distraction
It is during the insertion of the impression and while the material is setting that it is particularly important to distract the patient's attention from what is going on. This may be achieved by the clinician talking about something that is known to be of particular interest to the patient, or by reinforcing the requirement that the patient continues to breathe slowly and steadily through the nose. It has even been suggested that the patient be asked to raise one leg and to concentrate on not lowering it until the impression has set!

The severe gagging reflex

The first challenge when treating a patient who has this problem is to obtain an accurate impression so that a well-fitting denture base can be constructed. The second challenge is to provide a prosthesis that can be worn by the patient for a reasonable length of time. The following approaches to the management of this difficult problem have been found to be useful:

The training denture
The training denture approach may be of value when treating any patient with a long history of difficulties which suggest frank denture intolerance, including gagging. The rationale for this approach is that as new stimuli are introduced gradually, the patient has to cope with only one small step at a time and does not advance to the next stage in treatment until the previous stage has been mastered. The rate of progress is therefore under the patient's control, a feature which can increase patient confidence. This approach whereby intra-oral stimuli are gradually increased is known as

desensitisation (Bassi et al. 2004). A possible clinical progression is as follows:

(i) The impressions may be obtained by one of the techniques outlined above. Alternatively, primary impressions can often be successfully produced using impression compound because insertion, border moulding and removal of this type of impression can be completed so quickly that the gagging reflex does not have time to develop. As the compound is still soft on removal from the mouth it must be chilled immediately and thoroughly under cold water to prevent distortion. Training bases are constructed on the models obtained from the compound impressions and their fit is refined in the mouth using a chair side relining material. The close fit and small dimensions of the bases are much more easily tolerated than a conventional impression.

(ii) The upper training base is constructed with a posterior extension judged to be appropriate for a particular patient. This will vary from the minimum extension of a horseshoe, palateless design to conventional extension to the vibrating line. To help the patient to control the lower base, a spine of a polybutylmethacrylate resin may be added in the mouth so that the muscles of the tongue and cheeks rest against it.

(iii) It is often advisable for the patient to start by wearing just one of the bases. The base should be worn for as long as the patient can tolerate, but should be removed from the mouth before gagging occurs. This is because the objective of treatment is to extinguish the gag reflex, but if the patient is too heroic and persists in wearing the prosthesis until frank gagging occurs the reflex may in fact be reinforced. After a rest period, the base should be reinserted and an attempt made to increase the period of wear. This process is repeated until the pa-

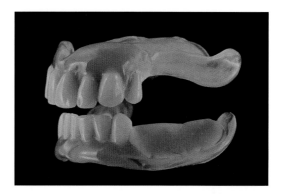

Figure 16.10 Training bases with the addition of anterior teeth and a spine of cold-curing polybutyl-methacrylate resin.

tient reports that the base can be worn successfully. Some patients find that it helps them get through this difficult early stage if they suck a boiled sweet while wearing the training base.

(iv) Once the first major challenge of wearing the initial training base for reasonable periods of time has been met successfully, further additions can be progressively introduced. For example, more courageous extensions can be developed with chair side relining materials and anterior teeth can be added (Fig. 16.10). Eventually, if progress is maintained, the complete dentures are developed and because the multiple additions make these look rather like a patchwork quilt, a copying technique may be used to produce the replacement prostheses. The training base approach to complete denture treatment is inevitably a complicated and long drawn-out affair. However, if all other more conventional techniques have failed, the approach may be the one remaining chance of providing a successful outcome.

Relative analgesia

Relative analgesia has been found to be a helpful technique in that it will allow the clinician to obtain a satisfactory impression whilst at the same time reducing patient embarrassment (Packer et al. 2005). However, the technique will only put off the evil hour; although it may indeed be possible to obtain a reasonable impression, ultimately the patient must meet the challenge of wearing a denture in an unsedated state. Of particular importance, though, are the regulations that govern this method of pain and anxiety control. The regulations in force in the particular country must be followed precisely.

Acupuncture

The gag reflex has been shown to be capable of being controlled by acupuncture (Fiske & Dickinson 2001; Rosted et al. 2006).

Hypnosis

Hypnosis has been used in the treatment of severe cases (Barsby 1994). Its success is dependent upon the patient being well motivated and being able to practise self-hypnosis, thus enabling a denture to be worn outside the dental surgery.

Gagging is a serious problem in a minority of patients only. From the foregoing account the reader will appreciate that treatment can be lengthy and that a great deal of patience and perseverance are required by both clinician and patient. Further details on aetiology and management can be obtained elsewhere (Bassi et al. 2004; Dickinson & Fiske, 2005).

The burning mouth syndrome

The burning mouth syndrome (BMS) can be very troublesome to the sufferer, presents problems of diagnosis and often involves prolonged treatment (Basker et al. 1978; Maresky et al. 1993). The symptoms occur in 5–7% of the adult population. Of those who seek treatment, there is a predominance of women, with a mean age of approximately 60 years. The most common sites of the complaint are the tongue and the upper denture-bearing tissues. Rather less common are the lips and lower denture-bearing tis-

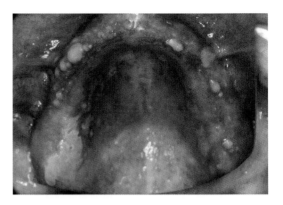

Figure 16.11 Severe blistering of the mucosa resulting from a residual monomer content of 3.2%.

sues. The oral mucosa typically appears normal. However, those cases due to a high level of residual monomer are the exception as the mucosa is inflamed (Fig. 16.11).

Many BMS patients have consulted numerous health care professionals before seeking help from the clinician or dental specialist. They rarely know of others with the complaint and can therefore feel quite isolated. If several professionals have stated that the mouth looks normal the patient may feel that 'it is all in the mind'. The level of anxiety is commonly raised and cancerophobia may develop.

Classification

Three types of BMS have been described (Lamey & Lewis 1989). The classification is useful as it points the way towards appropriate treatment and a probable prognosis.

Type 1

There are no symptoms on waking. A burning sensation then commences and becomes worse as the day progresses. This pattern occurs every day. Approximately 33% of patients fall into this category and are likely to include those with haematinic deficiencies and defects in denture design.

Type 2

Burning is present on waking and persists throughout the day. This pattern occurs every day. About 55% of patients are placed in this category, a high proportion of who have chronic anxiety and are the most difficult to treat successfully.

Type 3

Patients have symptom-free days. Burning occurs in less usual sites such as the floor of the mouth, the throat and the buccal mucosa. This category is made up of the remaining 12% of patients. A study of this group has shown that the main causative factors are allergy and emotional instability (Lamey et al. 1994). The investigation of these patients is likely to include patch testing.

Aetiology

BMS has been attributed to a multitude of causes which may be placed conveniently into three groups:

1. Local irritants, including denture faults
2. Systemic factors
3. Psychogenic factors

Local irritation

Denture faults

Errors in denture design which cause a denture to move excessively over the mucosa, which increase the functional stress on the mucosa or which interfere with the freedom of movement of the surrounding muscles may initiate a complaint of burning rather than frank soreness. Denture design errors have been discovered in 50% of BMS patients.

Residual monomer

High levels of residual monomer in the denture base have been reported and the tissue damage produced is considered to be the result of chemical irritation rather than a true allergy (Fig. 16.11) (Austin & Basker 1980). It is possible that high levels of residual monomer, which have ranged from three to ten times the normal value, are due to errors inadvertently introduced into the short curing cycles which are popular with manufacturers and dental laboratories. If the requisite curing temperature of 100°C is not achieved in the relevant part of the short curing cycle, there is a marked increase in residual monomer content (Austin & Basker 1982). This content can be measured by specialised analytical techniques such as gas chromatography and high-pressure liquid chromatography. Recent work (Zissis et al. 2008) has confirmed that higher levels of residual monomer are found in cold-curing as opposed to heat-curing resins. The cold-curing materials release significant amounts of residual monomer in the first few weeks of storage in water.

Some authorities may not consider a reaction to residual monomer to be an example of BMS where, classically, the mucosa looks normal. However, a patient who reacts to a high level of the chemical complains of a burning sensation and so we feel justified in including it.

Microorganisms

The role of microorganisms in burning mouth syndrome is controversial and studies have not shown a link between the presence of *Candida albicans* and the complaint.

Smoking and mouthwashes

Smoking and the regular use of some mouthwashes are irritants that have been implicated in BMS.

Systemic causes

Nutritional deficiencies

Contributions from nutritional deficiencies such as iron, vitamin B complex and folic acid

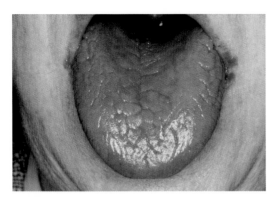

Figure 16.12 A burning tongue: note the smooth surface of the dorsum.

should be highlighted. An example of BMS caused by a deficiency is shown in Fig. 16.12.

Iron deficiencies have been found in 8% and folic acid deficiencies in 6% of BMS patients. Low blood levels of vitamin B_1 and B_6 were found in 40% of patients (Lamey 1998).

Endocrine disorders

What is apparent is the relative unimportance of the climacteric as a causative factor, a contemporary viewpoint which is at variance with past clinical opinion.

On rare occasions, the symptoms are found to be linked with an undiagnosed diabetes mellitus. Treatment of the medical condition results in resolution of BMS.

Xerostomia

Xerostomia, frequently associated with BMS, has many causes as mentioned earlier in this chapter. One that should be highlighted here is drug-induced xerostomia. Recent investigations have produced evidence of a link between Type 2 BMS, antidepressant medication and reduced parotid gland function (Lamey et al. 2001).

It should be recognised that the presence of a dry mouth is capable of accentuating the symptoms initiated by any of the causes of local irri-

tation. This is an example of the multifactorial nature of BMS.

Hypersensitivity

True hypersensitivity to constituents of denture base polymer is rare and typically results in local symptoms such as burning or itching. In one instance where there were systemic symptoms of nausea, dizziness and general malaise the patient was found to have reacted to dyes used to colour the polymer. Dentures made of clear polymer proved successful (Barclay et al. 1999).

In a study of Type 3 patients the avoidance in the diet of such food additives as benzoic acid, propylene glycol and cinnamon products rendered a significant number of patients asymptomatic. Interestingly, those patients who were not cured had higher levels of psychiatric illness (Lamey et al. 1994).

Parkinson's disease

It has been reported that the prevalence of BMS was 24% in people suffering from Parkinson's disease; this is five times that found in surveys of general populations (Clifford et al. 1998).

Psychogenic causes

The more common psychiatric disorders associated with BMS are anxiety, depression, cancerophobia and hypochondriasis. The associated parafunctional activities such as bruxism and abnormal and excessive tongue movements are capable of inducing mucosal irritation. One study showed that parafunctional habits were present in 61% of patients with BMS (Paterson et al. 1995).

Management

Faced with a multitude of causative factors, it will be recognised that the process of diagnosis and treatment is usually a time-consuming affair. It is beyond the scope of this book to discuss management in any detail, but the point should be made that establishing a diagnosis entails a very careful and systematic approach to history-taking and examination, and usually involves the need for a battery of special tests. The establishment of a multi-disciplinary clinic comprising a dental clinician, doctor, dermatologist and psychiatrist, together with expert technical assistance, is desirable in order to effectively follow the regimen outlined in the following:

   (i) Initial assessment (history/examination/ special tests)
 (ii) Provisional diagnosis
(iii) Initial treatment (e.g. elimination of local irritants and investigating and treating haematinic deficiencies)
 (iv) Assessment of initial treatment
  (v) Definitive diagnosis
 (vi) Definitive treatment (local/systemic correction/psychological therapy)
(vii) Follow-up

Outcome

With regard to outcome, analysis of various studies suggests that about two-thirds of BMS patients are either cured or improved to such an extent that the burning sensation is no longer an overwhelming problem. There remains a group of patients for whom the current state of knowledge can offer relatively little benefit. Some in this small group remain totally resistant to treatment. However, it should be remembered that even in these refractory cases BMS is not necessarily a life sentence as spontaneous remissions can eventually occur for no apparent reason.

The above account is a simplification of much work undertaken over the years. A detailed resumé may be found elsewhere (Klasser et al. 2008).

Disturbance of speech

The presence of complete dentures can modify speech by affecting articulation and by altering the degree of oral resonance (Lawson & Bond 1968, 1969; Carr et al. 1985; Seifert et al. 1999). A number of sounds are articulated by contact of the tongue with the palate and with the teeth. A change in speech that may be quite marked when the dentures are first inserted will usually disappear completely within a few days. However, if changes in the position or shape of contact surfaces on the denture require a modification of tongue behaviour that is beyond the adaptive capability of an individual patient, a speech defect will persist. It should also be remembered that the tongue of a patient who is wearing complete dentures has a dual function to take part in speech articulation and to control the dentures. If the dentures are loose, the demands of this latter function may be so great that there is a general deterioration in the quality of speech. As mentioned on p. 232, a dry mouth is likely to result in looseness of dentures and will also affect speech due to the loss of surface lubrication of the oral mucosa. The following relationships are particularly important to the production of clear speech.

Tip of the tongue to the palate

Contact between the tip of the tongue and the palate is required in the production of /s/, /z/, /t/, /d/ and /n/. Consequently, a change in the shape or thickness of the denture contact surface resulting from the fitting of new dentures will require a modification of tongue behaviour in order to produce sounds which are the same as before. In the vast majority of cases, the necessary modification occurs without any difficulty in a relatively short period of time.

The sound most commonly affected in this way is /s/, a sound which is generally produced with the tongue tip behind the upper anterior teeth. A narrow channel remains in the centre of the palate through which air hisses (Fig. 16.13). If the palate is too thick at this point, or if the incisors are positioned too far palatally, the /s/ may become a /th/. If the denture is shaped so that it is difficult for the tongue to adapt itself

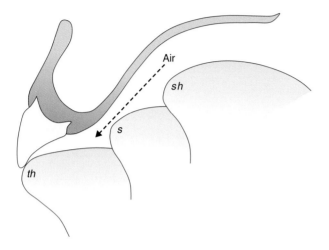

Figure 16.13 The position of the tongue for producing the sounds /th/, /s/ and /sh/.

closely to the palate, a channel narrow enough to produce the /s/ sound will not be produced and a whistle or /sh/ sound may result. This is most likely to be the consequence of excessive palatal thickening laterally in the canine region (Fig. 16.14)

Lower lip to incisal edges of upper anterior teeth

The lower lip makes contact with the incisal edges of the upper anterior teeth when the sounds /f/ and /v/ are produced. If the position of these teeth on a replacement denture is dra-

matically different from that on the old denture there is likely to be a disturbance in speech.

Lateral margin of the tongue to posterior teeth

Contact between the lateral margins of the tongue and the posterior teeth is necessary to produce the English consonants /th/, /t/, /d/, /n/, /s/, /z/, /sh/, /zh/ (as in measure), /ch/, /j/ and /r/ (as in red). Air is directed forwards over the dorsum of the tongue and may be modified by movement of the tongue against the teeth or anterior slope of the palate to produce the final sound. If the contact can only be achieved with

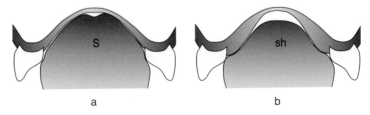

a   b

Figure 16.14 (a) The polished surface of the denture palatal to UR3 and UL3 is correctly shaped so that the tongue can form a narrow channel in the midline for producing the /s/ sound. (b) Excessive thickening of the palate laterally prevents close adaptation of the tongue to the palate so that the /s/ becomes /sh/.

difficulty, movement of the tip of the tongue may be restricted with consequent impairment of speech. This difficulty arises if the posterior contact surfaces are too far from the resting position of the tongue as a result of the occlusal plane being too high, the occlusal vertical dimension too great or the posterior teeth placed too far buccally. In extreme cases, it may not be possible for the tongue to produce a complete lateral seal so that air leaks out laterally during the production of /s/ and /z/ resulting in what is sometimes known as a lateral sigmatism.

The relationship of mandible to maxilla

The mandible moves closest to the maxilla during speech when the sounds /s/, /z/, /ch/ and /j/ are made. Normally, at this time, there will be a small space between the occlusal surfaces of the teeth. However, if the occlusal vertical dimension of the dentures is too great, the teeth may actually come into contact so that the patient complains that the teeth clatter.

References and additional reading

Almstahl, A., Wikstrom, M. & Fagerberg-Mohlin, B. (2008) Microflora in oral ecosystems in subjects with radiation-induced hyposalivation. *Oral Diseases*, 14, 541–9.

Austin, A.T. & Basker, R.M. (1980) The level of residual monomer in acrylic denture base material. *British Dental Journal*, 149, 281–6.

Austin, A.T. & Basker, R.M. (1982) Residual monomer levels in denture bases: the effects of varying short curing cycles. *British Dental Journal*, 153, 424–6.

Barbosa D.B., Monteiro D.R., Barao V.A., Pero A.C. & Compagnoni M.A. (2009) Effect of monomer treatment and polymerisation methods on the bond strength of resin teeth to denture base material. *Gerodontology*, 26, 225–31.

Barclay, S.C., Forsyth, A., Felix, D.H. & Watson, I.B. (1999) Case report – hypersensitivity to denture materials. *British Dental Journal*, 187, 350–52.

Barsby, M.J. (1994) The use of hypnosis in the management of 'gagging' and intolerance to dentures. *British Dental Journal*, 176, 97–102.

Basker, R.M., Sturdee, D.W. & Davenport, J.C. (1978) Patients with burning mouths. *British Dental Journal*, 145, 9–16.

Bassi, G.S, Humphris, G.M & Longman, L.P. (2004) The aetiology and management of gagging: a review of the literature. *Journal of Prosthetic Dentistry*, 91, 459–67.

Baysan, A., Whiley, R. & Wright, P.S. (1998). Use of microwave energy to disinfect a long-term soft lining material contaminated with *Candida albicans or Staphylococcus aureus. Journal of Prosthetic Dentistry*, 79, 454–8.

Bhat, J. & Wright, P.S. (2001) The clinical acceptability of chairside soft lining materials. *European Journal of Prosthodontics and Restorative Dentistry*, 9, 46.

Braden, M., Davey, K.W.M., Parker, S., Ladizesky, N.H. & Ward, I. (1988) Denture base poly(methyl methacrylate) reinforced with ultra-high modulus polyethylene fibres. *British Dental Journal*, 164, 109–13.

Brånemark, P.-I., Zarb, G.A., & Albrektsson, T. (eds) (1985) *Tissue integrated prostheses.* Quintessence, Chicago.

Buergers, R., Rosentritt, M., Schneider-Brachert, W., Behr, M., Handel, G. & Hahnel, S. (2008) Efficacy of denture disinfection methods in controlling *Candida albicans* colonization in vitro. *Acta Odontologica Scandinavica*, 66, 174–80.

Büyükyilmaz, S. & Ruyter, I.E. (1997) The effects of polymerization temperature on the acrylic resin denture base-tooth bond. *International Journal of Prosthodontics*, 10, 49–54.

Carlsson, G. (1998) Clinical morbidity and sequelae of treatment with complete dentures. *Journal of Prosthetic Dentistry*, 79, 17–23.

Carr, L., Wolfaardt, J.F. & Haitas, G.P. (1985) Speech defects in prosthetic dentistry. Part II – Speech defects associated with removable prosthodontics. *Journal of the Dental Association of South Africa*, 40, 387–90.

Chung K.H., Chung C.Y., Chung C.Y. & Chan D.C.N. (2008) Effect of pre-processing surface treatments of acrylic teeth on bonding to the denture base. *Journal of Oral Rehabilitation*, 35, 268–75.

Clifford, T.J., Warsi, M.J., Burnett, C.A. & Lamey, P.J. (1998) Burning mouth in Parkinson's disease sufferers. *Gerodontology*, 15, 73–8.

Cunningham, J.L. & Benington, I.C. (1997) A survey of the pre-bonding preparation of denture teeth and the efficiency of dewaxing methods. *Journal of Dentistry*, 25, 125–8.

Cunningham, J.L. & Bennington, I.C. (1999) An investigation of the variables which may affect the bond between plastic teeth and denture base resin. *Journal of Dentistry*, 27, 129–35.

Dalal, A., Juszczyk, S., Radford, D.R. & Clark, R.F.K (2009). Effect of curing cycle on the tensile strength of the bond between heat cured denture base acrylic resin and acrylic resin denture teeth. *European Journal of Prosthodontics and Restorative Dentistry*, 17, 146–9

Darbar, U.R., Huggett, R. & Harrison, A. (1994) Denture fracture – a survey. *British Dental Journal*, 176, 342–5.

Davenport, J.C. (1970) An adverse reaction to a silicone rubber soft lining material. *British Dental Journal*, 128, 545–6.

Davenport, J.C., Wilson, H.J. & Spence, D. (1986) The compatibility of soft lining materials and denture cleansers. *British Dental Journal*, 161, 13–17.

Dickinson CM & Fiske J. (2005). A review of gagging problems in dentistry: 1. Aetiology and classification. *Dental Update*, 32, 26–32

Dickinson, C.M. & Fiske J. (2005) A review of gagging problems in dentistry: 2. Clinical assessment and management. *Dental Update*, 32, 74–80.

Dootz, E.R., Koran, A. & Craig, R.G. (1993) Physical property comparison of 11 soft denture lining materials as a function of accelerated aging. *Journal of Prosthetic Dentistry*, 69, 114–19.

Ferreira, M.A., Pereira-Cenci, T., Rodrigues de Vasconcelos, L.M., Rodrigues-Garcia, R.C. & Del Bel Cury, A.A. (2009). Efficacy of denture cleansers on denture liners contaminated with *Candida* species. *Clinical Oral Investigations*, 13, 237–42.

Field, E.A., Fear, S., Higham, S.M., Ireland, R.S., Rostron, J. & Willetts, R.M. (2001) Age and medication are significant risk factors for xerostomia in an English population, attending general dental practice. *Gerodontology*, 18, 21–4.

Fiske, J. & Dickinson, C. (2001) The role of acupuncture in controlling the gagging reflex using a review of ten cases. *British Dental Journal*, 190, 611–13.

Flink, H., Bergdahl, M., Tegelberg A., Rosenblad, A. & Lagerlof, F. (2008) Prevalence of hyposalivation in relation to general health, body mass index and remaining teeth in different age groups of adults. *Community Dentistry & Oral Epidemiology*, 36, 523–31.

General Dental Council. *Maintaining Standards*. General Dental Council, London.

Goiato M.C., Pesqueira A.A., Vedovatto E., dos Santos D.M. & Gennari F.H. (2009) Effect of different repair techniques on the accuracy of repositioning the fractured denture base. *Gerodontology*, 26, 237–41

Guggenheimer G. & Moore P. (2003) Xerostomia. Etiology, recognition and treatment. *Journal of the American Dental Association*, 134, 61–9

Gutteridge, D.L. (1988) The effect of including ultrahigh-modulus polyethylene fibre on the impact strength of acrylic resin. *British Dental Journal*, 164, 177–80.

Handa, R.K., Jagger, D.C. & Vowles, R.W. (2008) Denture cleansers, soft lining materials and water temperature: what is the effect? *Primary Dental Care*, 15, 53–8.

Hargreaves, A.S. (1975) Polymethyl methacrylate as denture base material in service. *Journal of Oral Rehabilitation*, 2, 97–104.

Harrison, A., Basker, R.M. & Smith, I.S. (1989). Compatibility of temporary soft lining materials with immersion denture cleansers. *International Journal of Prosthodontics*, 2, 254–8.

Hayakawa, I., Hirano, S., Takahashi, Y. & Keh, E.N. (2000) Changes in the masticatory function of complete denture wearers after relining the mandibular denture with a soft denture liner. *International Journal of Prosthodontics*, 13, 227–31.

Haywood, J. Basker, R.M. Watson, C.J. & Wood, D.J. (2003) A comparison of three hard chairside reline materials. Part I. Clinical evaluation. *European Journal of Prosthodontics and Restorative Dentistry*, 11, 157–163.

Haywood, J. Wood, D.J. Gilchrist, A. Basker, R.M., & Watson, C.J. (2003). A comparison of three hard chairside reline materials. Part II. Changes in colour and hardness following immersion in three commonly used denture cleansers. *European Journal of Prosthodontics and Restorative Dentistry*, 11, 165–9.

Hemmings, K.W., Schmitt, A. & Zarb, G.A. (1994) Complications and maintenance requirements in the edentulous mandible. *International Journal of Oral and Maxillofacial Implantology*, 9, 191–6.

Jagger, D.C., Harrison, A. & Jandt, K.D. (1999) The reinforcement of dentures. *Journal of Oral Rehabilitation*, 26, 185–94.

Jepson, N.J.A., McCabe, J.F. & Storer, R. (1993). Age changes in the viscoelasticity of permanent soft lining materials. *Journal of Dentistry*, 21, 171–8.

Jepson, N.J.A., McCabe, J.F. & Storer, R. (1994) The clinical serviceability of two permanent denture soft linings. *British Dental Journal*, 177, 11–16.

Jepson N.J., McGill, J.T. & McCabe, J.F. (2000) Influence of dietary simulating solvents on the viscoelasticity of temporary soft lining materials. *Journal of Prosthetic Dentistry*, 83, 25–31.

Johansson, A.K., Johansson, A., Unell L, Ekback, G., Ordell, S. & Carlsson, G. E. (2009) A 15-yr longitudinal study of xerostomia in a Swedish population of 50-yr-old subjects. *European Journal of Oral Sciences*, 117, 13–19.

Karacaer, O., Dogan, O.M., Tincer, T. & Dogan, A. (2001). Reinforcement of maxillary dentures with silane-treated ultra high modulus polyethylene fibers. *Journal of Oral Science*, 43, 103–7.

Kawano, F., Dootz, E.R., Koran, A. & Craig, R.G. (1997b) Bond strength of six soft denture liners processed against polymerised and unpolymerised poly(methyl methacrylate). *International Journal of Prosthodontics*, 10, 178–82.

Kawano, F., Koran, A., Nuryanti, A. & Inoue, S. (1997a) Impact absorption of four processed soft denture liners as influenced by accelerated aging. *International Journal of Prosthodontics*, 10, 55–60.

Kim, S.H. & Watts, D.C. (2004). The effect of reinforcement with woven E-glass fibers on the impact strength of complete dentures fabricated with high-impact acrylic resin. *Journal of Prosthetic Dentistry*, 91, 274–80.

Kimoto, S., Kitamura, M., Kodaira, M., Yamamoto, S., Ohno, Y., Kawai, Y., Kawara, M. & Kobayashi, K (2004) Randomized controlled clinical trial on satisfaction with resilient denture liners among edentulous patients. *International Journal of Prosthodontics*, 17, 236–40.

Klasser, G.D., Fischer, D.J. & Epstein J.B. (2008) Burning mouth syndrome: recognition, understanding, and management. *Oral and Maxillofacial Surgery Clinics of North America*, 20, 255–71.

Kostoulas I.E., Kavoura V.T., Frangou M.J. & Polyzois G.L. (2008) The effect of length parameter on the repair strength of acrylic resin using fibres or metal wires. *General Dentistry*, 56, 51–5.

Lamey, P.J. (1998) Burning mouth syndrome: approach to successful management. *Dental Update*, 25, 298–300.

Lamey, P.J. & Lamb, A.B. (1988) Prospective study of aetiological factors in burning mouth syndrome. *British Medical Journal*, 296, 1243–6.

Lamey, P.J., Lamb, A.B., Hughes, A., Milligan, K.A. & Forsyth, A. (1994) Type 3 burning mouth syndrome: psychological and allergic aspects. *Journal of Oral Pathology & Medicine*, 23, 216–19.

Lamey, P.J. & Lewis, M.A.O. (1989) Oral medicine in practice: burning mouth syndrome. *British Dental Journal*, 167, 197–200.

Lamey, P.J., Murray, B.M., Eddie, S.A. & Freeman, R.E. (2001) The secretion of parotid saliva as stimulated by 10% citric acid is not related to precipitating factors in burning mouth syndrome. *Journal of Oral Pathology & Medicine*, 30, 121–4.

Lawson, W.A. & Bond, E.K. (1968) Speech and its relation to dentistry. Speech and speech defects. *Dental Practitioner and Dental Record*, 19, 75–81.

Lawson, W.A. & Bond, E.K. (1968) The influence of oral structures on speech. *Dental Practitioner and Dental Record*, 19, 113–18.

Lawson, W.A. & Bond, E.K. (1969) The effects on speech of variations in the design of dentures. *Dental Practitioner and Dental Record*, 19, 150–6.

Lechner SK, Champion, H. & Tongue, T.K. (1995) Complete denture problem solving – a survey. *Australian Dental Journal*, 40, 377–80.

Leung, K.C.M., McMillan, A.S., Cheung, B.P.K & Leung, W.K. (2008) Sjögren's syndrome sufferers have increase oral yeast levels despite regular oral care. *Oral Diseases*, 14, 163–73.

Lewis, M. (2009) An essential guide to xerostomia. *Oral Health Report*, 2, 2–6.

Locker, D. (1995) Xerostomia in older adults: a longitudinal study. *Gerodontology*, 12, 18–25.

Loney, R.W. & Moulding, M.B. (1993). The effect of finishing and polishing on surface roughness of a processed resilient denture liner. *International Journal of Prosthodontics*, 6, 390–6.

Lynch, C.D. & Allen, P.F. (2006) Management of the flabby ridge: using contemporary materials to solve an old problem. *British Dental Journal*, 200, 258–261.

Maresky, L.S., van der Bijl, P. & Gird, I. (1993) Burning mouth syndrome. Evaluation of multiple variables among 85 patients. *Oral Surgery, Oral Medicine, Oral Pathology*, 75, 303–7.

Marton, K., Madlena, M., Banoczy, J., Varga, G., Fejerdy, P., Shreebny, L.M. & Nagy, G. (2008) Unstimulated whole saliva flow rate in relation to sicca symptoms in Hungary. *Oral Diseases*, 14, 472–7.

McCabe, J.F., Basker, R.M., Murata, H. & Wollwage, P.G.F. (1996) The development of a simple test method to characterise the compliance and viscoelasticity of long-term soft lining materials. *European Journal of Prosthodontics and Restorative Dentistry*, 4, 77–81.

Murata, H. Kawamura, M., Hamada, T., Saleh, S., Kresnoadi, U. & Toki, K. (2001) Dimensional stability and weight changes of tissue conditioners. *Journal of Oral Rehabilitation*, 28, 918–23.

Murata, H., Murakami, S., Shigeto, N. & Hamada, T. (1994) Viscoelastic properties of tissue conditioners – influence of ethyl alcohol content and type of plasticizer. *Journal of Oral Rehabilitation*, 21, 145–56.

Mutluay, M.M. & Ruyter, I.E. (2005) Evaluation of adhesion of chairside hard relining materials to denture base polymers. *Journal of Prosthetic Dentistry*, 94, 445–52.

Mutluay, M.M., Ogus, S., Floystrand, F., Saxegaard, E., Dogan, A., Bek, B. & Ruyter, I.E. (2008) A prospective study on the clinical performance of polysiloxane soft liners: one-year results. *Dental Materials Journal*, 27, 440–7.

Narva, K.K., Vallittu, P.K., Helenius, H. & Yli-Urpo, A. (2001) Clinical survey of acrylic resin removable denture repairs with glass-fiber reinforcement. *International Journal of Prosthodontics*, 14, 219–24.

Niedermeier, W., Huber, M., Fischer, D., Beier, K., Müller, N., Schuler, R., Brininger, A., Fartasch, M., Diepgen, T., Matthaeus, C., Meyer, C. & Hector, M.P. (2000) Significance of saliva for the denture-wearing population. *Gerodontology*, 17, 104–18.

Oh, D.J., Lee, J.Y., Kim, Y.K. & Kho, H.S. (2008) Effects of carboxymethylcellulose (CMC-based) artificial saliva in patients with xerostomia. *International Journal of Oral and Maxillofacial Surgery*, 37, 1027–31.

Osborne, J. (1960) The full lower denture. *British Dental Journal*, 109, 481–97.

Packer M.E., Joarder, C. & Lall, B.A. (2005) The use of relative analgesia in the prosthetic treatment of the 'gagging' patient. *Dental Update*, 32, 544–6.

Paterson, A.J., Lamb, A.B., Clifford, T.J. & Lamey, P.J. (1995) Burning mouth syndrome: the relationship between the HAD scale and parafunctional habits. *Journal of Oral Pathology & Medicine*, 24, 289–92.

Rosted, P., Bundgaard, P., Fiske, J. & Pedersen, A.M.L. (2006) The use of acupuncture in controlling the gag reflex in patients requiring an upper alginate impression: an audit. *British Dental Journal*, 201, 721–5.

Scott, J. & Baum B.J. (1990) Oral effects of ageing. In: *Oral Manifestations of Systemic Disease*, 2nd ed., (eds J.H. Jones & D.K. Mason), pp. 311–38. Balliere Tindall, London.

Seifert E., Runte, C., Riebandt, M., Lambrecht-Dinnesen, A. & Bollmann, F. (1999) Can dental prostheses influence voice parameters? *Journal of Prosthetic Dentistry*, 81, 579–85.

Seo R.S., Neppelenbroek K.H. & Filho J.N. (2007) Factors affecting the strength of denture repairs. *Journal of Prosthodontics*, 16, 302–10.

Shim, J.S. & Watts, D.C. (2000) An examination of the stress distribution in a soft-lined acrylic resin mandibular complete denture by finite element analysis. *International Journal of Prosthodontics*, 13, 19–24.

Shimizu, H., Kakigi, M., Fujii, J., Tsue, F. & Takahashi, Y. (2008) Effect of surface preparation using ethyl acetate on the shear bond strength of repair resin to denture base resin. *Journal of Prosthodontics*, 17, 451–5.

Shimizu, H., Mori, N. & Takahashi, Y. (2008) Use of metal conditioner on reinforcement wires. *New York State Dental Journal*, 74, 26–8.

Ship, J.A., McCutcheon, J.A., Spivakovsky, S. & Kerr, A.R. (2007) Safety and effectiveness of topical dry mouth products containing olive oil, betaine and xylitol in reducing xerostomia for polypharmacy-induced dry mouth. *Journal of Oral Rehabilitation*, 34, 724–32.

Soh, K.I., Lee, J.Y., Chung, J.W., Kim, Y.K. & Kho H.S. (2007) Relationship between salivary flow rate and clinical symptoms and behaviours in patients with dry mouth. *Journal of Oral Rehabilitation*, 34, 739–44.

Svensson, P. & Kaaber, S. (1995) General health factors and denture function in patients with burning mouth syndrome and matched control subjects. *Journal of Oral Rehabilitation*, 22, 887–95.

Takahashi, Y., Chai, J., Takahashi, T. & Habu, T. (2000) Bond strength of denture teeth to denture base resins. *International Journal of Prosthodontics*, 13, 59–65.

Turner, M., Jahangiri, L. & Ship, J.A. (2008) Hyposalivation, xerostomia and the complete denture: a systematic review. *Journal of the American Dental Association*, 139, 146–50.

van der Waal, I. (1990) *The burning mouth syndrome*. Munksgaard, Copenhagen.

Verran, J. & Maryan, C.J. (1997) Retention of *Candida albicans* on acrylic resin and silicone of different surface topography. *Journal of Prosthetic Dentistry*, 77, 535–9.

von Bultzingslowen, I., Sollecito, T.P., Fox, P.C., Daniels, T., Jonsson, R., Lockhart, P.B., Wray, D., Brennan, M.T., Carrozzo, M., Gandera, B., Fujibayashi, T., Navazesh, M., Rhodus, N.L. & Schiodt, M. (2007) Salivary dysfunction associated with systemic diseases: systematic review and clinical management recommendations. *Oral Sugery, Oral Medicine, Oral Pathology, Oral Radiology & Endodontics*, 103, Suppl S57, e1–15.

Wilson, H.J. & Tomlin, H.R. (1969) Soft lining materials: some relevant properties and their determination. *Journal of Prosthetic Dentistry*, 21, 244–50.

Wright, P.S. (1984) The success and failure of denture soft lining materials in clinical use. *Journal of Dentistry*, 12, 319–27.

Wright, P.S. (1994) Observations on long-term use of a soft-lining material for mandibular complete dentures. *Journal of Prosthetic Dentistry*, 72, 385–92.

Wright, P.S., Young, K.A., Riggs, P.D., Parker, S. & Kalachandra, S. (1998) Evaluating the effect of soft lining materials on the growth of yeast. *Journal of Prosthetic Dentistry*, 79, 404–9.

Wright, S.M. (1979) An examination of factors associated with retching in dental patients. *Journal of Dentistry*, 7, 194–207.

Yemm, R. (1972) Stress-induced muscle activity: a possible etiologic factor in denture soreness. *Journal of Prosthetic Dentistry*, 28, 133–40.

Yilmaz, H., Aydin, C., Bal, B.T. & Ozcelik, B. (2005) Effects of disinfectants on resilient denture-lining materials contaminated with *Staphylococcus aureus*, *Streptococcus sobrinus* and *Candida albicans*. *Quintessence International*, 36, 373–81.

Zissis, A., Yannikakis, S., Polyzois, G. & Harrison, A. (2008) A long term study on residual monomer release from denture materials. *European Journal of Prosthodontics and Restorative Dentistry*, 16, 81–4.

Index

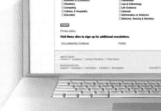
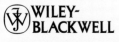